CLINICAL TEACHING STRATEGIES IN NURSING

Teresa Shellenbarger, PhD, RN, CNE, CNEcl, ANEF, FAAN is executive director, National League for Nursing (NLN) Commission for Nursing Education Accreditation. She is a Distinguished University Professor Emerita and was previously the founding Doctoral Nursing Program Coordinator, Indiana University of Pennsylvania, Indiana, Pennsylvania. During her 30 years of classroom and clinical teaching, she has established a reputation as an expert educator, mentor, and respected leader in academia. She was an invited member of the NLN work-group that developed the Academic Clinical Nurse Educator competencies that serve as the basis for the NLN clinical nurse educator certification exam. Dr. Shellenbarger recently published two books, *Clinical Nurse Educator Competencies: Creating an Evidence-Based Practice for Academic Clinical Nurse Educators* and *Academic Clinical Nurse Educator Review*. Dr. Shellenbarger frequently presents and publishes on topics related to innovative teaching, faculty role development, clinical teaching, and technology in nursing education.

Jennie C. De Gagne, PhD, DNP, RN, NPD-BC, CNE, ANEF, FAAN, is a professor of nursing and director of the Nursing Education Specialty at Duke University School of Nursing. With extensive experience in nursing education, she has provided consultation to nursing schools worldwide, including in South Korea, Ghana, India, Tanzania, Saudi Arabia, Oman, and Lebanon, focusing on curriculum and faculty development. Dr. De Gagne is an expert in educational technology and online education, particularly in the effective use of instructional technology and cybercivility across the curriculum. She has authored or coauthored over 250 publications, including more than 130 peer-reviewed journal articles and several nursing education textbooks in both English and Korean. A fellow of both the National League for Nursing Academy of Nursing Education and the American Academy of Nursing, Dr. De Gagne is nationally and internationally recognized for her contributions to advancing nursing education.

Marilyn H. Oermann, PhD, RN, ANEF, FAAN, is the Thelma M. Ingles Professor of Nursing at Duke University School of Nursing, Durham, North Carolina. She is the author or coauthor of 35 books and many articles on teaching in nursing, evaluation, and studies of the nursing literature. She is the Editor-in-Chief of *Nurse Educator.* Dr. Oermann received the National League for Nursing (NLN) Award for Excellence in Nursing Education Research, the Sigma Theta Tau International Elizabeth Russell Belford Award for Excellence in Education, the American Association of Colleges of Nursing Scholarship of Teaching and Learning Excellence Award, the Margaret Comerford Freda Award for Editorial Leadership in Nursing from the International Academy of Nursing Editors, and the NLN President's Award. The NLN established an award in her honor, the Marilyn H. Oermann Award for Distinguished Research in Nursing Education, to recognize an individual or team who has generated an evidentiary base for the science of nursing education.

Kathleen B. Gaberson, PhD, RN, CNOR, CNE, ANEF, is professor of nursing by courtesy at Duquesne University, and owner of and principal nursing education consultant for OWK Consulting, both in Pittsburgh, Pennsylvania. She has over 40 years of teaching and administrative experience in graduate and undergraduate nursing programs. She is coauthor of 13 nursing education books and author or coauthor of numerous articles on nursing education topics. Dr. Gaberson has received many teaching awards, and she presents and consults extensively on assessment and evaluation, clinical teaching, and research instrument development.

CLINICAL TEACHING STRATEGIES IN NURSING

Seventh Edition

Teresa Shellenbarger, PhD, RN, CNE, CNEcl, ANEF, FAAN
Jennie C. De Gagne, PhD, DNP, RN, NPD-BC, CNE, ANEF, FAAN
Marilyn H. Oermann, PhD, RN, ANEF, FAAN
Kathleen B. Gaberson, PhD, RN, CNOR, CNE, ANEF

SPRINGER PUBLISHING

First Springer Publishing edition 9780826112781 (1999); subsequent edition 2006, 2010, 2014, 2017, 2023

Springer Publishing Company, LLC
902 Carnegie Center/Suite 140, Princeton, NJ 08540
www.springerpub.com
connect.springerpub.com

Acquisitions Editor: Joseph Morita
Development Editor: Brenna Croker
Director, Production Project Management: Kris Parrish
Compositor: Amnet

ISBN: 978-0-8261-9151-9
e-book ISBN: 978-0-8261-8941-7
DOI: 10.1891/9780826189417

SUPPLEMENTS

SPRINGER PUBLISHING CONNECT™

A robust set of instructor resources designed to supplement this text is located at http://connect.springerpub.com/content/book/978-0-8261-8941-7. Qualifying instructors may request access by emailing textbook@springerpub.com.

Instructor Materials:
LMS Common Cartridge With All Instructor Resources ISBN: 978-0-8261-7608-0
Instructor's Manual ISBN: 978-0-8261-9726-0
Instructor Chapter PowerPoints ISBN: 978-0-8261-7564-9
Mapping to AACN Essentials ISBN: 978-0-8261-5452-1
Transition Guide: Sixth Edition to Seventh Edition ISBN: 978-0-8261-7196-2

26 27 28 29 / 5 4 3 2

Library of Congress Control Number: 2025037637

Printed in the United States of America.

Contents

SECTION III: EVALUATION STRATEGIES IN CLINICAL TEACHING

Contributors to Previous Editions

Eric Bauman, PhD, RN

Suzanne Hetzel Campbell, PhD, WHNP-BC, IBCLC

Christine Lind Colella, DNP, APRN-CNP, FAANP

Kimberly Day, DNP, RN

Mickey Gilmore-Kahn, CNM, MN

Katie Anne Haerling, PhD, RN, CHSE

Debra Hagler, PhD, RN, ACNS-BC, CNE, CHSE, ANEF, FAAN

Meigan Robb, PhD, RN

Elizabeth Speakman, EdD, RN, FNAP, ANEF, FAAN

Susan E. Stone, DNSc, CNM, FACNM

Diane M. Wink, EdD, FNP, ARNP

Contributor to the Seventh Edition

Brandon (Kyle) Johnson, PhD, RN, CHSE, ANEF, Executive Director Texas Tech University Health Sciences Center Simulation Program and Professor, Texas Tech University Health Sciences Center, School of Nursing, Lubbock, Texas

Preface

Teaching in clinical settings presents nurse educators with challenges that are different from those encountered in the classroom and in online environments. In nursing education, the classroom and clinical environments are closely linked because students apply in clinical practice what they have learned in the classroom, online, laboratory, and through other experiences. However, clinical settings require different approaches to teaching. The clinical environment is complex and rapidly changing, with a variety of new settings and roles in which nurses must be prepared to practice.

The seventh edition of *Clinical Teaching Strategies in Nursing* examines concepts of clinical teaching and provides a comprehensive framework for planning, guiding, and evaluating learning activities for prelicensure and graduate nursing students. It is a comprehensive source of information for full- and part-time faculty members whose responsibilities center largely on clinical teaching, for adjuncts and clinical nurse educators whose sole responsibility is clinical teaching, and for preceptors. The book also is useful when teaching nurses and other healthcare providers in the clinical setting. Although the focus of the book is clinical teaching in nursing, the content is applicable to teaching students in other healthcare professions.

The book describes clinical teaching strategies that are effective and practical in a rapidly changing healthcare environment. It presents a range of teaching, learning, and evaluation strategies useful for courses in which the teacher is on site with students, in courses using preceptors and similar models, and in distance education environments while describing roles and responsibilities associated with clinical teaching and providing guidance in the selection of teaching methods and learning activities. The book also examines innovative uses of simulation and technologies used in clinical education and discusses ethical and legal issues that arise with clinical teaching.

Each chapter includes a list of the content from the Certified Academic Clinical Nurse Educator (CNE®cl) Examination Test Blueprint that relate to the chapter content. In addition to the book, we have prepared Instructor Materials with a course syllabus; a complete online course (with modules for each chapter that include a chapter summary, student learning activities, discussion questions, online resources for students, and assessment strategies); and chapter-based PowerPoint presentations (for use in an online course or in-person classes). To obtain an electronic copy of these teaching materials, contact Springer Publishing Company (textbook@springerpub.com).

The book is organized into three sections. The first section, Foundations of Clinical Teaching, comprises six chapters that provide a background for clinical teaching and guide the teacher's planning for clinical learning activities. Chapter 1 describes the nurse educator shortage, faculty ranks and tracks, types of positions for clinical teachers and educational requirements, transition from clinician to educator, and certification. The chapter presents a philosophy that provides a framework for planning, guiding, and evaluating clinical learning activities. Chapter 2 discusses outcomes of clinical teaching; it emphasizes the importance of cognitive, psychomotor, and affective outcomes that guide clinical teaching and evaluation. It also discusses strategies to mitigate challenges in clinical learning and the role of faculty and student diversity in preparing nursing graduates for diverse healthcare environments.

Chapter 3 describes the process of clinical teaching—identifying clinical competencies, assessing learning needs, planning learning activities, guiding and supporting students in clinical practice, and evaluating performance. This chapter also addresses important characteristics of clinical teachers. Various clinical teaching models are described, including traditional, in which one teacher guides the learning of a small group of students; preceptor; and partnership including dedicated education units and other partnerships.

Clinical education can be provided in a wide variety of clinical sites, as explained in Chapter 4. Examples are provided of clinical learning opportunities in specialized patient care areas not used regularly for clinical learning, community-based settings, clinical learning at distant sites, and international settings. Chapter 5 describes the roles and responsibilities of faculty members, clinical staff, and other individuals involved in preparing learners in clinical settings. The chapter also offers practical methods for student preparation including the cognitive, affective, and psychomotor domains of learning while also addressing approaches faculty can implement to ensure smooth transition into clinical practice.

Chapter 6 addresses the ethical and legal issues in clinical teaching, focusing on how moral reasoning and accountability shape the ethical landscape. It also discusses practical guidance for faculty in reinforcing ethical standards and legal awareness, with an emphasis on equity and inclusivity in decision-making.

The second section of the book, titled Strategies for Effective Clinical Teaching, addresses important responsibilities of the clinical educator: selecting teaching methods and learning activities that are related to the competencies to be developed, appropriate to students' levels of knowledge and skill, and challenging enough to motivate learning. Chapter 7 presents clinical teaching methods—patient assignments and options for these assignments (student–patient ratio options, management activities, observation, and service learning); discussion; clinical conferences; written assignments; and various types of cases (short case, case study, and unfolding case). The chapter provides a framework for planning clinical assignments for learners.

Chapter 8 focuses on clinical simulation. The chapter includes a discussion of the use of clinical simulation as a learning activity. It discusses how the Healthcare Simulation Standards of Best Practice™ can be used to enhance clinical teaching and simulation. The chapter also explains how faculty can prepare, prebrief, facilitate, debrief, and evaluate simulation. Chapter 9 examines different technologies that can be used in clinical education, including artificial intelligence, to prepare nursing students for the evolving demands of healthcare. This chapter includes various technologies, such as simulated electronic health records, telepresence, telehealth, and virtual gamification, and explores strategies for integrating these tools into clinical teaching practices. The chapter also includes suggestions for selecting appropriate technologies and emphasizes the importance of aligning technology choices with the intended learning outcomes. Chapter 10 is devoted to the use of preceptors in clinical teaching in prelicensure through advanced practice nursing programs. The selection, preparation, role, evaluation of preceptors, and the advantages and disadvantages of using preceptors, are discussed.

The final section, Section III: Evaluation Strategies in Clinical Teaching, has two chapters. Chapter 11 examines clinical teaching in distance education, focusing on structured mentorship, apprenticeship models, and the integration of technology to enhance both student learning and preceptor support. The chapter examines strategies for developing partnerships with preceptors and clinical sites, clarifying the roles and responsibilities of faculty, preceptors, and students. Additionally, it discusses methods for evaluating student clinical performance, including site visits, virtual assessments, and preceptor evaluations, as well as approaches for assessing preceptor effectiveness and clinical site quality to maintain high standards in distance-based clinical education. Chapter 12 describes the process of clinical evaluation in nursing, use of competencies and entrustable professional activities for assessment of performance, and giving feedback to students. Multiple methods for evaluating clinical performance are described: observation, checklists, varied rating scales, simulations, standardized patients, objective structured clinical examinations, writing assignments, cases, e-portfolios, conferences, group projects, and self-assessment. How to grade students in clinical courses, examples of grading systems, and principles to follow in evaluating and grading clinical practice also are discussed in the chapter.

We acknowledge Joseph Morita, Executive Acquisitions Editor at Springer Publishing Company, for his continued support. We also thank Springer Publishing Company for its commitment to nursing education and for publishing our books for many years.

Teresa Shellenbarger
Jennie C. De Gagne
Marilyn H. Oermann
Kathleen B. Gaberson

Instructor Resources

SPRINGER PUBLISHING CONNECT™

A robust set of instructor resources designed to supplement this text is located at http://connect.springerpub.com/content/book/978-0-8261-8941-7
Qualifying instructors may request access by emailing textbook@springerpub.com.

- LMS Common Cartridge With All Instructor Resources
- Instructor's Manual
- Instructor Chapter PowerPoints
- Mapping to AACN Essentials: Core Competencies for Professional Nursing Education
- Transition Guide: Sixth Edition to Seventh Edition

SPRINGER PUBLISHING

Visit https://connect.springerpub.com and look for the **"Show Additional Resources"** button on the **book homepage**.

I

Foundations of Clinical Teaching

Role of the Clinical Nurse Educator and Context for Clinical Teaching

1

OBJECTIVES:

1. Describe the varied roles and educational preparation of nurse educators including clinical teachers.
2. Explore the philosophical context for clinical teaching and how these beliefs guide teaching and evaluating learning outcomes and competencies.
3. Discuss the context of clinical teaching, each component, and implications for clinical educators.

Effective clinical teaching and learning are influenced by several factors. Clinical teaching is performed by an educator within a curriculum that is planned and offered in response to professional, societal, environmental, and educational expectations and demands, using available human, intellectual, physical, and financial resources—the context of the curriculum. Considering the educational context, however, is not enough: Clinical teachers also need to consider the healthcare context to adequately prepare qualified nurses to be capable of responding to the needs and challenges of rapidly changing healthcare systems.

This chapter describes the nurse educator shortage, faculty ranks and tracks, types of positions for clinical teachers and educational requirements, transition from clinician to educator, and certification. It is important for clinical nurse educators to know where the clinical practicum they are teaching is positioned within the curriculum so they can build on students' previous knowledge and guide clinical learning. The chapter examines different terms used to describe clinical teaching and the philosophical context of clinical teaching. This context includes beliefs about the nature of the professional practice, importance of clinical teaching, role of the student as a learner, need for learning time before grading performance, climate for learning, need to focus on essential clinical competencies, espoused curriculum versus curriculum-in-use, and importance of quality over quantity of clinical activities.

SHORTAGE OF NURSE EDUCATORS

Many reports have highlighted the need for more nurse educators. Nursing shortages are cyclical and affected by economic conditions, population growth, the aging of the population, retirements of nurses, and other factors. The U.S. Department of Labor's Bureau of Labor Statistics (2023) projects a 6% growth of registered nurses (RNs) through 2032, but this is not enough of a growth to meet the need for nurses, particularly with older nurses retiring. At the national level, shortages are projected for RNs and licensed practical nurses/licensed vocational nurses (LPN/LVNs) through 2036. The Health Resources and Services Administration (HRSA, 2024) estimates that the demand for RNs in 2036 will exceed supply by 9%, a shortage of 337,970 full-time equivalent RNs. To maintain an adequate supply of nurses, schools of nursing need qualified faculty and clinical nurse educators to teach those students.

FACULTY RANKS AND TRACKS

For academic faculty positions in schools of nursing, beginning faculty are hired typically as instructors or assistant professors depending on the institution. As beginning faculty meet the criteria in the school of nursing for promotion to a higher rank, they progress to associate professor and professor ranks. Schools of nursing generally have two academic tracks: tenure and non tenure tracks, each with its own expectations for faculty performance and criteria for promotion (Oermann, 2025). Tenure-track positions provide job security. In the tenure track, once a faculty member meets certain requirements, they are granted tenure, which is a permanent position in the school and college or university. Most schools also have non tenure tracks (sometimes called clinical or teaching tracks), which have different requirements and performance expectations for faculty. With non tenure tracks, faculty have renewable contracts for employment versus a permanent position. Typically, the non tenure track role focuses on teaching. Educators who teach students in the clinical setting are typically non tenure track. **Table 1.1** provides a summary of differences between tenure and non tenure tracks.

TYPES OF POSITIONS FOR CLINICAL NURSE EDUCATORS AND REQUIREMENTS

There are many different positions and labels used to identify clinical nurse educators. In some programs, academic faculty from the school of nursing also teach

TABLE 1.1 COMPARISON OF TENURE AND NON TENURE TRACKS FOR FACULTY

Tenure	Non Tenure
Permanent position awarded after probationary period	Not permanent, by contracted length of time
Job security	No job security, contract might not be renewed Continued employment based on teaching needs in the school, numbers of students needing instruction in the clinical setting
Probationary period (usually 7 or 10 years depending on the university/college; 5 years in some schools). Includes pretenure review at 3 or 5 years	Annual or multiyear contracts for faculty Hiring is based on needs
Protects academic freedom (faculty can share own views and opinions and can engage in intellectual debate with students without fear of retaliation)	No protection of academic freedom
Need to demonstrate contributions to research/scholarship, teaching, and service	Need to demonstrate contributions to teaching and service, with some scholarship For clinical nurse educators, teaching only
Criteria for tenure (and promotion) and procedures determined by school of nursing consistent with university/college guidelines	Criteria for non tenure reappointments (and promotion) and procedures determined by school, college, and/or university Clinical nurse educator contracted per semester, term, or year as needed
Time allotted in workload for research/scholarship	No time allotted for research/scholarship Higher teaching load than tenure track
Number of tenure track positions is limited	Number of non tenure track positions fluctuates based on teaching needs of school

Source: Adapted from De Gagne, J. C., & Oermann, M. H. (2025). *Teaching in nursing and role of the educator: The complete guide to best practice in teaching, evaluation, and curriculum development* (4th ed., p. 6). Springer Publishing Company.

groups of students in the clinical setting or provide guidance to clinicians in dedicated education units and similar models. In other programs, adjunct or part-time educators are hired for clinical teaching, or advanced practice RNs (APRNs) and managers assume responsibility for teaching students through collaborative arrangements with the school such as joint appointments and shared positions through academic–practice partnerships.

For accreditation, there needs to be a sufficient number of faculty in a school of nursing to achieve its mission, goals, and program outcomes, and faculty need to be academically and experientially prepared for the areas in which they teach. For clinical teaching, educators need to meet the qualifications required by the school of nursing, for accreditation, and by the state board of nursing. For clinical teaching in associate degree in nursing (ADN) and LPN/LVN programs, a BSN may be needed. In BSN programs, educators should have a graduate degree or have a baccalaureate degree in nursing, have significant clinical experience, be enrolled in a graduate program (or be qualified through other means such as completing relevant graduate-level courses or continuing education), and have formal oversight by a graduate-prepared faculty member in the school. For teaching in the clinical setting, educators need to have clinical expertise in the relevant area of practice and maintain that expertise, for example, through their current practice. When teaching in an APRN program, there are additional requirements to be met; for example, the educator needs to have a graduate degree, be currently licensed or authorized to practice, and be nationally board certified as a nurse practitioner in the population focus of the major (National Organization of Nurse Practitioner Faculties [NONPF], 2022b). The degree required for clinical teaching varies based on board of nursing requirements in the state where they want to teach and the type of nursing program (e.g., certified nursing assistant, LPN/LVN, ADN, BSN, or APRN).

Academic credentials for nurse educators employed in postsecondary institutions are determined by state boards of nursing and accreditation agencies (Oermann, 2025). There are three agencies that accredit nursing programs: the Commission on Collegiate Nursing Education (CCNE), which accredits baccalaureate and higher-degree nursing programs (CCNE, 2024); the Accreditation Commission for Education in Nursing (ACEN), which accredits all levels of nursing programs, including doctor of nursing practice (DNP), master's/postmaster's certificate, baccalaureate, associate, diploma, and practical nursing programs (ACEN,

2023); and the National League for Nursing (NLN) Commission for Nursing Education Accreditation (CNEA), which also accredits all program levels (NLN CNEA, 2021). These agencies all indicate that the nurse educator needs to be qualified for their role through their education, professional credentials, and experience for their assigned teaching responsibilities.

TRANSITION FROM CLINICIAN TO EDUCATOR

Regardless of the type of nursing program in which they are teaching, nurses should be well prepared as educators (Hansbrough et al., 2023; Ross et al., 2024; Young-Brice et al., 2022). This preparation can be gained by completing a graduate degree or certificate program in nursing education, taking nursing education courses, or through continuing education.

Although the transition from clinician to educator presents challenges, Schoening and Rusch (2025) identified three predominant strategies to facilitate this transition. First, all clinical educators should have a formal, structured orientation to their role as a teacher. They need to understand the responsibilities of the clinical teacher, courses related to their clinical teaching assignment (how the clinical practicum fits within the course and curriculum), competencies to be developed by students, lines of communication between the clinical educator and school of nursing (e.g., with the course lead), clinical evaluation tool, and policies and procedures that impact clinical teaching.

Second, each clinical teacher needs effective mentoring. A mentor can guide and support clinicians as they learn about their role as educator. The third area critical to transition to the educator role is the development of instructional skills. These skills can be gained through faculty development offerings, workshops, continuing education courses, online modules, and other types of educational programs. These programs prepare clinicians for assessing students' learning needs, making patient assignments and developing clinical learning activities, guiding and supporting students, demonstrating procedures and technologies, assessing and evaluating performance, and giving feedback to learners. The role of the clinical educator and responsibilities are described further in Chapter 3.

CERTIFICATION FOR NURSE EDUCATORS

As nurse educators develop their knowledge and expertise, they can pursue certification as an educator. This certification, offered by the NLN, provides a way for educators to demonstrate their specialized knowledge, skills, and expertise and also contributes to their professional and career development (NLN, 2024). There are three certifications for nurse educators: Certified Nurse Educator (CNE®), Certified Academic Clinical Nurse Educator (CNE®cl), and Certified Novice Nurse Educator (CNE®n). Information about each of these certifications can be found at https://www.nln.org/awards-recognition/nln-certification. The chapters in this book are mapped to the competencies for the CNE®cl.

PHILOSOPHICAL CONTEXT FOR CLINICAL TEACHING

A philosophy is a system of shared beliefs and values held by members of an academic or practice discipline that helps to guide actions and curriculum implementation. A philosophy provides a framework for making curricular and instructional choices and decisions. Every clinical teacher has a philosophical approach to clinical teaching, whether the teacher realizes it or not. That philosophical context determines the teacher's understanding of their role, approaches to clinical teaching, selection of clinical learning activities, evaluation processes, and relationships with learners and others in the clinical environment. These beliefs serve as a guide to action, and they profoundly affect how clinical teachers practice, how students learn, and how learning outcomes and competencies are evaluated. Nurse educators are encouraged to articulate their philosophies of nursing education in general and clinical teaching in particular to guide their clinical teaching practices.

Students' clinical practice comprises an important part of the curriculum, offering opportunities for students to link the theory learned in the classroom, in online courses, in simulation, and through various learning activities (didactic part of the curriculum) to patient care. Clinical teachers should understand the curriculum so they can operationalize it consistently and align their teaching to guide students in applying their knowledge gained in the classroom to clinical practice.

A LEXICON OF CLINICAL TEACHING

Language has the power to shape thinking, and choice and use of words can affect the way a teacher thinks about and performs the role of clinical teacher. Terms related to clinical teaching are defined so educators share a common frame of reference for clinical teaching.

Clinical

The word *clinical* is an adjective, derived from the noun *clinic*. *Clinical* means involving direct observation of the patient. Like any adjective, the word clinical must modify a noun. Nurse educators sometimes say, "My students are in clinical today" or "I am not in clinical this week." Examples of correct use include clinical practice, clinical practicum, clinical instruction, and clinical evaluation.

Clinical Teaching or Clinical Instruction

The central activity of the teacher in the clinical setting is clinical instruction or clinical teaching. The teacher does not supervise students. Supervision implies administrative functions such as overseeing, directing, and managing the work of others. Supervision is a function that is more appropriate for professional practice situations, not the learning environment.

The appropriate role of the teacher is competent guidance. The teacher guides and supports students and facilitates their learning by designing appropriate learning activities in the clinical setting. An effective clinical teacher is a coach, focusing on promoting the student's development (van Ede et al., 2023). Similar to the clinical teacher, the preceptor (who is a clinician) guides students in the clinical practicum, new graduate nurses, and nurses new to the setting to develop their competencies and become socialized into the role for which they are preparing.

TABLE 1.2 DEFINITIONS OF TERMS

Term	Definition
Clinical	An adjective meaning involving direct observation of the patient. Examples include clinical practice, clinical practicum, clinical instruction, and clinical evaluation
Clinical Experience	Experienced by each student individually
Clinical Teacher, Clinical Nurse Educator, Adjunct Clinical Instructor, other similar roles	Individual who guides students in the clinical setting and facilitates their learning
Clinical Teaching or Instruction	Selection of learning activities to promote students' development of competencies
Preceptor	Clinician who guides students in the clinical practicum to develop their competencies and meet course outcomes, new graduate nurses, and nurses new to the clinical unit or setting. Preceptors work with learners for a set period of time

Clinical Experience

Learning is an active, personal process. The student is the one who experiences the learning. Teachers cannot provide the experience; they can only provide the opportunity for the experience. The teacher's role is to plan and provide appropriate activities that will facilitate learning. However, each student will experience activity in a different way. For example, a teacher can provide a guided observation of a procedure for a group of students. Although all students may be present in the room at the same time and all are observing the same procedure, each student will experience something slightly different. One of the reasons teachers require students to do written reflections or to participate in clinical conferences is to allow the teacher a glimpse of what students have derived from the learning activities.

Table 1.2 provides a summary of these terms. This allows clinical educators and faculty members to have a common frame of reference as they discuss clinical teaching with students, colleagues, and others involved in teaching students in practice settings.

THE CONTEXT FOR CLINICAL TEACHING

The philosophical context of clinical teaching includes beliefs about the nature of the professional practice, essential nurse educator competencies, the importance of clinical teaching, the role of the student as a learner, the need for learning time before evaluation and grading, the climate for learning, the essential versus enrichment curricula, the espoused curriculum versus curriculum-in-use, and the importance of quality over quantity of clinical activities. Each of these elements serves as a guide to action for clinical teachers in nursing.

Clinical Education Should Reflect the Nature of Professional Practice

Nursing is a professional discipline. Professional disciplines are differentiated from academic disciplines by their practice component. Clinical practice requires problem-solving abilities and clinical judgment, specialized psychomotor and technological skills, and a professional value system. These are essential competencies to be developed by nursing students consistent with the role for which they are preparing, for example, for transition into the role of a RN or as an APRN. Practice in clinical settings exposes students to the realities of professional practice that cannot be conveyed by a textbook or a simulation (Oermann et al., 2025). Clinical education should allow students to encounter real practice problems that they need to solve with guidance from and support of the clinical educator. Because healthcare professionals typically practice as members of interprofessional teams, clinical education should also include opportunities for interprofessional practice (Interprofessional Education Collaborative, 2023).

To prepare nursing students for their future professional practice, clinical practice needs to reflect the realities of healthcare and society. The National Academy of Medicine in *The Future of Nursing 2020–2030: Charting a Path to Achieve Health Equity* addresses nursing's role in reducing health inequities and improving health and well-being for the U.S. population (National Academies of Sciences, Engineering, and Medicine [NASEM], 2021). One of the roles of the clinical educator is to prepare students to engage in the essential work of advancing health equity, addressing social determinants of health, and meeting social needs of individuals and families (NASEM, 2021).

Clinical Teaching Is Important

Because nursing is a professional practice discipline, what nurses and nursing students do in clinical practice is important, and clinical educators have a critical role in the nursing program (Oermann, 2024). They need to be well prepared for their role as educators and preceptors (Griffiths et al., 2022; Wells-Beede et al., 2023). Clinical learning activities provide real-life opportunities for the transfer of knowledge to practice. Some learners who perform well in the classroom have difficulty applying their knowledge successfully in the clinical area. Clinical educators guide students in transferring this knowledge to clinical practice and developing essential competencies.

Clinical teaching is the most expensive element of any nursing curriculum. Lower student-to-teacher ratios in clinical settings usually require a larger number of clinical teachers than classroom teachers. Students and teachers spend numerous hours in clinical settings; those contact hours typically exceed the number of credit hours for which students pay tuition. Even if the tuition structure compensates for that intensive use of resources, clinical instruction remains an expensive enterprise. Therefore, classroom instruction (didactic) is used to prepare students for their clinical activities. Students learn prerequisite knowledge in the classroom and through other learning activities that they apply in simulation and clinical practice.

The Student in the Clinical Setting Is a Learner, Not a Nurse

In preparation for professional practice, the clinical setting is the place where students come in contact with patients, families, and other healthcare providers, within varied systems of care. The main goal in clinical education should be on students' learning. The student is not a nurse but a learner. Expectations of the nurse educator, clinicians in the setting, managers, and other healthcare professionals need to be consistent with the knowledge and skill level of the student. An important role of the clinical educator is ensuring individuals who work with nursing students understand the knowledge and skills students bring to the setting and not expect students to provide care at the level of an RN. For this reason, the term *nursing student* (emphasizing the noun *student*) is preferred rather than *student nurse* (emphasizing the noun *nurse*).

Sufficient Learning Time Should Be Provided Before Performance Is Evaluated for a Grade

If students enter the clinical area to learn, then it follows that students need to engage in activities that promote learning and to practice before their performance is evaluated for a grade. Many nursing students perceive that the main role of the clinical teacher is to evaluate, and some clinical educators spend more time on evaluation activities than on teaching. Learning in the clinical setting is a complex process that requires time for applying knowledge and concepts to care of patients, families, and communities and developing competencies. Clinical nurse educators and preceptors, who work one-to-one with students, should expect students to make mistakes and not hold perfection as the standard. Therefore, clinical teachers should allow learning time with ample feedback from the teacher (formative evaluation) before determining the grade for clinical practice (summative evaluation). Evaluation and grading are discussed in Chapter 12.

A Climate of Mutual Trust and Respect Is Needed for Effective Clinical Teaching

Another element of a philosophy of clinical teaching is the importance of creating and maintaining a climate of mutual trust and respect that supports learning and student growth. Educators should respect students as learners and trust their motivation and commitment to the profession they seek to enter. Students should respect the teacher's commitment to both nursing education and society and trust that clinical educators and clinicians in the setting will treat them with fairness and, to the extent that it is possible, not allow students to make mistakes that would harm patients.

The responsibilities for maintaining this climate are mutual, but teachers have the ultimate responsibility to establish these expectations in the nursing program. Nurse educators need to state clearly, early, and often that they view nursing education as a shared enterprise, that they sincerely desire student success, and that they will partner with students in achieving success. Clinical teaching, especially in providing feedback to students in the clinical setting, needs to take place in a climate of mutual trust and respect.

Clinical Teaching Should Focus on Essential Competencies

Every nursing curriculum comprises knowledge, skills, and values that are essential for safe, competent practice and those that would be nice to have but are not critical. In other words, there is an essential curriculum and an enrichment curriculum. No nursing program has the luxury of unlimited time for clinical teaching. Therefore, clinical teaching should focus on the essential knowledge and competencies to be developed and on the most common practice problems that nurses are likely to encounter.

Competencies are the observable abilities of the student: what the student can do (Oermann, 2022). The American Association of Colleges of Nursing (AACN) defines competency as the ability of a healthcare professional that integrates multiple components, including knowledge, skills, values, and attitudes (AACN, 2021). The AACN *The Essentials: Core Competencies for Professional Nursing Education* identify 10 domains or areas of nursing competence that include broad competencies and multiple subcompetencies. These are discussed further in Chapters 3 and 12. NONPF also has identified competencies and subcompetencies that APRNs must achieve for entry into practice regardless of their population focus (NONPF, 2022a). NONPF also provides guidelines to assist faculty and preceptors in implementing the AACN *Essentials* Level 2 Subcompetencies and NONPF Role Core Competencies (NONPF, 2024).

Competency-based education focuses on the end point and allows variable times for achievement (Jones-Schenk, 2025). In clinical practice, students and new graduates typically need varying amounts of time and learning activities to develop their competencies. The clinical educator and preceptor should not expect each student to achieve the competencies in the same amount of time; students may need additional learning activities. One of the responsibilities of the clinical teacher is to understand these differences across students, assess the needs of each student, and plan individualized learning activities to facilitate student development of the competencies.

The Espoused Curriculum Should Be the Curriculum-in-se

A nursing curriculum often operates on two levels. The espoused curriculum is the one that is described in nursing program documents, such as the bulletin, on the school of nursing website, in course syllabi, and in the self-study report for accreditation and state board approval of the program. However, the curriculum-in-use is what happens during teaching whether it is in the classroom, online environment, simulation, or clinical setting. A faculty member can include or exclude certain learning activities, goals, or evaluation methods in the curriculum, but when clinical teachers are in their own clinical settings, they often do what seems right to them at the time, in the context of changing circumstances and resources. Every clinical teacher needs to interpret the espoused curriculum in view of the clinical situation, resources in the clinical setting, and individual needs of students, patients, families, and staff at the time. In reality, nursing faculty cannot prescribe to the last detail what clinical teachers will teach (and when and how) and what learners will learn (and when and how) in clinical settings. Consequently, every student experiences the curriculum differently, hence the distinction between learning activity and learning experience made earlier.

Although there needs to be some flexibility for clinical educators in guiding students in applying concepts and knowledge they are learning to clinical practice, the integrity of the curriculum may be compromised if an individual clinical teacher diverges widely from the curriculum. While academic freedom is valued in nursing education, clinical educators need to teach consistently based on the program and course outcomes and where the clinical practicum fits within the overall curriculum, for example, a beginning course versus a course later in the program. Understanding the curriculum is important for all clinical educators to operationalize the curriculum with students they are teaching.

Quality Is More Important Than Quantity

The length of time spent in clinical activities is no guarantee of the amount or quality of learning that results. Both the learning activities and amount of time need to be individualized. Some faculty members worry too much about how many hours students spend in the clinical setting and too little about the quality of the learning that is taking place. A 2-hour activity that results in critical skill learning or development of clinical judgment is far more valuable than an 8-hour activity that merely promotes repetition of skills and habit formation. Nurse educators often worry there is not enough time to teach everything that students need to learn, but a rapidly increasing knowledge base and technologies in clinical practice ensure there will never be enough time. This is why focusing clinical learning activities on the specific competencies to be developed is essential. A few examples are provided in **Table 1.3.**

TABLE 1.3 EXAMPLES OF CLINICAL LEARNING ACTIVITIES PLANNED FOR SPECIFIC COMPETENCIES

AACN *Essentials* Subcompetency	Example Clinical Learning Activity
5.2a Describe the factors that create a culture of safety.	Entry level: Collect information on your unit (or in your assigned clinical setting) that is designed to improve safety and reduce risk of errors and harm. Complete a short paper with a summary of this information (2 pages or less). Interview the nurse manager or charge number and one RN on the unit/in the clinical agency and record how they describe the culture of safety and strategies for improving safety. Report in postclinical conference. Identify types of benchmark data collected on the unit and explain each benchmark and why it is important for patient safety. Report in a short paper (no more than 2 pages).
5.1d Interpret benchmark and unit outcome data to inform individual and microsystem practice.	Entry level: Review unit-based report cards. Compare the national benchmarks and unit specific data (e.g., the benchmarks for central line-associated bloodstream infections [CLABSI], falls, and others and unit rates). Complete a written report on the comparison of national benchmarks and unit data (no more than 3 pages). One student to interview risk management and its role in the healthcare system. Report in postclinical conference.
5.1 l Collaborate in analyzing organizational process improvement initiatives.	Advanced level: Analyze national benchmarks data with unit-specific data for two quality indicators and develop a quality improvement plan. Review your draft plan with your preceptor and, in collaboration with the preceptor, modify the plan as needed. Follow the instructions on this assignment and submit a paper to the course instructor.
5.2b Articulate the nurse's role within an interprofessional team in promoting safety and preventing errors and near misses.	Entry level: Participate in or observe a huddle. Summarize your observations, data shared, actions planned, and the nurse's role. Complete a short paper (1 page).
5.2h Lead analysis of actual errors, near misses, and potential situations that would impact safety. 5.2i Design evidence-based interventions to mitigate risk.	Advanced level: Interview a nurse or leader in the setting on actual errors or near misses they know about and actions taken post error or near miss. Critique system and organizational processes that might be modified. Include interventions to improve processes related to these errors/near misses with a rationale and evidence for support. Prepare a paper (no more than 5 pages) that includes support from related research.

USING A PHILOSOPHY OF CLINICAL TEACHING TO IMPROVE CLINICAL EDUCATION

Differences in philosophical approaches can profoundly affect how individuals enact the role of clinical teacher. Every decision about teaching strategy, setting, outcome, and role behavior should be grounded in the teacher's philosophical perspective. The core values inherent in an educator's philosophy of clinical teaching can serve as the basis for useful discussions with colleagues and evaluation of new teaching strategies. Reflection on one's philosophy of clinical teaching may uncover the source of incongruities between an individual's espoused theory of clinical teaching and the theory-in-use. When the outcomes of such reflection are shared with other clinical teachers, they provide a basis for the continual improvement of clinical teaching.

Nurse educators are encouraged to continue to develop their philosophies of clinical teaching by reflecting on how they view the goals of clinical education and how they carry out teaching activities to meet those goals. A philosophical approach to clinical education will thus serve as a guide to more effective practice and a means of ongoing professional development.

SUMMARY

This chapter described the nurse educator shortage, faculty ranks and tracks, types of positions for clinical teachers and educational requirements, transition from clinician to educator, and certification. It is important for clinical teachers to know where the clinical practicum they are teaching is positioned within the curriculum.

The context in which clinical teaching occurs is a major determinant of its effectiveness. A philosophical context for clinical teaching influences one's understanding of the role of the clinical teacher and the process of teaching in clinical settings. This philosophy includes fundamental beliefs about the value of clinical education, roles and relationships of teachers and learners, and how to achieve desired outcomes and competencies.

Terms related to clinical teaching were defined to serve as a common frame of reference. The adjective *clinical* means involving direct observation of the patient; its proper use is to modify nouns such as practicum, instruction, practice, or evaluation. The teacher's central activity is clinical teaching or clinical instruction rather than supervision, which implies administrative activities such as overseeing, directing, and managing the work of others. Because learning is an active, personal process, the student is the one who experiences the learning. Therefore, teachers cannot provide clinical experiences, but they can offer opportunities and activities that will facilitate learning. Each student will experience a learning activity in a different way.

The philosophy of clinical teaching described in this chapter comprises the authors' shared beliefs about clinical teaching and learning and the roles of teachers and students. Subsequent chapters operationalize this philosophical approach to clinical teaching.

Clinical education should reflect the nature of the professional practice. Practice in clinical settings exposes students to realities of professional practice that cannot be conveyed by a textbook or simulation. Most professional practice situations are complex, unpredictable, and unique. Therefore, clinical learning activities should expose students to problems that cannot be solved easily with existing knowledge and technical skills. Another element of the philosophy of clinical teaching concerns the importance of clinical teaching. Because nursing is a professional practice discipline, the quality of students' clinical practice is important. Clinical education provides opportunities for real-life experiences and the transfer of knowledge to practical situations. In the clinical setting, nursing students encounter patients for the purpose of applying knowledge and developing competencies. The central activity of the student in clinical education should be learning, not doing. Sufficient learning time should be provided before performance is evaluated. Students need to engage in learning activities and practice competencies before their performance is evaluated summatively. Teachers should allow sufficient learning time with ample opportunity for feedback before evaluating performance.

Another element of this philosophy of clinical teaching is the importance of a climate of mutual trust and respect that supports learning and student development. Teachers and learners share the responsibility for maintaining this climate, but teachers are ultimately accountable for establishing expectations that faculty and students will be partners in achieving success. Clinical teaching should focus on essential competencies for transition to practice, whether they are at the entry or advanced level. Because every nursing program has limited time for clinical teaching, this time is used to maximum advantage by focusing on the most common practice problems and examplars that learners are likely to encounter. Educators need to identify the knowledge, skills, and attitudes that are most essential for students to learn. Learners need to spend most of their time on this essential curriculum, with opportunities to participate in the enrichment curriculum as well.

In clinical settings, the espoused curriculum should be the curriculum-in-use. Although most educators would argue that there is one curriculum for a nursing program, in reality the espoused curriculum is sometimes interpreted differently by each clinical teacher. Consequently, every student experiences this curriculum-in-use differently. Faculty cannot prescribe every detail of what clinical educators will teach and what learners will learn in clinical settings. Instead, it is usually more effective to specify competencies to be developed and allow teachers and learners to meet them in a variety of ways. Finally, the distinction between quality and quantity of clinical learning is important. The quality of a learner's experience is more important than the amount of time spent in clinical activities. Both the activity and amount of time should be individualized.

CERTIFIED ACADEMIC CLINICAL NURSE EDUCATOR® (CNE®cl) EXAMINATION TEST BLUEPRINT COMPETENCIES

1. **Function within the Education and Healthcare Environments**
   - A. **Function in the Clinical Nurse Educator Role**
     1. Integrate theory and practice in the clinical setting
   - B. **Operationalize the Curriculum**
     1. Assess congruence of the clinical environment with curriculum, course outcomes, and learner needs when evaluating clinical sites
     3. Facilitate meaningful and relevant clinical learning activities to promote optimal learning
   - C. **Abide by Legal Requirements, Ethical Guidelines, Agency Policies, and Guiding Framework**
     3. Facilitate learning activities that support the mission, goals, and values of the academic institution and the clinical agency
2. **Facilitate Learning in the Healthcare Environment**
   - A. Implement a variety of clinical teaching strategies congruent with learner needs, desired learner outcomes, course outcomes, setting, and context (e.g., virtual, telehealth, in-person simulation)
   - B. Apply teaching strategies from educational theory and evidence-based teaching practices
   - F. Create a positive and caring learning environment
5. **Facilitate Learner Development and Socialization**
   - F. Create learning environments that promote socialization to the role of the nurse

Note: The Certified Academic Clinical Nurse Educator (CNE®cl) Competencies in this and subsequent chapters identify selected competencies that relate to the content in each chapter. The lettering and numbering of competencies correspond to the structure of the CNE®cl Examination Detailed Test Blueprint. The CNE®cl Handbook with the full list of competencies is available at https://www.nln.org/awards-recognition/nln-credentialing/cne-cl/Certification-for-Nurse-Educatorscnecl/cne-cl-handbook

Source: National League for Nursing (NLN). (2025). Certified Academic Clinical Nurse Educator (CNE®cl) 2024 Candidate Handbook. Copyright by NLN. Reprinted with permission.

LEARNING ACTIVITIES

CourseConnect

To access self-assessment questions and interactive, competency-based learning activities for this chapter, visit www.springerpub.com/courseconnect. See inside front cover and tear-out card for CourseConnect details.

REFERENCES

Accreditation Commission for Education in Nursing. (2023). *ACEN standards and criteria. Standard 2 – Faculty*. https://resources.acenursing.org/space/SAC/1825603701/STANDARD+2+-+Faculty

American Association of Colleges of Nursing (AACN). (2021). *The essentials: Core competencies for professional nursing education*. AACN.

Commission on Collegiate Nursing Education. (2024). *Standards for accreditation of baccalaureate and graduate nursing programs*. https://www.aacnnursing.org/Portals/0/PDFs/CCNE/CCNE-Education-Standards-2024.pdf

Griffiths, M., Creedy, D., Carter, A., & Donnellan-Fernandez, R. (2022). Systematic review of interventions to enhance preceptors' role in undergraduate health student clinical learning. *Nurse Education in Practice, 62*, 103349. https://doi.org/10.1016/j.nepr.2022.103349

Hansbrough, W., Dunker, K., Duprey, M., & Lawrence, A. (2023). Descriptive analysis of newly hired academic nurse educator onboarding practices. *Nurse Educator, 48*(4), 192–196. https://doi.org/10.1097/NNE.0000000000001402

Interprofessional Education Collaborative. (2023). *IPEC core competencies for interprofessional collaborative practice: Version 3*. https://ipec.memberclicks.net/assets/core-competencies/IPEC_Core_Competencies_Version_3_2023.pdf

Jones-Schenk, J. (2025). Competency-based education coming to a nursing program near you. *Journal of Continuing Education in Nursing, 56*(1), 8–9. https://doi.org/doi:10.3928/00220124-20241213-03

National Academies of Sciences, Engineering, and Medicine. (2021). *The future of nursing 2020–2030: Charting a path to achieve health equity*. The National Academies Press. https://doi.org/10.17226/25982

National League for Nursing. (2024). *Certification for nurse educators*. https://www.nln.org/awards-recognition/nln-certification

National League for Nursing Commission for Nursing Education Accreditation (CNEA). (2021). *Standards for accreditation*. https://cnea.nln.org/standards-of-accreditation

National Organization of Nurse Practitioner Faculties. (2022a). *National Organization of Nurse Practitioner Faculties' nurse practitioner role core competencies*. https://cdn.ymaws.com/www.nonpf.org/resource/resmgr/competencies/nonpf_np_role_core_competenc.pdf

National Organization of Nurse Practitioner Faculties, National Task Force. (2022b). *Standards for quality nurse practitioner education, A report of the national task force on quality nurse practitioner education* (6th ed.). https://cdn.ymaws.com/www.nonpf.org/resource/resmgr/ntfstandards/ntfs_final.pdf

National Organization of Nurse Practitioner Faculties. (2024). *Competency implementation guide for nurse practitioner faculty*. https://www.nonpf.org/page/DNP_NPCompetencies

Oermann, M. H. (2022). Some principles to guide assessment of competencies. *Nurse Educator, 47*(1), 1. https://doi.org/10.1097/NNE.0000000000001143

Oermann, M. H. (2024). Key role of clinical nurse educators and preceptors in competency-based education. *Nurse Educator, 49*(5), 289. https://doi.org/10.1097/nne.0000000000001691

Oermann, M. H. (2025). Role of the nurse educator. In J. C. De Gagne & M. H. Oermann (Eds.)., *Teaching in nursing and role of the educator: The complete guide to best practice in teaching, evaluation, and curriculum development* (4th ed., pp. 3–18). Springer Publishing Company.

Oermann, M. H., Gaberson, K. B., & De Gagne, J. C. (2025). *Evaluation and testing in nursing education* (7th ed.). Springer Publishing Company.

Ross, J. G., Dunker, K. S., Morrell, M., Duprey, M. D., Parson, T., & Kim, L. (2024). Clinical faculty orientation practices in the United States: A descriptive study. *Nurse Educator, 49*(5), 278–283. https://doi.org/10.1097/nne.0000000000001625

Schoening, A. M., & Rusch, L. M. (2025). The transition from clinician to educator. In J. C. De Gagne & M. H. Oermann (Eds.), *Teaching in nursing and role of the educator: The complete guide to best practice in teaching, evaluation, and curriculum development* (4th ed., pp. 19–34). Springer Publishing Company.

U. S. Department of Labor. Bureau of Labor Statistics. (2023). *Occupational outlook handbook*. https://www.bls.gov/ooh/healthcare/registered-nurses.htm

U. S. Department of Health and Human Services, Health Resources and Services Administration. (2024). *2022 National sample survey of Registered Nurses snapshot*. https://bhw.hrsa.gov/sites/default/files/bureau-health-workforce/Nurse-Survey-Fact-Sheet-2024.pdf

van Ede, A. E., Claessen, R., van Gils, M., van Hoogstraten, C., van den Berg, I., & van Gurp, P. J. M. (2023). The teacher as coach: An innovative, longitudinal training for (bio)medical educators. *Clinical Teacher, 20*(2), e13564. https://doi.org/10.1111/tct.13564

Wells-Beede, E., Sharpnack, P., Gruben, D., Klenke-Borgmann, L., Goliat, L., & Yeager, C. (2023). A scoping review of nurse educator competencies: Mind the gap. *Nurse Educator, 48*(5), 234–239. https://doi.org/10.1097/nne.0000000000001376

Young-Brice, A., Farrar-Stern, K., & Malin, M. (2022). Comprehensive onboarding and orientation to support newly hired faculty in a nursing program. *Nurse Educator, 47*(6), 347–351. https://doi.org/10.1097/NNE.0000000000001242

Outcomes of Clinical Teaching

2

OBJECTIVES:

1. Integrate competency-based education frameworks into clinical teaching to align educational processes with professional standards and enhance student outcomes across cognitive, psychomotor, and affective domains.
2. Evaluate strategies to mitigate unintended negative consequences in clinical learning, such as anxiety and exposure to poor role models, through supportive feedback, reflective practices, and role modeling.
3. Leverage faculty and student diversity to enrich clinical teaching, foster cultural competence, and prepare nursing graduates for effective practice in diverse and evolving healthcare environments.

Clinical education in nursing requires a significant investment of resources, making it essential for educators to establish clear, realistic expectations for the intended outcomes of clinical learning. Clinical settings provide students with unique opportunities to acquire essential nursing knowledge and skills beyond those generally attainable in traditional classrooms. Traditionally, clinical learning opportunities in nursing education have revolved around the logistics of determining and coordinating available appropriate settings, activities, and time allocations. However, current accreditation standards in higher education, especially in nursing, require demonstrable evidence that educational programs are achieving meaningful outcomes.

This chapter explores the broad outcomes that can be achieved through a competency-based approach to clinical teaching and learning. Competency-based education aligns educational processes with specific professional standards and is increasingly recognized as crucial for integrating theoretical knowledge with practical skills. This chapter also discusses the importance of adapting clinical education to meet the diverse and complex needs of nursing students and considers how faculty and student diversity can influence the dynamics of clinical teaching, enhance educational outcomes, and enrich the learning experience.

INTENDED OUTCOMES

Accrediting bodies in higher education are increasingly emphasizing the importance of measuring student and graduate performance by holding faculty and institutions accountable for the outcomes of their educational programs (i.e., the behaviors, characteristics, qualities, or attributes that learners exhibit at the conclusion of an educational program). Teachers are tasked with specifying outcomes of nursing education programs that align with both current and future societal needs. Influences such as changes in healthcare delivery systems, demographic trends, technological advances, and developments in higher education shape the competencies required for professional nursing practice. After establishing the philosophical context for their nursing education program, nursing faculty must consider these influences as they design a context-relevant, evidence-informed curriculum and articulate its outcome statements.

In nursing education, various terms are employed to denote the professional abilities expected of learners at a program's conclusion. The term *outcomes* may refer to specific abilities demonstrated by program graduates or denote intended or expected results of the education program described in *outcome statements*. Alternative terms for *outcomes* include *terminal objectives* (usually associated with a behaviorist philosophical approach) and *goals* (outcomes that are broadly stated). Performance expectations at the end of a curriculum level or course are often referred to as *competencies*. In this book, the term *outcomes* is used to describe the intended or expected results of clinical teaching.

The curriculum reform movement of the 1980s focused on the importance of outcomes rather than on processes in improving the quality of teaching and learning in nursing education. This movement recognized that curricular design must take into account learners' individual needs, abilities, and learning preferences, thereby allowing learners to reach the same goals using different strengths. Development of an outcome-driven curriculum begins with a definition of desired ends and selection of content, followed by a determination of teaching strategies aimed at achieving those ends. Therefore, planning for clinical teaching commences with the identification of learning outcomes necessary for safe, competent nursing practice. The resulting outcome statements will reflect the faculty's chosen philosophical approach to curriculum development, and thus they will encompass outcomes related to one or more of the three domains of learning: cognitive (knowledge and intellectual skills), psychomotor (skills and technological abilities), and affective (professional attitudes, values, and beliefs) (Oermann et al., 2024).

Cognitive Domain Outcomes

Clinical learning activities provide students with opportunities to transfer knowledge from the classroom and other learning settings to real-life situations. In clinical practice, theoretical knowledge and scientific evidence are applied in practice, enabling students to deepen their understanding and refine their application of concepts. Through clinical activities, students extend and build upon the knowledge acquired in the classroom, simulation labs, and self-directed learning. To ensure that resources are used effectively, clinical learning activities should prioritize the development of knowledge that cannot be obtained in nonclinical settings.

As nursing and healthcare knowledge rapidly expands, new content is frequently added to nursing curricula. Without deliberate evaluation and removal of outdated or nonessential content, curricula risk becoming congested and content-saturated, potentially diluting the focus on essential knowledge outcomes. Therefore, nurse educators must develop and employ evidence-based teaching skills to critically evaluate content additions and deletions, thus ensuring that the curriculum remains focused on knowledge essential for safe and competent nursing practice. Faculty members preparing students for licensure or certification can benefit from consulting relevant test plans, such as the National Council of State Boards of Nursing (NCSBN®) test plans for practical nurses (NCSBN-PN, 2023) and registered nurses (NCSBN-RN, 2023), as well as the American Association of Colleges of Nursing (AACN) publication *The Essentials: Core Competencies for Professional Nursing Education* (AACN, 2021). These resources provide valuable guidance for selecting and organizing essential content for undergraduate and graduate nursing programs.

The complex and dynamic environments of contemporary healthcare demand that students acquire the ability to think critically and adaptively to ensure high-quality care and patient safety. Newer teaching approaches, such as narrative pedagogy, emphasize the development of higher-level thinking abilities by focusing on the process of thinking rather than the accumulation of content. This shift in emphasis encourages students to engage deeply with the evolving contexts of nursing practice and develop the ability to consider multiple perspectives.

To practice nursing effectively, students must develop higher-level cognitive abilities such as *problem solving, critical thinking, clinical reasoning, decision making,* and *clinical judgment*. Although these terms are often used interchangeably, they represent distinct skills that have implications for how they are taught and assessed (Pérez-Perdomo & Zabalegui, 2024). Understanding these distinctions is crucial as traditional pedagogical approaches that emphasize memorization and straightforward application of content are insufficient for fostering these advanced cognitive skills. When faculty aim to cultivate these higher-level cognitive skills, they should use strategies that actively involve students in questioning, interpreting, and reflecting on significant issues from various viewpoints. By adopting teaching strategies that promote the development of each of these critical cognitive abilities, faculty ensures that students are prepared to navigate the complexities of contemporary nursing practice.

PROBLEM SOLVING

Clinical learning activities provide rich sources of realistic practice problems to be solved. Some problems are related to patients and their health needs; others arise from the clinical environment itself. Most clinical problems tend to be complex, unique, and ambiguous. The ability to solve clinical problems is an important outcome of clinical teaching and learning, and the nursing process itself is a problem-solving approach. Most nurses and nursing students have some experience in problem solving, but complex problems of clinical practice often require new methods of reasoning and problem-solving strategies. Nursing students may not yet have achieved the ability to solve problems on a cognitive level sufficient to address clinical problems effectively. To achieve this important outcome, clinical activities should expose the learner to realistic clinical problems of increasing complexity.

Many nurse educators and students might equate problem solving with critical thinking; however, the ability to solve clinical problems is insufficient on its own for professional nursing practice, as it tends to focus solely on finding solutions or outcomes rather than on fostering a comprehensive understanding of the situation within its broader context. Problem solving encompasses identifying and defining the problem, collecting relevant data, proposing and implementing solutions, and evaluating their effectiveness. Students cannot effectively solve problems about which they lack a deep understanding and relevant knowledge base. Thorough comprehension of a problem in its full context provides a framework for effective problem solving when the student encounters similar cases to which they can apply knowledge gained from previous experience (Oermann et al., 2024).

CRITICAL THINKING

Critical thinking remains a vital outcome of nursing education. Although it is no longer specified as an accreditation requirement for prelicensure programs, it continues to be a focal point in major standards, competencies, and reports, including *The Future of Nursing 2020–2030* (National Academies of Sciences, Engineering, and Medicine [NASEM], 2021), the Quality and Safety Education for Nurses (QSEN) Institute (2022a, 2022b), and the AACN (2021). These guidelines reinforce the value of critical thinking for enhancing patient safety and delivering cost-effective, high-quality care.

Given today's complex healthcare environment, nurses must handle extensive clinical information, meet diverse patient needs, and navigate frequent ethical challenges, all of which demand strong critical-thinking abilities (Oermann et al., 2024). Many healthcare employers expect new graduates to demonstrate competence in this area, recognizing that sound judgment is integral to professional nursing practice. Consequently, nurse educators bear the responsibility of developing learning activities that help students cultivate both the skills and disposition necessary for critical thinking. Through intentional instructional design and targeted clinical experiences, educators can better equip future nurses to excel in a constantly evolving healthcare landscape.

Multiple definitions of *critical thinking* exist, and faculty members must concur on a definition that is suitable for their program—consensus helps guide the teaching and assessment of critical thinking and facilitates clear communication of this concept to students. Critical thinking is an intellectual process involving analysis, logic, information seeking, discrimination between relevant and irrelevant data, application of standards, prediction of outcomes, and drawing valid conclusions. It is purposeful, outcome-directed, and evidence-based (Ignatavicius & Andersen, 2024). Students who think critically (a) ask questions and are curious and willing to search for answers, (b) consider alternate perspectives and explanations, (c) question current practices, and (d) are open-minded (Oermann et al., 2024).

Although most educators would classify critical thinking as a cognitive domain outcome, some definitions of critical thinking characterize it as a composite of attitudes, knowledge, and skills. It encompasses the ability to systematically seek and analyze truth with an open mind and includes attitudinal dimensions such as self-confidence, perseverance, flexibility, creativity, intellectual integrity, and inquisitiveness (De Gagne & Oermann, 2025; Ignatavicius & Andersen, 2024). Critical thinking transcends clinical situations, extending to professionals in every discipline and often creating challenges in measuring and evaluating crucial outcomes. Nonetheless, clinical learning activities are essential for helping learners develop discipline-specific critical thinking skills as they observe, participate in, and evaluate nursing care in an increasingly complex and uncertain healthcare environment.

CLINICAL REASONING

Clinical reasoning is an essential feature of nursing competence. As a discipline-specific skill applied in clinical settings, it is often demonstrated by experienced nurses. In nursing, clinical reasoning entails a rigorous process of evaluating the quantity, quality, and reliability of available evidence; analyzing patient information comprehensively; and making informed professional judgments about patient management. The outcome of effective clinical reasoning is clinical judgment (i.e., the inference or conclusion drawn through the process of clinical reasoning) (Ignatavicius & Andersen, 2024).

Effective clinical reasoning mirrors the broader skill of critical thinking and hinges on a profound understanding of each patient's specific context. It involves the ability to understand the changing nature of patients' needs over time and adapt reasoning as clinical situations evolve. This dynamic aspect of clinical reasoning requires a responsive and flexible thought process that enables the nurse to adjust their judgment and actions according to immediate patient needs and conditions. The development of robust clinical reasoning skills in nursing students is highly dependent on their exposure to diverse and complex clinical scenarios. Clinical experience—characterized not just by its duration but also by its diversity and quality—is essential for cultivating these skills. Such experiences help students to integrate theoretical knowledge with practical application, thereby enhancing their ability to navigate the nuances of patient care effectively. Fostering environments that encourage questioning, critical analysis, and reflective practice can also significantly enhance the clinical reasoning abilities of nursing students, thus preparing them for the complexities of modern healthcare settings.

CLINICAL DECISION-MAKING

Professional nursing practice necessitates making informed decisions about patient care through identifying problems and potential solutions and selecting the best approach to address a specific situation. Decision-making also extends to managing the clinical environment, care delivery, and related activities (Oermann et al., 2024). The decision-making process entails gathering, analyzing, weighing, and valuing information in order to select the most appropriate course of action from several alternatives. However, nurses sometimes face situations in which not all possible alternatives, benefits, and risks are known, and thus a degree of uncertainty is introduced into their clinical decision-making. For this reason, clinical decision-making should be guided by national and specialty organization standards of nursing practice, such as the American Nurses Association's (ANA) *Scope and Standards of Practice* (2021). Additionally, it should be informed by evidence-based practice (EBP) guidelines, such as those from the American Society of PeriAnesthesia Nurses, *Perianesthesia Nursing Standards, Practice Recommendations, and Interpretive Statements* (2025), alongside healthcare organization standards of care, policies, and procedures, and critical paths. A critical component of decision-making, however, involves recognizing when standards and guidelines may not apply to a specific clinical context (Ignatavicius & Andersen, 2024).

Decisions are also shaped by individual values, biases, and cultural norms that influence how situations are perceived and analyzed. Nurses must be able to understand and address these personal and cultural factors in order to make nuanced decisions that respect diverse perspectives and patient backgrounds. In nursing, clinical decision-making is not only a technical skill but a collaborative and participatory process involving patients and staff members. A collaborative approach fosters supportive environments that value shared decision-making, thus enhancing the likelihood that decisions will meet with full acceptance and adherence. To build competencies, clinical learning activities should provide learners with numerous realistic decision-making opportunities that enable them to practice and refine their skills in a controlled yet challenging setting. Such hands-on experiences are essential for preparing nursing students to handle the complexities of real-world clinical scenarios and ensuring that they are equipped to make informed, effective decisions under pressure.

CLINICAL JUDGMENT

Clinical judgment is a cornerstone of nursing practice which significantly impacts patient outcomes and healthcare quality. According to a 2013–2014 NCSBN Practice Analysis, newly licensed nurses are frequently tasked with complex decision-making situations that critically affect patient care. In response, the NCSBN has developed a comprehensive Clinical Judgment Model (CJM) designed to measure and enhance competence in clinical judgment during the nursing licensure examination. This model integrates critical thinking and decision-making skills into a dynamic process involving the following abilities: recognition and interpretation of clinical cues, generation and evaluation of hypotheses, engagement in evidence-based actions, and assessment of outcomes. The NCSBN CJM underscores the need to adapt according to internal factors (e.g., the nurse's knowledge and experience) and external factors (e.g., task complexity, environmental pressures) (Dickison et al., 2019).

The Lasater Clinical Judgment Rubric (LCJR) offers a detailed framework for assessing the development of clinical judgment skills across 11 dimensions (Lasater, 2011). Based on Tanner's (2006) foundational work, this rubric facilitates structured feedback, enabling students to reflect effectively on their clinical experiences. It serves both formative and summative purposes by guiding educators in designing assessment tools that accurately measure clinical judgment capabilities (Hensel & Billings, 2020; Lasater, 2011). Recent research has validated the LCJR's effectiveness for scoring learners' clinical judgment in asynchronous simulation-based activities, highlighting the rubric's reliability and practicality in assessing written reflections and in supporting its broader application across educational settings (Rogers & Franklin, 2023).

Virtual simulations have also become an essential component of clinical judgment education, providing scalable, controlled environments that mimic real-life scenarios. As they allow students to practice and refine their judgment skills safely, these simulations align with Tanner's (2006) Model of Clinical Judgment and offer a structured way to apply theoretical knowledge in practical settings (Legge et al., 2024). The integration of these innovative teaching methods marks a significant evolution in nursing education and a movement toward more interactive and experiential learning experiences.

A comprehensive methodology allows educators to instill essential competencies for safe and effective patient care, thereby enhancing their students' clinical judgment abilities in preparation for the challenges of modern healthcare settings and equipping them with the critical skills necessary for licensure and their future professional roles. This alignment of educational outcomes with industry standards and expectations ensures that graduates are thoroughly prepared to apply their clinical judgment skills effectively in real-world settings.

Psychomotor Domain Outcomes

Skills are an important outcome of clinical learning. Nurses must possess adequate psychomotor, communication, technological, and organizational skills to practice effectively in an increasingly complex healthcare environment. Although these skills often incorporate cognitive and attitudinal dimensions, clinical teaching primarily emphasizes performance.

PSYCHOMOTOR SKILLS

Psychomotor skills are vital to effective nursing practice. These skills enable nurses to perform proficiently in situations that demand neuromuscular coordination. Characterized by purposeful, complex, movement-oriented activities, psychomotor skills require an overt physical response. The concept of *skill* in this context refers to the ability to execute physical movements with efficiency, speed, and accuracy. Consequently, psychomotor proficiency extends beyond mere capability; it encompasses the ability to perform actions proficiently, smoothly, and consistently under diverse conditions and within specific time constraints. Learning these skills involves substantial practice accompanied by feedback, which is crucial for refining performance until the desired outcomes are achieved. Clinical learning activities should provide abundant opportunities for practicing these skills as well as timely feedback to enhance the learning process.

The development of psychomotor skills entails more than achieving technical proficiency, however. When performing technical tasks, nursing students and practitioners must also demonstrate caring behaviors, engage in critical thinking, apply clinical reasoning, solve problems, and make clinical decisions. These further competencies typically can be integrated after the technical aspects of the skill have been mastered to the extent that the learner practices them without a conscious effort. At this advanced stage of skill development, learners can fully comprehend situations and focus holistically both on the patient and on the technical execution of their skills.

INTERPERSONAL SKILLS

Interpersonal skills are fundamental to nursing practice; they play a pivotal role in assessing patient and family needs, planning and implementing care, evaluating outcomes, and effectively communicating and documenting all aspects of patient care. These skills encompass a broad spectrum of activities including proficient communication, the therapeutic use of self, and the educational engagements that are critical in healthcare settings. Interpersonal skills entail not only mastery of verbal and written communication but also of nuanced expression through (and interpretation of) nonverbal cues such as facial expressions, body posture, movement, and touch. Clinical learning environments provide nursing students with diverse opportunities to develop these skills through direct patient interactions, collaborative team involvement, and detailed care documentation. These activities help students form therapeutic relationships, foster teamwork with health professionals, and engage in meaningful educational exchanges with patients and their families.

In addition to foundational interpersonal skills, the development of emotional intelligence is crucial for managing the personal and professional challenges that nurses face, particularly the delivery of bad news to patients and their families. Nnate and Nashwan (2023) highlight the critical role of emotional intelligence in enhancing a nurse's ability to handle stressful communications effectively. Emotional intelligence allows nurses to manage their reactions and maintain professionalism during difficult conversations, thus ensuring more compassionate and effective patient care. Moreover, emotional intelligence fosters stronger nurse–patient relationships and holistic care by enabling nurses to recognize and respond appropriately to patients' emotional cues. This aspect of nursing practice is vital in ensuring that communication transcends mere transactional exchanges and evolves into supportive, empathetic interactions that respect patient and family experiences and preferences (Nnate & Nashwan, 2023).

To support the development of these competencies and ensure that nurses are not only clinically proficient but also adept at navigating the interpersonal dynamics inherent in healthcare settings, nursing programs should integrate targeted training that emphasizes emotional intelligence, conflict resolution, and advanced communication strategies. This comprehensive approach can enhance patient satisfaction, improve clinical outcomes, and support the overall well-being of both patients and healthcare providers.

ORGANIZATIONAL SKILLS

Nurses must have excellent organizational skills to effectively navigate the complex healthcare environment and deliver high-quality patient care. These foundational skills encompass time management, priority setting, and efficient task sequencing. Delegation is a particularly critical skill, as it enables nurses to manage diverse tasks and responsibilities within healthcare settings efficiently.

Effective delegation requires nurses to make precise judgments regarding which tasks to delegate and to whom and under what circumstances they can be delegated safely. This essential skill is based on a firm understanding of legal and ethical guidelines, strong communication skills, and the ability to manage team dynamics effectively. A scoping review by Clarke (2021) highlights the importance of delegation in nursing practice, noting that proficiency in this area is essential for both novice and experienced nurses. The study reveals that effective delegation is closely linked with leadership, critical thinking, decision-making, and interpersonal skills, all of which are cultivated through both theoretical learning and practical application.

To ensure that nursing students develop strong delegation skills, educational programs must provide numerous opportunities for practical experience, including creating clinical and simulated environments in which students engage in detailed scenarios involving task assignment, method specification, and setting feedback expectations. Simulation exercises that replicate real-life clinical situations allow students to test and refine their delegation strategies within a safe and controlled setting (Clarke, 2021).

Clinical activities provide opportunities for learners at various levels of nursing education (e.g., graduate, undergraduate) to develop essential leadership and management skills. These activities aim to enhance the learner's ability to manage patient care collectively, evaluate personal and team performance, allocate and coordinate resources, collaborate within healthcare teams, and maintain patient safety and quality of care. Clinical teachers, along with staff members and preceptors in clinical settings, play a pivotal role in modeling these skills. They provide visible examples of effective delegation and decision-making, such as serving on practice committees, addressing safety concerns or healthcare errors, and demonstrating strategic delegation. Because these activities may not always be apparent to students, educators and clinical staff should make their strategic thinking accessible to students by openly discussing their decision-making processes and sharing the rationale behind their actions. Research by Unsworth et al. (2021) underscores the importance of structured learning experiences in developing these competencies, which are critical as students transition into their roles as registered nurses, and supports the need for effective training in prioritization, resource management, and risk management to enhance patient care and safety.

Affective Domain Outcomes

Clinical learning significantly contributes to developing affective outcomes (i.e., beliefs, values, attitudes, and dispositions) that are essential components of professional nursing practice (Oermann et al., 2024) because they encompass the profession's humanistic and ethical dimensions. Nurses are expected to uphold and demonstrate core values such as respect for patient uniqueness, support for patient autonomy and the right to make informed choices, and maintenance of the confidentiality of patient information.

The values integral to professional nursing are articulated in the American Nurses Association's *Code of Ethics for Nurses* (2025). Nursing faculty should introduce this code early in educational programs and consistently reinforce its values through clinical learning activities designed to help students internalize these principles. Furthermore, professional nurses must engage in moral reasoning, values clarification, and values inquiry in order to navigate the ethical complexities of modern healthcare (Hamaideh et al., 2024).

In an era marked by rapid advances in knowledge and technology, nursing education programs are tasked with producing graduates who are committed lifelong learners, dedicated to their continued professional development. The professional nurse persona is shaped in clinical settings where accountability is emphasized and the impact of decisions and actions is immediately evident, thus offering students a platform on which to develop, practice, and evaluate affective outcomes. Effective clinical education should provide exposure to exemplary role models, including nursing faculty and practicing nurses who embody professional values. Additionally, it should offer structured opportunities for value development to support students in their professional role formation.

Integrated Domain Outcomes

In the previous discussion, outcomes were classified within the cognitive, psychomotor, or affective domains; however, some intended outcomes of clinical learning include elements of all three domains. Two examples of such integration are cultural competence, and healthcare quality and patient safety competence.

CULTURAL COMPETENCE

Recent demographic shifts underscore the increasing racial and ethnic diversity of the United States and highlight the importance of cultural competence in nursing education. According to the 2020 U.S. Census, 61.6% of the population self-identifies as non-Hispanic White, 12.4% as Black or African American, 6.0% as Asian, 18.7% as Hispanic or Latino, and 8.4% with two or more races (U.S. Census Bureau, 2021). Projections indicate that by 2060, the proportion of non-Hispanic White Americans may fall to roughly 44% of the total population, while the proportion of Hispanic or Latino Americans could approach nearly 29% (U.S. Census Bureau, 2021). These trends reflect a growing need for nurses who can provide culturally sensitive, patient-centered care.

The AACN continues to emphasize the importance of integrating cultural competence throughout baccalaureate, master's, and doctoral programs. In *The Essentials: Core Competencies for Professional Nursing Education* (AACN, 2021), educators are encouraged to promote the development of cultural humility, awareness, and skills in order to address patients' varying values, beliefs, and health practices effectively. By actively preparing students to recognize and respond to cultural differences, nursing programs foster care practices that acknowledge social determinants of health and reduce healthcare disparities.

Culturally competent care aligns with broader priorities in healthcare such as achieving social justice, promoting health equity, and ensuring effective interprofessional collaboration. Nursing faculty can reinforce these priorities by designing learning activities that challenge students to explore diverse cultural perspectives and cultivate empathetic, respectful communication skills. Immersive clinical experiences, simulations, and reflective dialogue help nursing students to gain the insights and abilities needed to practice in a global environment while upholding the highest standards of patient-focused care.

HEALTHCARE QUALITY AND PATIENT SAFETY COMPETENCIES

A primary goal of clinical teaching involves fostering evidence-based, interprofessional practice within a framework focused on quality improvement (QI) and patient safety. These competencies are critical for preparing all healthcare professionals; in nursing, a pivotal initiative in this area is the QSEN project, which began in 2005 (QSEN, 2023). The QSEN project highlights the importance of equipping future nurses with the knowledge, skills, and attitudes (KSAs) required to continually enhance the quality and safety of healthcare systems (QSEN, 2023). These KSAs are organized around six core competencies: patient-centered care, teamwork and collaboration, EBP, QI, safety, and informatics (QSEN, 2023). Nursing programs commonly integrate these concepts into prelicensure, graduate, and nurse residency curricula.

Patient-Centered Care

Patient-centered care involves viewing patients or their chosen representatives as key partners in compassionate, coordinated care that respects personal preferences, values, and needs (QSEN, 2022b). For prelicensure students, related KSAs include recognizing the diverse cultural, ethnic, and social backgrounds that influence patient, family, and community values; delivering care that acknowledges this diversity; and offering support to patients whose values differ from one's own (QSEN, 2022b). At the graduate level, KSAs include synthesizing multiple models of pain and suffering, ensuring that these factors are addressed according to patient preferences, and valuing patients' expertise in their own health (QSEN, 2022a). Instructors can help learners develop these competencies through authentic or simulated clinical situations that prompt them to reflect on differences between routine practice and practice that truly addresses patients' values, needs, and preferences.

Teamwork and Collaboration

Teamwork and collaboration entail functioning effectively with nursing and interprofessional colleagues and emphasizing open communication, mutual respect, and collaborative decision-making (QSEN, 2022b). Prelicensure KSAs include understanding the roles and scopes of practice of various team members, demonstrating competence within one's own role as a team member, and recognizing the patient's pivotal role in the healthcare team (QSEN, 2022b). Graduate students further develop these KSAs by identifying systemic barriers and facilitators to teamwork, contributing to structures that support effective collaboration, and appreciating how system-level solutions can improve team functioning (QSEN, 2022a). Assigning learners to clinical settings where interprofessional collaboration is routine (e.g., operating rooms) can greatly enhance their ability to acquire these KSAs.

Evidence-Based Practice

Evidence-based practice refers to integrating the best available evidence with clinical expertise as well as patient and family values and preferences to deliver optimal healthcare (QSEN, 2022b). For prelicensure students, relevant KSAs include recognizing credible evidence-based guidelines, consulting with clinical experts prior to deviating from established protocols, and valuing ongoing QI informed by emerging research (QSEN, 2022b). Graduate students develop further by pinpointing gaps in specialty practice, employing systematic literature searches to address clinical questions, and emphasizing ethical considerations in both research and QI (QSEN, 2022a). Depending on each learner's level, clinical experiences offer abundant opportunities to practice delivering high-quality patient care guided by evidence and best practices appropriate to generalist or advanced roles.

Quality Improvement

QI focuses on using data to measure care outcomes and employing systematic methods to design and evaluate changes, thereby continuously enhancing healthcare quality and safety (QSEN, 2022b). Prelicensure KSAs include understanding why measurement is critical to assessing care quality, contributing to root cause analyses following sentinel events, and recognizing the impact of unwanted care variations (QSEN, 2022b). Graduate-level KSAs involve identifying relevant quality metrics in a particular specialty, overseeing ethical processes for managing QI projects, and valuing the role of metrics in maintaining high standards of patient care (QSEN, 2022a). Faculty can enable students to develop QI competencies by assigning them to gather or review data on care quality and participate in or lead QI initiatives, as deemed appropriate for their level.

Safety

Safety involves minimizing the risk of harm to patients and providers by ensuring that systems are efficient and individuals perform effectively (QSEN, 2022b). Prelicensure KSAs include describing factors that foster a culture of safety, employing methods to reduce reliance on memory, and acknowledging personal responsibility in preventing errors (QSEN, 2022b). Graduate students learn to outline best practices for specialty-related patient and provider safety, adopt a systems-based perspective rather than blaming individuals for errors, and appreciate the value of organizational reporting systems (QSEN, 2022a). Faculty reinforce this competency by modeling an understanding of human cognitive and physical limitations, promoting a just culture in nursing education, and encouraging students to openly discuss and learn from errors or near-misses. Incorporating national patient safety resources, actively partnering with patients and families to ensure safe care, and applying a systemic viewpoint are all vital to students' progression in meeting safety KSAs.

Informatics

Informatics focuses on the use of information and technology to communicate effectively, manage knowledge, minimize errors, and guide decision-making (QSEN, 2022b). As electronic health records (EHRs) become more prevalent, students must learn to access and apply patient information, plan care, and document interventions using these systems. In *The Future of Nursing 2020–2030: Charting a Path to Achieve Health Equity*, NASEM (2021) reaffirm the importance of leveraging innovative technologies and complex informatics to promote health equity, improve care delivery, and expand access—particularly in underserved communities. This perspective highlights the need for nurses to value the meaningful use of health data and embrace standardized nursing terminologies that enhance interoperability.

Consequently, nursing students need to appreciate the meaningful use of health information, value standardized nursing terminologies, and contribute to interoperability within healthcare technology systems. At the prelicensure level, essential KSAs include recognizing how technology and information management contribute to patient safety and quality outcomes, employing EHRs appropriately, and committing to ongoing informatics education (QSEN, 2022b). Graduate students further develop by critically evaluating taxonomic systems that ensure data consistency, taking part in designing clinical decision support tools, and appreciating the necessity of collaboration when developing informatics solutions (QSEN, 2022a). Programs that incorporate health information technology concepts throughout multiple courses help learners cultivate these competencies more effectively than reliance on a single informatics course alone.

UNINTENDED OUTCOMES

Nurse educators typically design clinical learning activities with specific intended outcomes, yet these activities can have unintended consequences, both positive and negative. A positive outcome could be a student's realization of their preferred career choice due to a clinical experience that helped them gauge their interest and competency in a specific specialty. For instance, exposure to postanesthesia care units during clinical rotations can prompt students to consider or dismiss postanesthesia nursing based on their suitability and interest in that specialty.

On the other hand, clinical learning activities can yield negative outcomes, such as the adoption of poor practice habits observed and copied from experienced nurses. Students often imitate workarounds and shortcuts they observe, even when these practices deviate from evidence-based standards taught in the classroom. It is crucial that clinical instructors not only recognize the influential power of role models but engage students in discussions about poor practices they observe to help them critically evaluate and learn from these experiences.

One significant unintended outcome of clinical education is the anxiety commonly experienced by nursing students, which can adversely impact their learning, effectiveness in teamwork, and overall ability to deliver safe and compassionate care. Research by Vo et al. (2023) highlights how high levels of anxiety are prevalent among nursing students in clinical settings, affecting both their mental and physical well-being. This research suggests that although various interventions have aimed to reduce this anxiety (e.g., student-led strategies such as expressive writing, faculty-led behavioral interventions), the evidence supporting their effectiveness remains limited. These findings underscore the need for continued research into diverse and potentially effective methods to mitigate anxiety and enhance the clinical learning environment for nursing students (Vo et al., 2023).

Another negative unintended outcome of clinical learning may be academic dishonesty. Academic dishonesty involves intentional participation in deceptive practices such as lying, cheating, or misrepresenting one's academic work. These behaviors are often associated with classroom learning, but in clinical settings, they may entail serious or dangerous misconduct such as falsifying assessment findings, breaching patient confidentiality, or failing to report errors. Clinical instructors may inadvertently contribute to this issue by promoting a culture in which perfection is the expected standard, inadvertently suggesting that good nurses do not make errors. This expectation is not only unrealistic but also detrimental, especially for nursing students whose learning process naturally involves making and learning from mistakes. The emphasis on perfection can lead students to conceal their errors or their lack of knowledge and skills to avoid punitive measures such as low grades or negative evaluations, which are typically ineffective in preventing future mistakes.

A scoping review on academic dishonesty among nursing students (He et al., 2024) highlights that fostering a learning environment based on mutual trust and respect, setting a standard of excellence rather than of perfection, acknowledging the inevitability of errors, and ensuring respectful treatment when students admit their shortcomings can significantly reduce tendencies towards dishonest behaviors. Moreover, by modeling academic and professional integrity and creating opportunities for open discussion about errors, clinical educators can help students learn valuable lessons from their mistakes, thereby enhancing safety and integrity in clinical practice. This approach not only prevents dangerous consequences for patients but also prevents lost learning opportunities for students (He et al., 2024).

IMPACT OF DIVERSITY ON CLINICAL TEACHING AND LEARNING

A diverse mix of faculty and students can play an integral role in shaping the nature of clinical teaching and realizing desired educational outcomes. Diversity in this context spans an array of attributes, including but not limited to cultural, ethnic, gender, and socioeconomic differences. Such multiplicity enriches the learning environment by reflecting the realities of modern healthcare and prepares students to provide culturally responsive care.

Diverse faculty bring a range of perspectives, teaching styles, and life experiences, which can lead to more inclusive methods of instruction. By addressing varied learning needs and preferences, these educators help students remain engaged, ultimately promoting academic success. Additionally, when faculty model culturally competent behaviors, students gain insights into how to interact respectfully and effectively with individuals from different backgrounds—an essential skill in clinical practice. Students from diverse backgrounds can learn from one another's experiences, perspectives, and problem-solving approaches. Exposure to peers who differ in culture, language, or worldview cultivates open-mindedness and encourages critical thinking; it also equips learners to better recognize and address health disparities, thus enhancing communication and empathy—qualities crucial for patient-centered care (De Gagne & Oermann, 2025).

The impact of diversity becomes particularly evident in clinical settings. Students who practice alongside colleagues and mentors from various backgrounds become more adept at tailoring care to meet each patient's unique needs and preferences. These real-world interactions foster the development of cultural humility, refine clinical judgment, and promote teamwork in situations that mirror the multifaceted demands of complex healthcare. Ensuring equitable opportunities to learn from and within diverse groups helps reduce educational disparities. By designing clinical learning activities that account for learners' cultural, linguistic, and socioeconomic contexts, nurse educators create more inclusive environments in which all students can thrive. This approach not only advances fairness but also strengthens future nursing workforces that reflect and respond to the communities they serve.

Clinical educators are pivotal in modeling inclusive practices through respectful communication and acknowledgment of individual differences. Their professional conduct transcends the teaching of clinical skills, instilling in students the professional values needed to succeed in diverse healthcare contexts. Consequently, developing and embracing diversity in clinical education fosters robust teamwork, creative problem-solving, and culturally competent care—ultimately shaping nursing graduates who are well-prepared to meet the evolving needs of diverse patient populations. By examining how diversity among faculty and students influences the dynamics of clinical teaching, nurse educators can better align curricula, mentorship, and program design with the goal of producing culturally aware professionals who are equipped to deliver high-quality, patient-centered care.

SUMMARY

Clinical teaching is designed to develop nursing students' knowledge, skills, and values across cognitive, psychomotor, and affective domains. Accreditation standards and professional guidelines emphasize the importance of producing meaningful, measurable outcomes that demonstrate capabilities essential for safe, evidence-based practice, such as problem-solving, critical thinking, clinical decision-making, clinical reasoning, and clinical judgment. Students develop these skills through realistic clinical experiences, guided by reflective practices and supported by faculty who model best practices. Psychomotor skills, integral to effective patient care, are complemented by robust interpersonal competencies. Students learn to prioritize tasks, manage time, delegate responsibilities, communicate therapeutically, and resolve conflicts—skills that are fundamental to leadership and effective teamwork. Equally important are the affective outcomes, such as the development of professional values, ethical reasoning, and cultural competence, which enable nurses to deliver compassionate, personalized care and promote equity in diverse healthcare environments.

Clinical learning not only leads to positive outcomes like enhanced self-awareness and informed career choices but also poses risks of unintended negative consequences. For instance, anxiety can significantly affect performance and learning, and observing poor role models may compromise safe practice and ethical conduct. To mitigate these risks, educators must set realistic expectations, foster academic integrity, and provide supportive, constructive feedback. Furthermore, educators must recognize the pivotal role of diversity in enriching clinical teaching and preparing graduates to effectively navigate and thrive in complex, multicultural healthcare settings. By understanding and integrating this diversity, clinical education not only meets traditional goals but also adapts to the evolving demands of global healthcare environments.

CNE®cl EXAMINATION TEST BLUEPRINT CORE COMPETENCIES

1. **Function Within the Education and Health Care Environments**
   A. Function in the Clinical Nurse Educator Role
      1. Integrate theory and practice in the clinical setting
      2. Foster professional growth of learners (e.g., coaching, reflection, and debriefing)
      4. Act as a role model of professional nursing within the clinical learning environment
      5. Create a diverse, equitable, and inclusive learning environment

   B. Operationalize the Curriculum
      2. Identify learners' goals and outcomes
      4. Prepare learners for clinical experiences (e.g., facility, clinical expectations, equipment, and technology-based resources)
      6. Provide opportunities for learners to develop clinical judgment related to course outcomes

   C. Abide by Legal Requirements, Ethical Guidelines, Agency Policies, and Guiding Framework
      1. Apply ethical and legal principles to create a safe clinical learning environment (e.g., privacy laws, confidentiality, error/near-miss situation reporting, remediation, negligence, liability, scope/standards of practice)
2. **Facilitate Learning in the Healthcare Environment**
   D. Create opportunities for learners to develop clinical judgment
   E. Promote a culture of safety and quality in the delivery of healthcare
   F. Create a positive and caring learning environment
3. **Demonstrate Effective Interpersonal Communication and Collaborative Interprofessional Relationships**
   D. Support an environment of frequent, respectful, and civil communication within the healthcare team
   G. Respond to learner concerns, needs, or questions in a supportive manner
   K. Demonstrate culturally sensitive communication in clinical learning environments
4. **Apply Clinical Expertise in the Healthcare Environment**
   A. Maintain clinical skills relevant to the learning environment
   C. Provide client care using evidence-based practice and standards of care
   E. Adjust learner assignments based on client care needs to assure a culture of safety
5. **Facilitate Learner Development and Socialization**
   A. Mentor learners in professional nursing behaviors
   B. Promote professional integrity and accountability
   H. Encourage the use of self-care techniques to promote wellbeing (e.g., relaxation, meditation, mindfulness)
6. **Implement Effective Clinical and Assessment Evaluation Strategies**
   A. Employ a variety of strategies to determine achievement of learning outcomes

LEARNING ACTIVITIES

CourseConnect

To access self-assessment questions and interactive, competency-based learning activities for this chapter, visit www.springerpub.com/courseconnect. See inside front cover and tear-out card for Course Connect details.

REFERENCES

American Association of Colleges of Nursing. (2021). *The essentials: Core competencies for professional nursing education*. Author.

American Nurses Association. (2021). *Nursing: Scope and standards of practice* (4th ed.). Author.

American Nurses Association. (2025). *Code of ethics for nurses*. https://codeofethics.ana.org

American Society of PeriAnesthesia Nurses. (2025). *2023–2024 Perianesthesia nursing standards, practice recommendations, and interpretive statements*. Author.

Clarke, H. (2021). How pre-registration nursing students acquire delegation skills: A systematic literature review. *Nurse Education Today*, *106*, 105096. https://doi.org/10.1016/j.nedt.2021.105096

De Gagne, J. C., & Oermann, M. H. (2025). *Teaching in nursing and role of the educator: The complete guide to best practice in teaching, evaluation, and curriculum development* (4th ed.). Springer Publishing Company.

Dickison, P., Haerling, K. A., & Lasater, K. (2019). Integrating the national council of state boards of nursing clinical judgment model into nursing educational frameworks. *Journal of Nursing Education*, *58*(2), 72–78. https://doi.org/10.3928/01484834-20190122-03

Hamaideh, S., Abuhammad, S., Abu Khait, B., Al-Modallal, H., Hamdan-Mansour, A., Masa'deh, R., & Alrjoub, S. (2024). Levels and predictors of empathy, self-awareness, and perceived stress among nursing students: A cross sectional study. *BMC Nursing*, *23*(1), 131. https://doi.org/10.1186/s12912-024-01774-7

He, F. X., Fanaian, M., Zhang, N. M., Lea, X., Geale, S. K. Gielis, L., Razaghi, K., & Evans, A. (2024). Academic dishonesty in university nursing students: A scoping review. *International Journal of Nursing Studies*, *154*, 104752. https://doi.org/10.1016/j.ijnurstu.2024.104752

Hensel, D., & Billings, D. M. (2020). Strategies to teach the national council of state boards of nursing clinical judgment model. *Nurse Educator*, *45*(3), 128–132. https://doi.org/10.1097/NNE.0000000000000773

Ignatavicius, D. D., & Andersen, S. (2024). *Alfaro's clinical judgment in nursing: A how-to practice approach* (8th ed.). Elsevier.

Lasater, K. (2011). Clinical judgment: The last frontier for evaluation. *Nurse Education in Practice*, *11*(2), 86–92. https://doi.org/10.1016/j.nepr.2010.11.013

Legge, T. R., Holthaus, A., Hallmark, B., & Alexander, K. (2024). Preparing for the Next Generation NCLEX using a virtual simulation. *Journal of Nursing Education*, *63*(7), 485–489. https://doi.org/10.3928/01484834-20230713-01

National Academies of Sciences, Engineering, and Medicine. (2021). *The future of nursing 2020–2030: Charting a path to achieve health equity*. National Academies Press. https://doi.org/10.17226/25982

National Council of State Boards of Nursing. (2023). *Next generation national council licensure examination for practical nurses (NCLEX-PN®) test plan*. https://www.ncsbn.org/public-files/2023_PN_Test%20Plan_FINAL.pdf

National Council of State Boards of Nursing. (2023). *Next generation national council licensure examination for registered nurses (NCLEX-RN®) test plan*. https://www.ncsbn.org/public-files/2023_RN_Test%20Plan_English_FINAL.pdf

Nnate, D. A., & Nashwan, A. J. (2023). Emotional intelligence and delivering bad news in professional nursing practice. *Cureus*, *15*(6), e40353. https://doi.org/10.7759/cureus.40353

Oermann, M. H., Gaberson, K. B., & De Gagne, J. C. (2024). *Evaluation and testing in nursing education* (7th ed.). Springer Publishing Company.

Pérez-Perdomo, A., & Zabalegui, A. (2024). Teaching strategies for developing clinical reasoning skills in nursing students: A systematic review of randomised controlled trials. *Healthcare*, *12*(1), 90. https://doi.org/10.3390/healthcare12010090

Quality and Safety Education for Nurses Institute. (2022a). *Graduate QSEN competencies*. https://www.qsen.org/competencies-graduate-ksas

Quality and Safety Education for Nurses Institute. (2022b). *Pre-licensure KSAs*. https://www.qsen.org/competencies-pre-licensure-ksas

Quality and Safety Education for Nurses Institute. (2023). *Project overview: The evolution of the quality and safety education for nurses initiative*. https://www.qsen.org/post/project-overview

Rogers, B. A., & Franklin, A. E. (2023). Lasater clinical judgment rubric reliability for scoring clinical judgment after observing asynchronous simulation and feasibility/usability with learners. *Nurse Education Today*, *125*, 105769. https://doi.org/10.1016/j.nedt.2023.105769

Tanner, C. A. (2006). Thinking like a nurse: A research-based model of clinical judgment in nursing. *Journal of Nursing Education*, *45*(6), 204–211. https://doi.org/10.3928/01484834-20060601-04

Unsworth, J., Melling, A., & Porteous, D. (2021). Development and evaluation of the validity and reliability of the leading and managing care pre-registration nursing student assessment tool. *SAGE Open Nursing*, *7*, 23779608211000259. https://doi.org/10.1177/23779608211000259

U.S. Census Bureau. (2021). *2020 census data*. https://www.census.gov

Vo, T. N., Chiu, H. Y., Chuang, Y. H., & Huang, H. C. (2023). Prevalence of stress and anxiety among nursing students: A systematic review and meta-analysis. *Nurse Educator*, *48*(3), E90–E95. https://doi.org/10.1097/NNE.0000000000001343

Process and Models of Clinical Teaching

3

OBJECTIVES:

1. Describe the clinical teaching process, key steps involved, and their interrelationships.
2. Examine characteristics of an effective clinical teacher and essential teaching skills.
3. Compare models of clinical teaching (traditional, preceptor, and partnership), including the advantages, disadvantages, and outcomes for students, educators, and healthcare systems.

Clinical teaching is a complex interaction between students and educators. Various factors influence this process, including the characteristics of the teacher and learner, the clinical environment, the nature of practice within that environment, the patients and families involved in care, other healthcare providers, and the inherent uncertainties of clinical practice. This chapter outlines the process of clinical teaching and provides a framework for planning learning activities appropriate for the competencies to be achieved, for guiding and supporting students in the practice setting, and for evaluating clinical performance.

The process of clinical teaching begins with identification of the competencies to be achieved and proceeds through assessing the learner's knowledge and skills, planning clinical learning activities, developing a supportive learning environment, guiding students in the clinical setting, and evaluating performance. The clinical competencies, outcomes to be met in the course, and expectations of students should be communicated clearly to students, be in written form, and be understood by them. Similarly, the teacher has an important responsibility in discussing these competencies and related clinical activities with clinical site personnel. Models of clinical teaching—traditional (in which one teacher guides the learning of a small group of students), preceptor, and partnership—are also explained in this chapter.

TEACHING AND LEARNING

Teaching is a complex process intended to facilitate learning. While the goal of teaching is to lead students in discovering knowledge for themselves, the teacher encourages this discovery through deliberate teaching actions that lead in that direction. Clinical teaching involves a sharing and mutual experience on the part of both teacher and student and is carried out in an environment of support and trust. Teaching is not telling, it is not dispensing information, and it is not merely demonstrating skills. Instead, teaching is *involving* the student as an active participant in this learning. The teacher is a resource person with knowledge and skills to share to facilitate learning.

Learning is a process through which people change as a result of their experiences. Some of these changes are observable and measurable; for example, the student can explain the evidence base of an intervention or can accurately perform a procedure. In clinical practice, however, new insights and perspectives may be as critical to the student's learning and development as measurable competencies. Learning, therefore, may also reflect a new insight into patient care.

The teaching–learning process is a complex interaction of these processes. When students are actively involved in their learning and perceive a positive teacher–student relationship, they can be honest about their learning needs and seek guidance from clinical educators to help them develop their competencies. Active learning may also foster students' higher-level thinking as they reflect on patient problems and possible approaches and consider multiple options. In a systematic review and meta-analysis, Xiaoyan et al. (2024) compared the outcomes of team-based learning, which emphasizes group work and active student participation, with conventional teaching practices that rely on lectures and more passive teaching strategies. The findings indicated that team-based learning not only enhanced nursing students' knowledge and practical skills, but also promoted self-directed learning and critical thinking. Other studies on team-based and problem-based learning support these results, confirming that student-centered methods foster critical thinking, clinical performance, student engagement, and other positive learning outcomes (Burton et al., 2024; Jenkins Barnard et al., 2024; Wei et al., 2024). However, whether these methods improve retention remains unclear (Alizadeh et al., 2024).

PROCESS OF CLINICAL TEACHING: FIVE STEPS

The process of clinical teaching includes five steps:

1. identifying the clinical competencies;
2. assessing learning needs;
3. planning clinical learning activities;
4. guiding and supporting learners; and
5. evaluating clinical learning and performance.

This process is not linear; rather, each step influences others. For example, clinical evaluations provide data on the further learning needs of students, which in turn suggest new learning activities. Similarly, as the teacher works with students, observations of performance may alter the assessment and suggest different learning activities.

Identifying the Clinical Competencies

The first step in clinical teaching is to identify the clinical competencies to be achieved in the course or practicum. These competencies guide the educator in determining the learning activities that should be planned for students and the focus of clinical evaluation. Competencies are the observable abilities of the student: what the student can *do* in clinical practice (Oermann, 2022). The American Association of Colleges of Nursing (AACN) defines competencies as the observable abilities of students—their knowledge, skills, and attitudes (AACN, 2021). In some nursing programs, rather than clinical competencies, faculty identify the outcomes of learning or objectives to be achieved by students in the clinical course or at the end of a specific clinical practicum or set of learning activities.

In Chapter 12, Table 12.1 provides examples of clinical competencies with their relationship to the AACN *The Essentials: Core Competencies for Professional Nursing Education*, which identify competencies and subcompetencies at two levels (entry and advanced). The clinical competencies should be observable and achievable by students, considering their prior knowledge, skills, and experiences. Learning opportunities should be available in the clinical setting, simulation, or through other experiences. The competencies should be communicated clearly to students, be in written form, and be understood by them. Similarly, the teacher has an important responsibility in *discussing* these competencies and related clinical activities with agency site personnel, not *telling* them. Agency personnel need input into decisions about clinical learning activities. With this input, the teacher may need to alter the planned clinical activities and other types of learning opportunities for students.

It is important for all clinical nurse educators—full and part time, adjunct, and preceptors—to understand the competencies students should develop in a course or clinical practicum. The faculty member (from the school of nursing) is responsible for ensuring that all clinical educators, preceptors, and others participating in a course, no matter what their role, use the competencies to guide their selection of patients and other learning activities for students and to assess performance.

Assessing Learning Needs

Teaching begins at the level of the learner. The teacher's goal, therefore, is to assess the student's present level of knowledge and skill and other characteristics that may influence achieving the competencies. The first area of assessment involves collecting data on whether the student has the prerequisite knowledge and skills for the clinical situation and for completing the learning activities. For instance, if the learning activities focus on interventions for health promotion, students first need some understanding of health and wellness. Similarly, changing a sterile dressing requires an understanding of principles of asepsis. The teacher's role in assessment is important so that students engage in learning activities that build on their current knowledge and skills and competencies already attained. When students lack the prerequisites, then the instruction can remedy these and more efficiently move students forward in their learning.

Because not every student will enter the clinical practicum with the same level of competence, assessment helps identify the point at which the instruction should begin. It does not imply poor performance, but rather highlights those learners who may need different types of learning activities. Assessment may also indicate that some students have already attained certain clinical competencies and can progress to new areas of learning. Recognizing students' previous experiences, identifying current needs, and making learning resources available are important areas of assessment (Gcawu & van Rooyen, 2022).

Planning Clinical Learning Activities

Following assessment, the teacher plans learning activities. The main considerations are the competencies to be developed in the clinical practicum and individual learner needs.

If the competencies focus on communication skills, then the learning activities may involve interviews with patients and others, papers analyzing those interactions, and analysis of patient–nurse interactions in a postclinical conference. While the competencies provide the framework for planning the learning activities, the other main consideration is the needs of the student. Some students may have already met some of the competencies and can then progress to other types of learning activities. The activities should build on the student's present competencies and take into consideration other learner characteristics. Each student does not have to complete the same learning activities; the educator is responsible for individualizing the clinical activities so that they best meet each student's needs while promoting achievement of the competencies. Learning activities also build on one another. Planning includes organizing the activities to provide for the progressive development of knowledge, skills, and values for each learner.

Characteristics of the clinical site including its size also influence the learning activities planned for students. In a clinic, a physician office, or an outpatient setting, it is likely that only one advanced practice registered nursing (APRN) student can be placed in the setting for their precepted experience. Similarly, in many community settings, only a limited number of students can be assigned there because of the number of available clients and nurses to guide student learning. Even in acute care settings, the size of the unit has an impact on the number of students who can be placed there. The patient population, the educational level and preparation of nurses, the types and numbers of other healthcare providers, the availability and interest of nurses and other providers in working with students, and other characteristics of the clinical environment should be considered in planning the learning activities.

If the traditional model of clinical instruction is used in the nursing program, in which one clinical nurse educator or clinician is responsible for a group of nursing students, the size of the student group is important to consider. The educator or preceptor working with prelicensure or APRN students needs to be available to guide students' learning. The level of prelicensure students in a clinical group, for instance, also will influence the type of learning activities planned for a course. Beginning students and nurses new to a clinical practice area may require more time and guidance from the teacher than experienced students and nurses.

Guiding and Supporting Learners in Clinical Practice

The next step in the process of clinical teaching is guiding learners' practice. Guiding is a facilitative and supportive process that leads the student toward achievement of the competencies. It is a process of supporting and coaching students in their learning. Guiding is not supervision; supervision is a process of overseeing. Effective clinical teaching requires that educators model professional practice and guide students in their learning, not oversee their work.

This is the instructional phase in the clinical teaching process—the actual teaching of students in the clinical setting either on site or at a distance. For distance education courses, the instructional phase may be carried out by preceptors, APRNs in the clinical setting, and other healthcare providers depending on the competencies. With some learning activities, the teacher has a direct instructional role—for instance, demonstrating an intervention to students and questioning them to expand their understanding. Other teaching activities, though, may be indirect, such as giving feedback on papers and preparing preceptors for their role, among others.

In the process of guiding learners, the teacher needs to be skilled in: (a) observing clinical performance, arriving at sound judgments about that performance, and planning additional learning activities if needed, and (b) questioning students to promote higher-level thinking and development of clinical judgment. Observing students as they learn to care for patients, families, and community members and to interact with others allows the teacher to identify continued areas of learning. This information, in turn, suggests new learning activities for clinical practice.

Observations of students may be influenced by the teacher's values and biases, which may affect *what they see* as they observe a student's performance and their *impressions* of the quality of that performance. All educators should know their own values and biases that might influence their observations of student performance in clinical practice and judgments about student performance of the competencies. Guidelines for observing students are summarized in **Exhibit 3.1**.

Another skill needed by the educator to effectively guide clinical learning activities is an ability to ask thought-provoking questions without making students feel interrogated. The ability to think critically and make

EXHIBIT 3.1 Guidelines for Observing Students in Clinical Practice

Examine your values and biases that may influence observations of students in clinical practice and judgments about clinical performance.

Do not rely on first impressions for these might change significantly with further observations of the student.

Make a series of observations before drawing conclusions about clinical performance.

Share with students on a continual basis observations made of clinical performance and judgments about whether students are meeting the clinical competencies.

Focus observations on the competencies to be achieved.

When the observations reveal aspects of performance that need further development, share these with students and use the information as a way of providing feedback on performance.

Discuss observations with students, obtain their perceptions of performance, and be willing to modify judgments when a different perspective is offered.

sound clinical judgments is integral to providing quality care. These skills can be encouraged by asking students to clarify, relate, think beyond the obvious, and connect theory to practice (Ho et al., 2023; Maffucci et al., 2024; Makhene, 2019; Seibert, 2023). Open-ended questions about students' thinking and the rationale underlying their clinical judgments foster the development of higher-level cognitive skills. For example, Kim et al. (2025) evaluated the outcomes of a program using reflective questions on newly graduated nurses' (n = 153) clinical judgment skills. Nurses who completed the program had significantly higher scores in clinical judgment.

When questioning students in clinical practice, the educator should assess understanding of related knowledge and concepts and how they apply to patient care. Other questions can ask students about different approaches and decisions possible in a clinical situation, consequences of each decision, what they would do, and their rationale; possible problems, interventions, and their evidence base; and assumptions underlying their thinking. Questions should encourage learners to think beyond the obvious.

The way in which questions are asked is also significant. The goal of questioning is to encourage students to consider other perspectives and possibilities, not to drill them or create added stress. In the beginning of a clinical course, and particularly in the beginning of the nursing program, the educator should discuss the purpose of questioning and its relationship to developing thinking and clinical judgment skills. The teacher can demonstrate the type of questions that will be asked in the course and emphasize that the goal is to help students learn and begin to think like a nurse.

Because questioning serves instructional purposes, students need to feel assured that their responses will not influence their clinical grades. Instead, the questions asked and the answers given are an essential part of the teaching process, aimed at promoting learning and the development of higher-level thinking skills, rather than for grading purposes. Only with this framework will students be comfortable in responding to questions and evaluating alternative perspectives, using the teacher as a resource.

Evaluating Clinical Learning and Performance

The remaining component of the clinical teaching process is evaluation. Clinical evaluation serves two purposes: formative and summative. Through formative evaluation, the teacher monitors student progress toward achieving the competencies for clinical practice. Formative evaluation provides information about further learning needs of students and where additional clinical instruction is needed. Clinical evaluation that is formative is not intended for grading purposes; instead, it is designed to diagnose learning needs as a basis for further instruction.

Summative evaluation, in contrast, takes place at the completion of the clinical practicum to assess whether the student developed the essential competencies or achieved the outcomes (Oermann et al., 2025). Summative evaluation provides the basis for determining grades in clinical practice or certifying competency. This type of clinical evaluation determines what *has been* learned rather than what *can be* learned. There are many clinical evaluation strategies that can be used in nursing courses. These are discussed and examples are provided in Chapter 12.

Table 3.1 provides a summary of the clinical teaching process. The table includes questions for the clinical educator to evaluate their own skills and preparation for engaging in this process. Answers to these questions suggest to the educator areas where further development is needed for effectiveness as a clinical nurse educator.

TABLE 3.1 PROCESS OF CLINICAL TEACHING

Steps of Process	Questions to Guide Teaching
Clinical Competencies	What are the clinical competencies to be attained and evaluated in the clinical practicum?
Individual Learning Needs	Does the student have the prerequisite knowledge and skills for achieving the competencies? Does the student have the prerequisite competencies? What competencies has the student already achieved? Is the student ready for this new learning? What are the student's individual learning needs?
Clinical Learning Activities	What learning activities would: ■ Facilitate students' development of the clinical competencies? ■ Help students gain the prerequisite knowledge and skills or competencies? ■ Meet students' individual learning needs? What are characteristics of the clinical setting that influence potential learning activities (e.g., size, patient population, availability of nurses and other providers, and their interest in working with students)? If using a traditional model of clinical education, how many students are in the group, and what is their level of knowledge and experience related to the patient population? In a preceptor model, what are characteristics of the patients and setting that may impact the availability of the preceptor to work with and guide students?

(continued)

TABLE 3.1 PROCESS OF CLINICAL TEACHING (CONT.)

Steps of Process	Questions to Guide Teaching
Clinical Learning Activities	What concepts are students learning in the curriculum to be applied in clinical practice? What are possible exemplars of those concepts (relevant to the clinical setting)?
Educator Role	What is your role with students in the clinical setting? What competencies do you need to be effective in your role, and do you have them? If not, what are strategies and professional development opportunities to prepare yourself for your clinical teaching role?
Evaluation of Performance	Is the aim of the evaluation to provide feedback to learners (formative) or to assess performance to determine competence (summative)? Are you prepared to give feedback, both positive and negative? Are you prepared to have difficult conversations with students, if necessary?

QUALITIES OF EFFECTIVE CLINICAL TEACHERS

Clinical teaching requires an educator who is knowledgeable about the clinical practice area, is clinically competent, knows how to teach, relates effectively to students, and is enthusiastic about clinical teaching. The teacher also serves as a role model for students or selects clinicians who will model important professional behaviors. Hull (2024) found through a concept analysis that defining attributes of clinical nurse educator competence includes the knowledge, skills, attitudes, and behaviors to educate, mentor, and evaluate nursing students. Every clinical teacher should be aware of behaviors that promote learning in the practice setting and ones that impede student learning.

Knowledge

Nurse educators, as in any field, need to have expertise in the subject they are teaching. In clinical teaching, this means that educators are knowledgeable about patient conditions and populations, interventions, new treatments and technologies in patient care, and related research. Teachers must be up to date in the area of clinical practice in which they are working with students. This is particularly true in the traditional model of clinical teaching.

Clinical Competence

Teachers cannot guide student learning in clinical practice without being competent themselves. They need to be experts in the area of clinical practice in which they are teaching, maintain their clinical skills, be able to explain and demonstrate nursing care in a real situation, and be competent in the technology being used in the setting. This area of teaching competence may be problematic for faculty members who teach predominantly in the classroom or change practice settings frequently and do not keep current in an area of clinical practice. However, it is up to the teacher to maintain expertise through ongoing professional development, mentorship, and a commitment to lifelong learning (Hull, 2024).

Competence in Clinical Teaching

Effective teaching in the clinical setting requires a wide range of skills. Ye et al. (2022), through a literature review; focus group interviews with nurse managers, clinical nurse educators, staff nurses, and nursing students; and a Delphi study, identified four broad competency areas needed by nurse educators: (a) clinical teaching competency, (b) clinical nursing skills, (c) management and leadership competencies, and (d) innovation and research competency. Clinical educators need to know *how to teach*, which, while seemingly obvious, is not always the case. In some settings, clinical teachers, preceptors, and others working with students are not prepared educationally for their roles. They have limited knowledge about how to guide students' learning in the clinical setting and assess their performance. Being an expert clinician alone is not enough. Effective teachers are fair in their evaluations of students, correct student errors without belittling students and diminishing their self-confidence, and give prompt feedback that promotes further learning and development. Essential teaching skills are outlined in **Exhibit 3.2**.

Interpersonal Relationships With Students

The ability of the clinical teacher to interact with students, both on a one-to-one basis and in a group, is another important teacher behavior. Qualities of an effective teacher in this area are showing confidence in students, respecting students, being honest and direct, supporting students and demonstrating caring behaviors, being approachable, and encouraging students to ask questions and seek guidance when needed.

EXHIBIT 3.2 Clinical Teaching Skills

Assesses prerequisite knowledge, skills, and competencies of students, recognizing individual differences.
Identifies students' learning needs in collaboration with students.
Plans patient assignments and other learning activities that help in transfer of learning to clinical practice, meet learning needs, and promote development of competencies.
Communicates clearly to students (and others) the clinical competencies to be achieved and expectations of students in practice.
Considers student goals and needs in planning the clinical activities.
Structures clinical learning activities so they build on one another.
Explains clearly related knowledge, concepts, and theories applicable to patient care.
Demonstrates effectively clinical skills, procedures, and use of technology.
Provides opportunities for practice of competencies, clinical skills, procedures, and technology, and recognizes differences among students in the amount of practice needed.
Is well prepared for clinical teaching.
Develops clinical teaching strategies that encourage students to problem solve and make sound clinical judgments.
Asks higher level questions that assist students in thinking through complex clinical situations.
Encourages students through teaching and assessment to think independently and beyond accepted practices and to try out new interventions.
Varies clinical teaching strategies and learning activities to stimulate student interest and meet individual needs of students.
Is available to students in clinical practice when they need assistance.
Serves as a role model for students.
Demonstrates leadership skills and ability to manage clinical teaching responsibilities.
Provides specific, timely, and useful feedback on student progress.
Shares observations of clinical performance with students on a continual basis.
Encourages students to assess their own performance.
Corrects mistakes without belittling students.
Exhibits fairness in evaluation.

Students have reported that their interpersonal relationship with the teacher was the most important characteristic (Buanz et al., 2024). Considering the demands on students as they learn to care for patients, students need to view the teacher as someone who supports them in their learning.

Personal Characteristics of the Clinical Teacher

Personal characteristics of the teacher also influence teaching effectiveness. These include the teacher's enthusiasm, a sense of humor, willingness to admit limitations and mistakes honestly, patience, and flexibility. Students often describe an effective teacher as someone who is friendly and provides an opportunity for them to share feelings and concerns about patients. Clinical educators are role models for students: In clinical practice, students mirror the behaviors of the educator who is professional and competent (Natesan et al., 2020). The teacher should develop an atmosphere of trust and support for students to engage in open discussions about care and clinical situations. For these discussions to occur, the student needs to feel safe to share views and opinions.

In clinical teaching, educators need to self-assess and recognize areas of teaching to be improved. They should be willing to reflect on their teaching and evaluation practices and consider better ways of designing clinical activities and guiding students in their learning. Good teachers strive to perfect their teaching skills over time and avoid stagnation in their teaching approaches.

STRESSES OF STUDENTS IN CLINICAL PRACTICE

Clinical practice is stressful for both prelicensure nursing students and graduate students preparing for advanced nursing practice. Findings of an umbrella review of 12 articles, which included 189 studies, indicated that nursing students experienced moderate to high levels of stress during their nursing program (Labrague, 2024; Zheng et al., 2022). In the clinical setting, students face uncertainties and unique situations that they may not have encountered in their prior learning. For some students, clinical practice is stressful because they are unsure about approaches and interventions to use. Interacting with the teacher, other healthcare providers, the patient, and family members may also contribute to the stress that students experience in clinical practice.

Other stresses, from the students' perspective, relate to the changing nature of patient conditions, a lack of knowledge and skill to provide care to patients, excessive workload, unfamiliarity in the clinical setting, working with difficult patients, lack of technological skills, inadequate professional skills, and being observed and evaluated by the teacher (Bhurtun et al., 2019; Mohamed et al., 2024; Wang et al., 2019). In a study of 93 undergraduate nursing students in the final year of their nursing program, students reported three situations that were most anxiety producing in the clinical practicum: fear of making a mistake, being observed by the clinical instructor, and their initial clinical experience on a unit (Wang et al., 2019). Learning in clinical practice occurs in public under the watchful eye of the teacher, the patient, and others in the setting. By keeping the nature of clinical learning in mind and using supportive behaviors when interacting with students, the teacher can reduce some of the stress that students naturally feel in clinical practice.

STRESSFUL NATURE OF CLINICAL TEACHING

Clinical teaching can be stressful for the teacher. First, it is time consuming. In many schools, a three-credit theory or online course requires 3 hours per week of instruction, with 50 minutes for each credit hour, excluding preparation time. However, a three-credit clinical course may require 6 to 9 hours of clinical teaching each week, or 2 to 3 clinical practice hours per credit hour, and even more in some nursing education programs. This time commitment can create stress for faculty, who are also responsible for academic advisement, conducting research, writing for publication, serving on committees, providing community service, and maintaining clinical practice. In addition to the demands of multiple roles, other aspects of clinical teaching may contribute to stress, including:

- coping with the many expectations associated with clinical teaching;
- a heavy workload;
- pressure to maintain clinical competence or clinical practice without sufficient time;
- difficulty satisfying the demands of students, clinical agency personnel, patients, and others;
- teaching inadequately prepared students; and
- feeling unprepared for one's role as a clinical nurse educator.

For new clinical teachers, stress often stems from a lack of preparation for the role. While clinicians have expert knowledge and skills in their specialty area, they may have limited knowledge of how to teach. As clinicians are recruited to academic positions, schools of nursing should provide an orientation for these educators. Most schools of nursing, however, hire clinicians who are new to teaching without organizational structures to develop their teaching skills and support them (Hansbrough et al., 2023). Ross et al. (2024) found that the orientation of clinical teachers varied widely across schools. In their study involving 113 novice clinical instructors, 70.8% reported that they were not provided a formal orientation. Among multiple topics, they stated that they needed to learn *how to be a clinical nurse educator* and how to promote students' clinical judgment. Not only is it important to orient new educators to ensure they are prepared to teach, but this orientation can serve as a recruitment and retention strategy (Young-Brice et al., 2022). Novice educators and faculty members who are new to a nursing program should find a mentor in the school who can support them as they learn the educator role in that setting. Mentors can be good sources of guidance on how to balance clinical teaching with other roles. Adjunct and part-time clinical educators also need a mentor to help them develop as effective clinical teachers. The mentor can be a resource for the clinical teacher and provide a link to the nursing program.

MODELS OF CLINICAL TEACHING

There are different models of clinical teaching: traditional, in which the teacher is directly responsible for guiding a group of students in the clinical setting; preceptor; and partnership, including dedicated education units (DEUs). In the preceptor and partnership models, preceptors and others in the clinical setting provide the clinical instruction, with the faculty member (from the school of nursing) responsible for overall planning and coordinating the experience, supporting the clinician, grading clinical practice, and assuming other course-related responsibilities.

Traditional Model

In the traditional model of clinical teaching, the educator is typically on site during the clinical experience. Students learn to provide care as they engage in practice themselves. A benefit of this model is the opportunity to select patient assignments and plan other learning activities to assist students in applying the knowledge and concepts learned in class to patient care. If the clinical educator is also involved with the course and curriculum overall, the clinical activities can be carefully selected to provide exemplars of the concepts that students are learning in the course. Although this is the most commonly used model, surprisingly there are few studies that document the outcomes of this model (Leighton et al., 2021).

Disadvantages are the large number of students for whom the clinical educator may be responsible; not being accessible to students when needed because of demands of other students in the group; teaching procedures, clinical skills, and technologies for which the educator may lack expertise; time commitment of providing on-site clinical instruction for faculty members with multiple other roles; and high costs for the nursing program. Clinical nurse educators who are adjunct may not be sufficiently familiar with the philosophy and goals of the program, overall curriculum, clinical competencies developed prior to and following the course in which they are teaching, and other program characteristics, which may affect their planning of clinical activities for students and their expectations of students in the course. It is critical for the full-time faculty to prepare and orient part-time and adjunct clinical educators so they are not only aware of their role and responsibilities but also understand how their course relates to the overall nursing curriculum.

In the traditional model, students may have unproductive time waiting for the educator or another clinician to answer their questions and guide their learning. In the community, patients and families may not be available at the time students have their assigned clinical practice. Patients' conditions may deteriorate, resulting in students lacking the requisite knowledge and skills to care for them.

Another disadvantage is that the educator and students may not be part of the healthcare system in which students have clinical practice. They are outsiders to the clinical setting and may not understand the system of care in that setting and its culture. In these situations, educators should work closely with the managers and staff to ensure an effective clinical experience for students. It is up to the clinical educator to develop working relationships with the staff, which is essential to create an environment for learning and take advantage of activities that could be available for students in the setting. In the traditional model, educators who are not also practicing in the clinical setting often invest extensive time in developing and maintaining these relationships.

Preceptor Model

In the preceptor model, an expert nurse in the clinical setting works with the student usually on a one-to-one basis. Preceptors are clinicians (nurses, APRNs, and other healthcare providers) employed by the clinical setting who, in addition to their ongoing patient care responsibilities, provide clinical instruction for students and new graduate nurses. In addition to one-to-one teaching, the preceptor guides and supports learners and serves as a role model. In this model, the faculty member from the nursing program serves as the coordinator, liaison between the nursing program and clinical setting, and resource person for the preceptor. The faculty member, however, is typically not on site during the clinical practicum. The preceptor model involves sharing clinical teaching responsibilities between nursing program faculty and expert clinicians from the practice setting.

One strength of the preceptor model is the one-to-one relationship of the student and preceptor, providing an opportunity for the student to work closely with a role model. This close relationship promotes professional socialization and enables students to gain an understanding of how to function in the role for which they are being prepared. By working closely with a clinical expert in the field, students improve their critical thinking and decision-making skills, develop clinical competencies, gain confidence, and improve readiness for practice as an RN or APRN (Abdelaliem et al., 2025; Fowler et al., 2018; Kantar, 2021; Thomas et al., 2023). Due to a lack of preceptors for APRN students and potential inconsistencies when evaluating students, Burns et al. (2024) developed the Dyad/Precepting to Optimize Development (POD) model. In this model, a consistent team of students, preceptors, and faculty participate in the preceptorship. Two students rotate in pairs every 4 to 8 weeks with the group of preceptors over the course of their program. In a mixed-methods study, students, preceptors, and faculty reported satisfaction with this model.

Potential disadvantages of the preceptor model include the lack of integration between didactic learning and clinical practice, limited flexibility in reassigning students to other preceptors when needed, and the time and other demands placed on preceptors. Preceptors must be well prepared for their roles and demonstrate competence in both clinical teaching and patient care. Ulrich et al. (2025) define the preceptor as an individual with expertise to guide, assess, and validate the knowledge, skills, and attitudes needed by a nurse (preceptee) to transition to a new role, specialty, or environment. They identified seven preceptor role domains: role model, teacher/coach, facilitator, protector, socialization agent, leader/influencer, and evaluator; essential attributes for preceptors; and 66 competencies across these domains. **Table 3.2** defines each of these role domains.

Partnership Model

There are varied types of academic–practice partnerships in nursing education. Some of these are the result of nursing programs searching for ways to cope with a lack of available clinical sites and to maintain student enrollment when faced with budgetary constraints and a nursing faculty shortage. Other partnerships are intended to address the gap in preparation for practice readiness (Buron et al., 2024; Greenwood, 2025; Luckenbach & L'Ecuyer, 2023; Luckenbach et al., 2021; Mennenga et al., 2021).

Partnerships vary widely across schools of nursing. In some programs, the partnership model is a collaborative relationship between a clinical site and nursing program that involves sharing a clinician and academic faculty member. The clinician teaches students in the clinical setting, with the faculty member serving as course coordinator and in turn, contributing to the clinical agency—for example, by conducting research and serving as a consultant, or practicing as an APRN in the agency. Expertise and services are shared between the partners. In this type of partnership, the clinician may work with a prelicensure or

TABLE 3.2 DEFINITIONS OF PRECEPTOR ROLE DOMAINS

Role Domains	Definitions
Preceptor	An individual with demonstrated competence in a specific area who guides, assesses, and validates the knowledge, skills, and attitudes needed to transition to a new role, specialty, or environment
Preceptor Role Domain	*Role Definition: The Preceptor. . .*
Role model	Models professionalism and role competence to positively influence the preceptee
Teacher/coach	Expands the knowledge, skills, and competence of the preceptee with sensitivity to the preceptee's individual strengths and learning needs
Facilitator	Finds, negotiates, and creates positive and rich experiential learning opportunities and environments
Protector	Ensures the safety of the preceptee and the patient by creating a safe and supportive learning environment and providing preceptee oversight
Socialization agent	Facilitates assimilation of the preceptee into the work environment and relationships by helping the preceptee understand social and cultural norms
Leader/influencer	Inspires and guides the actions of others and conveys professional values in the practice setting
Evaluator	Continuously assesses the preceptee's performance and competence for job readiness with ongoing feedback for performance improvement

Source: Ulrich, B. T. (2024). The preceptor role. In: B. T. Ulrich (Ed.), *Mastering precepting* (3rd ed., pp. 1–28). Sigma; Harper, M. G., Maloney, P., Ulrich, B., Warren, J. I., MacDonald, R., & Whiteside, D. (2023). *Summary findings from the 2023 preceptor competency consensus study*. Association for Nursing Professional Development. https://www.anpd.org/Portals/0/Files/ANPD_1127571-23_PreceptorCompetencies_Report.pdf. Ulrich, B., Harper, M. G., Maloney, P., Warren, J. I., Whiteside, D., & MacDonald, R. (2025). National preceptor competency consensus study. *JONA: The Journal of Nursing Administration, 55*(1), 18. https://doi.org/10.1097/nna.0000000000001523. Reprinted by permission of Wolters Kluwer Health, February 3, 2025.

APRN student on a one-to-one basis or may teach a small group of students, as in the traditional model.

Buron et al. (202[illegible]) developed a clinical cohort model within their academic–practice partnership. In this model, all nursing students are placed in the healthcare system for their clinical courses under the guidance of an adjunct nursing instructor employed by the healthcare system. The model led to a significant reduction in the cost of clinical education; the 2-year retention rate postgraduation for RNs who were part of the cohort model was 100%, and nursing students were highly satisfied with this practice model.

In another type, an affiliate faculty model, staff nurses teach clinical students 1 day per week (as an affiliate faculty member) but continue to maintain full-time status in the healthcare system. This partnership model allowed the school of nursing to decrease its student-to-faculty ratio and orientation for clinical nurse educators because they are already employees of the health system (Luckenbach et al., 2021). In an evaluation of the model, students agreed that affiliate faculty prepared them to provide safe care, helped them connect classroom learning to clinical practice, were effective educators, supported them at the bedside, and enjoyed teaching.

DEDICATED EDUCATION UNIT

Another type of partnership is the DEU, which is a unit within a clinical setting that is dedicated to teaching nursing students. A DEU is a triad of students, clinicians, and faculty members who collaborate to create a learning environment for students. While there are varied DEU models in the United States and other countries, a common element is the active engagement of nursing and other staff in the education of students. In these models, clinicians teach the students with academic faculty members in the role as liaison, guiding the clinician to ensure a quality learning experience and that course outcomes are met (Greenwood, 2025; Musallam et al., 2021).

DEUs are used across varied types of healthcare systems including ambulatory care settings (Benike et al., 2023). With DEUs students learn to practice with the guidance of a clinical expert, improving students' clinical knowledge and skills, ability to manage varied patient care demands, leadership skills, and clinical judgment (Cooper et al., 2025; De Juan Pardo et al., 2022; Pedregosa et al., 2024). Benefits for the clinical partner are reduced orientation and onboarding time for new graduate nurses who had their DEU experiences in the setting and improved retention.

SELECTING A CLINICAL TEACHING MODEL

There is no one model that meets the needs of every nursing education program, clinical course, or group of students. The faculty should select a model considering these factors:

- educational philosophy of the nursing program;
- philosophy of the faculty about clinical teaching;
- clinical competencies to be developed;
- intended outcomes of the clinical course;

- level of nursing student;
- type of clinical setting;
- availability of preceptors, clinicians, and others in the practice setting who can provide clinical instruction; and
- willingness of clinical partners to participate in teaching students.

SUMMARY

The process of clinical teaching begins with identification of the competencies to be achieved and proceeds through assessing the learner, planning clinical learning activities, guiding and supporting students, and evaluating clinical performance. The competencies, outcomes to be met in the course, and expectations of students should be communicated clearly to students, provided in written form, and understood by them. Similarly, the teacher has an important responsibility in discussing these competencies and related clinical activities with clinical site personnel.

Teaching begins at the level of the learner. The teacher's goal, therefore, is to assess the student's present level of knowledge and skill and other characteristics that may influence developing the clinical competencies. After assessing learner needs, the teacher plans learning activities that guide learners in acquiring the essential knowledge, skills, and values needed to perform the competencies. In guiding learners, the teacher must be skilled in observing clinical performance, making sound judgments about that performance, and adjusting learning activities when necessary. Additionally, the teacher should ask thought-provoking questions that encourage higher-level thinking, but without making the students feel interrogated. The final step in the clinical teaching process is evaluation, which involves constructive feedback and assessing students' readiness to meet clinical competencies. Effective teaching in the clinical setting, therefore, requires an educator who is not only knowledgeable and clinically competent but also skilled in teaching, able to relate effectively to students, and enthusiastic about clinical teaching. Research in nursing education has substantiated that these qualities are essential for effective clinical teaching.

Clinical practice is inherently stressful for students. Common sources of anxiety include fear of making mistakes that could harm patients, difficulty interacting with patients, teachers, and healthcare providers, and uncertainty about patient conditions. Some students may also feel unprepared for the tasks required of them. Teachers play a critical role in mitigating these stressors by creating a supportive and caring environment, where students feel comfortable making mistakes and learning from them. Building trusting relationships between teachers and students is essential for fostering a positive learning climate.

The teacher chooses a model for clinical teaching, which may be traditional, preceptor-based, or partnership-based, including the DEU model. In the traditional model, the clinical educator teaches a group of students and is present on site for the practicum. In the preceptor model, an expert nurse works with a student on a one-to-one basis, providing direct guidance and mentorship. The partnership model varies with academic institutions but is generally a collaborative relationship between the nursing program and a clinical site. One example is the DEU, in which clinicians serve as clinical teachers with academic faculty members acting as liaisons to ensure a quality clinical experience and alignment with course outcomes.

This chapter explored the essential elements of clinical teaching, including the process, models, and qualities needed for effective teaching and student support. including the process, models, and qualities needed for effective teaching and student support. Because there is no single model that meets the needs of every nursing education program or group of students, the choice of model should be guided by factors such as the educational philosophy of the nursing program, the clinical competencies to be developed, the intended outcomes of the clinical course, the level of nursing students, the type of clinical setting, and the availability of preceptors and other clinical instructors.

CNE®cl EXAMINATION TEST BLUEPRINT CORE COMPETENCIES

1. **Function within the Education and Health Care Environments**
   A. Function in the Clinical Nurse Educator Role
      1. Integrate theory and practice in the clinical setting
      2. Foster professional growth of learners (e.g., coaching, reflection, and debriefing)
      4. Act as a role model of professional nursing within the clinical learning environment
      5. Create a diverse, equitable, and inclusive learning environment
   B. Operationalize the Curriculum
      1. Assess congruence of the clinical environment with curriculum, course outcomes, and learner needs when evaluating clinical sites
      2. Identify learner goals and outcomes
      3. Facilitate meaningful and relevant clinical learning activities to promote optimal learning
      6. Provide opportunities for learners to develop clinical judgment related to course outcomes
      7. Implement academic program's assigned models of clinical teaching consistent with course

outcomes (e.g., traditional, preceptor, simulation, dedicated education units)

C. Abide by Legal Requirements, Ethical Guidelines, Agency Policies, and Guiding Framework
   2. Assess learner readiness prior to clinical learning experiences
   3. Facilitate learning activities that support the mission, goals, and values of the academic institution and the clinical agency
   4. Inform others of program and clinical agency policies, procedures, and practices

2. Facilitate Learning in the Healthcare Environment

A. Implement a variety of clinical teaching strategies appropriate to learner needs, desired learner outcomes, content, and context (e.g., virtual, telehealth, in-person, simulation)

F. Create a positive and caring learning environment

G. Develop collegial working relationships with learners, faculty, and clinical environment personnel

H. Demonstrate enthusiasm for teaching, learning, and nursing to help inspire and motivate learners

3. Demonstrate Effective Interpersonal Communication and Collaborative Interprofessional Relationships

B. Foster the development of a collegial learning community

N. Communicate performance expectations to learners and clinical staff

5. Facilitate Learner Development and Socialization

F. Create learning environments that promote socialization to the role of the nurse

LEARNING ACTIVITIES

CourseConnect

To access self-assessment questions and interactive, competency-based learning activities for this chapter, visit www.springerpub.com/courseconnect. See inside front cover and tear-out card for CourseConnect details.

REFERENCES

Abdelaliem, S. M. F., Alsleem, D. K., Aladdad, S. K., Alqahtani, A. S., Alenazi, R. K., Alotaibi, M. G., Oqailan, H. K., & Almarshad, L. B. (2025). The relationship between practical skills confidence and readiness for transition to practice among nursing internship students: Exploring the mediating role of preceptorship. *Nurse Education Today, 147*, 106587. https://doi.org/10.1016/j.nedt.2025.106587

Alizadeh, M., Masoomi, R., Mafinejad, M. K., Parmelee, D., Khalaf, R. J., & Norouzi, A. (2024). Team-based learning in health professions education: An umbrella review. *BMC Medical Education, 24*(1), 1131. https://doi.org/10.1186/s12909-024-06147-x

American Association of Colleges of Nursing. (2021). *The essentials: Core competencies for professional nursing education*. https://www.aacnnursing.org/Portals/0/PDFs/Publications/Essentials-2021.pdf

Benike, L., Darst, E., Witwer, S., Enos, M., Flaten, C., Bartley, L. H., Kubat, B., & Foote, J. (2023). The Ambulatory Dedicated Education Unit (DEU): An important example of academic practice partnership in ambulatory care. *Journal of Professional Nursing, 45*, 64–70. https://doi.org/10.1016/j.profnurs.2023.01.009

Bhurtun, H. D., Azimirad, M., Saaranen, T., & Turunen, H. (2019). Stress and coping among nursing students during clinical training: An integrative review. *Journal of Nursing Education, 58*(5), 266–272. https://doi.org/10.3928/01484834-20190422-04

Buanz, S. F., Alsenayien, A. Y., Altharman, H. A., Alnaqi, R. I., Llaguno, M. B. B., Mousa, O., & Siraj, R. A. (2024). Nursing students, faculty, and preceptors perception of effective characteristics of clinical instructor: A cross-sectional study. *SAGE Open Nursing, 10*, 23779608241298427. https://doi.org/10.1177/23779608241298427

Burns, D., Breckenridge, L. A., Gregory, A., & Nye, C. (2024). Redesigning nurse practitioner clinical education with a Dyad/POD model: A feasibility study. *Journal of the American Association of Nurse Practitioners, 36*(12), 704–710. https://doi.org/10.1097/jxx.0000000000001013

Buron, B., Abbott Eng, C., & Eagleton, A. (2024). Reimagining the future of clinical nursing education: A cohort partnership model. *Nurse Educator, 49*(6), 321–326. https://doi.org/10.1097/nne.0000000000001681

Burton, R., Kellett, U., Mansah, M., & Sriram, D. (2024). A systematic review of online team based learning approaches in health professional education. *Nurse Education Today, 138*, 106156. https://doi.org/10.1016/j.nedt.2024.106156

Cooper, R., Musallam, E., & Warner, K. (2025). The effects of a dedicated education unit on baccalaureate nursing students' clinical judgment. *Journal of Nursing Education, 64*(1), 35–39. https://doi.org/10.3928/01484834-20240827-01

De Juan Pardo, M., Vissandjee, B., Guillaumet Olives, M., Cerezuela Torre, M., & Gallart Fernández-Puebla, A. (2022). Enhancing perceived leadership of nursing students through a student-led dedicated education unit in a community setting: A feasibility study. *Journal of Professional Nursing, 43*, 152–161. https://doi.org/10.1016/j.profnurs.2022.10.009

Fowler, S. M., Knowlton, M. C., & Putnam, A. W. (2018). Reforming the undergraduate nursing clinical curriculum through clinical immersion: A literature review. *Nurse Education in Practice, 31*, 68–76. https://doi.org/10.1016/j.nepr.2018.04.013

Gcawu, S. N., & van Rooyen, D. (2022). Clinical teaching practices of nurse educators: An integrative literature review. *Health SA, 27*, 1728. https://doi.org/10.4102/hsag.v27i0.1728

Greenwood, E. (2025). Academic-practice partnerships. In J. C. De Gagne & M. H. Oermann (Eds.), *Teaching in nursing and role of the educator: The complete guide to best practice in teaching, evaluation, and curriculum development* (4th ed., pp. 237–253). Springer Publishing Company.

Hansbrough, W., Dunker, K., Duprey, M., & Lawrence, A. (2023). Descriptive analysis of newly hired academic nurse educator onboarding practices. *Nurse Educator, 48*(4), 192–196. https://doi.org/10.1097/nne.0000000000001402

Ho, Y. R., Chen, B. Y., & Li, C. M. (2023). Thinking more wisely: Using the Socratic method to develop critical thinking skills amongst healthcare students. *BMC Medical Education, 23*(1), 173. https://doi.org/10.1186/s12909-023-04134-2

Hull, J. L. (2024). Competence of the academic clinical nurse educator: A concept analysis. *Journal of Professional Nursing, 55*, 146–151. https://doi.org/10.1016/j.profnurs.2024.10.004

Jenkins Barnard, P., Saylor, J., Graber, J., & Trinkaus, D. (2024). Educational outcomes in undergraduate nursing: A systematic review. *Journal of Nursing Education, 63*(6), 380–386. https://doi.org/10.3928/01484834-20240404-06

Kantar, L. D. (2021). Teaching domains of clinical instruction from the experiences of preceptors. *Nurse Education in Practice, 52*, 103010. https://doi.org/10.1016/j.nepr.2021.103010

Kim, A. R., Hong, J. H., Kim, K., Kim, Y., Lee, J. M., Lee, H., Yoon, J. H., & Kim, M. S. (2025). Clinical judgment model-based critical reflection program for newly graduated nurses: A nonrandomized controlled trial. *Research in Nursing and Health, 48*(2), 234–235. https://doi.org/10.1002/nur.22444

Labrague, L. J. (2024). Umbrella review: Stress levels, sources of stress, and coping mechanisms among student nurses. *Nursing Reports, 14*(1), 362–375. https://doi.org/10.3390/nursrep14010028

Leighton, K., Kardong-Edgren, S., McNelis, A. M., Foisy-Doll, C., & Sullo, E. (2021). Traditional clinical outcomes in prelicensure nursing education: An empty systematic review. *Journal of Nursing Education, 60*(3), 136–142. https://doi.org/10.3928/01484834-20210222-03

Luckenbach, A., & L'Ecuyer, K. (2023). The clinical academic partnership for excellence: Lessons learned from a clinical faculty onboarding program. *Nurse Educator, 48*(3), 147–152. https://doi.org/10.1097/NNE.0000000000001310

Luckenbach, A., Nelson-Brantley, H., & Ireland-Hoffmann, G. (2021). Affiliate faculty in nursing clinical education: Student and faculty perceptions. *Nurse Educator, 46*(4), 245–249. https://doi.org/10.1097/NNE.0000000000000925

Maffucci, J., Vanderzwan, K., & Burt, L. (2024). Evaluating a shared reflective practice to develop nursing student clinical judgment. *Nurse Educator, 49*(3), 147–151. https://doi.org/10.1097/nne.0000000000001570

Makhene, A. (2019). The use of the Socratic inquiry to facilitate critical thinking in nursing education. *Health SA Gesondheid, 24*, a1224. https://doi.org/10.4102/hsag.v24i0.1224

Mennenga, H. A., Brown, R. J., Horsley, T. L., Abuatiq, A. A., & Plemmons, C. (2021). Collaborating with rural practice partners to provide a primary care experience for prelicensure nursing students. *Nurse Educator, 46*(2), E14–E17. https://doi.org/10.1097/NNE.0000000000000876

Mohamed, N. A., Ali, S. O., Ehrahim, E. E. E., Ahmed, A. L., & Wahba, A. M. (2024). Predictors of academic and clinical stress among nursing students. *SAGE Open Nursing, 10*, 23779608241290392. https://doi.org/10.1177/23779608241290392

Musallam, E., Ali, A. A., & Nicely, S. (2021). The impact of dedicated education model on nursing students' outcomes: An integrative review. *Nurse Educator, 46*(5), E113–E116. https://doi.org/10.1097/nne.0000000000001022

Natesan, S., Bailitz, J., King, A., Krzyzaniak, S. M., Kennedy, S. K., Kim, A. J., Byyny, R., & Gottlieb, M. (2020). Clinical teaching: An evidence-based guide to best practices from the Council of Emergency Medicine Residency Directors. *Western Journal of Emergency Medicine, 21*(4), 985–998. https://doi.org/10.5811/westjem.2020.4.46060

Oermann, M. H. (2022). Some principles to guide assessment of competencies. *Nurse Educator, 47*(1), 1. https://doi.org/10.1097/NNE.0000000000001143

Oermann, M. H., Gaberson, K. B., & De Gagne, J. C. (2025). *Evaluation and testing in nursing education* (7th ed.). Springer Publishing Company.

Pedregosa, S., Zabalegui, A., Fabrellas, N., Risco, E., Pereira, M., Dmoch-Gajzlerska, E., Şenuzun, F., & Martin, S. (2024). Nurses, midwives and students' reports of effective dedicated education units in five European countries: A qualitative study. *Nursing Open, 11*(7), e2210. https://doi.org/10.1002/nop2.2210

Ross, J. G., Dunker, K. S., Morrell, M., Duprey, M. D., Parson, T., & Kim, L. (2024). Clinical faculty orientation practices in the United States: A descriptive study. *Nurse Educator, 49*(5), 278–283. https://doi.org/10.1097/nne.0000000000001625

Seibert, S. A. (2023). Scaffolding questions to foster higher order thinking. *Teaching and Learning in Nursing, 18*(1), 185–187. https://doi.org/10.1016/j.teln.2022.09.003

Thomas, K. J., Yeganeh, L., Vlahovich, J., & Willey, S. M. (2023). Midwifery professional placement: Undergraduate students' experiences with novice and expert preceptors. *Nurse Education Today, 131*, 105976. https://doi.org/10.1016/j.nedt.2023.105976

Ulrich, B., Harper, M. G., Maloney, P., Warren, J. I., Whiteside, D., & MacDonald, R. (2025). National preceptor competency consensus study. *JONA: The Journal of Nursing Administration, 55*(1), 14–21. https://doi.org/10.1097/nna.0000000000001523

Wang, A. H., Lee, C. T., & Espin, S. (2019). Undergraduate nursing students' experiences of anxiety-producing situations in clinical practicums: A descriptive survey study. *Nurse Education Today, 76*, 103–108. https://doi.org/10.1016/j.nedt.2019.01.016

Wei, B., Wang, H., Li, F., Long, Y., Zhang, Q., Liu, H., Tang, X., & Rao, M. (2024). Effectiveness of problem-based learning on development of nursing students' critical thinking skills: A systematic review and meta-analysis. *Nurse Educator, 49*(3), E115–e119. https://doi.org/10.1097/nne.0000000000001548

Xiaoyan, W., Lifeng, Y., & Jing, J. (2024). Effects of TBL teaching on nursing students' knowledge, practical skills and core ability: A systematic review and meta-analysis. *Nurse Education in Practice, 80*, 104125. https://doi.org/10.1016/j.nepr.2024.104125

Ye, J., Tao, W., Yang, L., Xu, Y., Zhou, N., & Wang, J. (2022). Developing core competencies for clinical nurse educators: An e-Delphi-study. *Nurse Education Today, 109*, 105217. https://doi.org/10.1016/j.nedt.2021.105217

Young-Brice, A., Farrar-Stern, K., & Malin, M. (2022). Comprehensive onboarding and orientation to support newly hired faculty in a nursing program. *Nurse Educator, 47*(6), 347–351. https://doi.org/10.1097/nne.0000000000001242

Zheng, Y.-x., Jiao, J.-R., & Hao, W.-N. (2022). Stress levels of nursing students: A systematic review and meta-analysis. *Medicine, 101*(36), e30547. https://doi.org/10.1097/md.0000000000030547

Developing Clinical Learning Sites: Prelicensure Through Advanced Practice

4

OBJECTIVES:

1. Justify the need for diverse and varied clinical sites for nursing students' clinical learning experiences from prelicensure through advanced practice.
2. Propose clinical learning experiences in specialized patient care sites, community-based clinical sites, and distant sites.
3. Plan for students' clinical learning experiences in international sites.

Nursing care occurs in diverse settings where there are patients (individuals, families, groups, and communities) who can benefit from the services of a professional nurse. Professional nurses assume multiple roles as they work with patients of all ages, races, ethnic groups, and cultures. These patients have the full scope of health promotion; health maintenance; and acute, chronic, and rehabilitation care needs.

In an ideal world, all nursing students would have clinical learning activities in all settings, with all patient populations, and in all professional nursing roles, and they would be prepared to adapt to rapid changes impacting patients, their health, and their care. Students would have opportunities to work with people in diverse settings and from cultures other than their own. The clinical setting and healthcare providers with whom students work would help promote the development of students' clinical reasoning and skill development so that graduates are adequately prepared to enter and contribute to the workforce.

Nursing education does not exist in such an ideal world. All students cannot participate in every learning activity, nor can every student provide care for all these diverse groups during their nursing education. Faculty must make difficult choices about clinical education with the hope that the breadth and depth of students' clinical learning activities result in the development of the core competencies and skills needed for safe and effective nursing practice. For students who are already licensed nurses and pursuing advanced degrees, their clinical experiences must help them grow as professionals as they move to more advanced levels of practice. Their clinical education should focus on a more autonomous role. They need to develop skilled decision making and use advanced assessment, diagnosis, planning, implementation, and evaluation skills.

This chapter explores options for providing clinical learning opportunities for undergraduate and graduate nursing students in a wide variety of clinical sites. Examples are provided of clinical learning opportunities in specialized patient care areas not used regularly for clinical learning, community-based settings, clinical learning at distant sites, and international settings.

NEED FOR DIVERSE AND VARIED CLINICAL SETTINGS

The traditional approach to prelicensure clinical nursing education involves a faculty member working with a group of students (approximately 6–12, although this can vary from program to program), typically on an acute care unit in a hospital for a portion of a clinical shift or in a public health setting. At the graduate level, the apprenticeship model using a preceptor–student teaching method has been the primary approach used for advanced practice nursing education (American Association of Colleges of Nursing [AACN], 2021a). These clinical teaching approaches, while frequently used in nursing education, may provide an unpredictable, rapidly changing, and haphazard learning environment and may no longer be sustainable given limited preceptor availability and growing competition for clinical sites (Gubrud-Howe, 2024).

Regardless if the clinical education is offered for prelicensure or advanced practice nurses, factors, such as changing patient demographics, variable diagnoses and acuity of patients, diverse care needs, and advances in medical technology, impact the clinical learning opportunities. Because of the high patient acuity and care complexity, some clinical sites do not permit engagement in the full scope of clinical learning. Collaboration with other disciplines, acting as a change agent, being a patient advocate, and the development of many key assessment and psychomotor skills can be difficult in a setting where all patients are so critically ill. Additionally, because of the increasingly specialized nature of many acute care units, it is challenging for prelicensure students to see a broad scope of patient problems and gain a generalist perspective of care when they have a finite number of clinical hours, a predetermined schedule, and practice in specialized areas. Programs preparing advanced practice nurses also face difficulties identifying and maintaining quality clinical learning opportunities and preceptors to guide graduate student learning (Bavis et al., 2024; Gigli & Gonzalez, 2022).

Due to the decreasing length of inpatient stays and economic pressures to provide care in outpatient and community settings, limited (and, in some cases, decreased) numbers of clinical learning activities take place on hospital units that provide care for children, individuals with psychiatric illnesses, and women and families during pregnancy and childbirth. Even with these challenges, faculty teaching prelicensure students may still believe that the longstanding traditional clinical teaching models with rotations that align with curriculum content through varying acute care clinical locations and sites and have specific numbers of clinical hours in those areas are important. A systematic review conducted by Leighton et al. (2021) found a lack of evidence that supported the traditional clinical teaching models and achievement of learning outcomes. Clinical teaching continues in the traditional approach with faculty teaching the way it has always been done. This traditional clinical educational approach may not align with emergent trends in nursing education focusing on outcomes-based competency frameworks. Contemporary clinical teaching approaches should allow learning opportunities that increase in complexity, progressively build on competencies, and enable learners to guide their own learning (AACN, 2023). To ensure this occurs, a wide variety of alternative settings may be necessary.

Even when traditional acute care placements are appropriate, implementing clinical learning activities in such settings can be challenging. High demand for clinical placements from nursing education programs (often with rapidly increasing enrollments) and other healthcare profession programs have overwhelmed many acute care agencies and limits program choices for clinical learning experiences. Both staff members and patients can be asked to interact with students 24 hours a day, 7 days a week. As a result, acute care agencies often place limitations on the numbers of students per unit or the days and times that students can be present. In some cases, the mandated clinical group size is so limited that some students in a clinical group must be scheduled for clinical learning activities elsewhere so that fewer students are present on the clinical unit. In other cases, the group size must be kept very small, a remedy that is usually neither economically feasible nor ideal for learning and meeting the educational goals of the course and the program. Engaging in these alternate clinical activities may decrease students' opportunity to actively participate in learning the professional nursing role and may also consume the time and resources of staff in these other areas. Faculty members must evaluate the appropriateness of observation activities, address concerns about student guidance in the absence of a clinical instructor, and support staff members as they encounter different students arriving for observation activities each day.

The growing aging population with increasing care needs, the lack of access to adequate and appropriate affordable healthcare for many individuals, and increases in chronic and behavioral health conditions has led to a national examination of healthcare delivery and nursing's role in addressing health equity and needed changes. The COVID-19 pandemic further illuminated gaps in community health that were already becoming apparent and forced educators to implement clinical learning in innovative and creative approaches, many of which were outside of the traditional educational model and acute care clinical settings. It became clear that past education approaches that have been used in clinical education for more than 40 years without significant changes were inadequate in preparing nurses for future practice roles (Jones-Schenk, 2021). As the pandemic resolved, the National Academies of Sciences, Engineering, and Medicine's (NASEM) *The Future of Nursing 2020-20230: Charting a Path to Achieve Health Equity* (2021) offered a needed guide for healthcare and nursing education transformation. Recommendations focused on the pivotal role of community and public health nursing and how nursing education can help prepare students at all educational levels to address and support health status issues, tackle social determinants of health concerns, and decrease health inequity. This national consensus report of healthcare leaders offers nurse educators a roadmap for educational changes.

Faculty have started to reexamine clinical nursing education and explore alternative approaches. They have shifted emphasis from acute care to primary care and increased the variety of clinical settings used for teaching to allow for a broader scope of experience for students. Even though national and international leaders have advocated for nursing education to provide enhanced education that integrates social determinants of health, these concepts are not adequately incorporated into nursing and clinical education (Colburn, 2022). Yet, addressing how social, economic, environmental, cultural, and political forces impact health provides for unique emerging clinical learning opportunities, many of which will take place outside of acute care settings.

Another driving force for the use of diverse settings for clinical learning is a call to increase the cultural competencies of graduates of nursing education programs. Through clinical learning experiences nursing students need to develop essential knowledge and skills that will allow them to deliver culturally competent care and practice from a global perspective. Examples of these experiences include:

- participation in a cultural immersion experience including international clinical placements;
- participation in community projects involving community members—for example, health fairs, community forums—to understand concerns, values, and beliefs about healthcare;
- development of academic partnerships with community organizations such as churches, businesses, schools, or community groups serving vulnerable populations; and
- service learning opportunities working with populations such as immigrants, migrants, underserved or Indigenous groups.

REIMAGINING CLINICAL LEARNING

Students can learn about nursing care wherever they have contact with patients. The required competencies and learning objectives do not prescribe a specific setting where the learning activities must take place. The core components of a clinical learning activity can be present in settings other than acute care hospital units. However, clinical learning settings must provide opportunities for students to have an active role in assessment, goal setting, planning, implementing, and evaluating care; clinical reasoning and problem-solving opportunities; team-based and interdisciplinary care; competent guidance (from the clinical teacher or someone designated to take on the teaching role in that site); and skill development (intellectual as well as psychomotor).

An emerging innovative alternative to the traditional clinical experience involves longitudinal placements. In this approach, students participate in immersive clinical experiences in a single healthcare agency throughout their entire nursing education rather than rotating to different clinical facilities. Using this longitudinal approach decreases the time needed for student orientation and helps build community engagement and student confidence. This approach benefits the healthcare agency by providing a work-ready applicant pipeline familiar and comfortable with the clinical facility. Although there is limited research available about this approach, this newer alternative offers a reenvisioning of clinical education (Buron et al., 2024; Goers et al., 2022).

Benefits

Reimagining and transforming clinical placements for nursing students have multiple benefits. These include preparing students to be a part of a healthcare team and a system in which the acute care hospital is but one part. Not only will students learn about the varied settings in which healthcare is provided, but they will also have opportunities to develop skills that these settings are best able to provide. For example, development of psychomotor skills such as initiation of IV therapy, including the clinical assessment and decision-making skills that go with this routine procedure, might be best learned in a perioperative setting. Development of therapeutic communication competencies might be best achieved in rehabilitation settings where it is possible to have sustained patient contact. The best opportunities to learn care planning, evaluation, and revision might be available in a home health setting where multidisciplinary care planning is fully integrated into patient services. Or, for advanced practice nursing students, development of care coordination skills may be best achieved through an experience in a nursing clinic.

Clinical learning activities in community-based settings allow nursing students to work with patients where they live and work. Students see the challenges that patients face as they implement self-care for health promotion and maintenance, as well as see the impact on family members. Collaboration with other members of the healthcare team is a natural, necessary, and active part of care delivery in community-based settings.

EXAMPLES OF ALTERNATIVE CLINICAL LEARNING SETTINGS

Clinical learning activities in alternative settings include opportunities for students to meet specific learning objectives while caring for patients. Four categories are used as examples of such activities. The first consists of specialized patient care areas that are not used regularly as clinical learning sites. Some of these patient care sites (e.g., the operating room [OR]) have been eliminated as clinical learning sites by many prelicensure nursing programs, while others (e.g., outpatient clinics, nursing homes) are underused, despite the rich learning opportunities provided for students in these settings. The second category includes community-based sites where the provision of healthcare may not be the prime focus of the site or agency but provide learning opportunities for clinical nursing students. Examples are schools, camps, or community agencies. An example of a learning activity in a community-based site is service learning. With the growth of technology and online nursing education, distance sites provide a third category of alternative clinical learning opportunities. The fourth category is the use of international clinical learning activities. Although these learning opportunities may be brief (often 1 week), students gain valuable experiences in diverse international settings while serving as part of a team providing health services. **Exhibit 4.1** provides examples of alternate clinical nursing learning opportunities.

EXHIBIT 4.1 Alternate Clinical Nursing Learning Opportunities

Addition Recovery Settings
Camps
Correctional Facilities
Day Care Centers (Children and Seniors)
Emergency Services and Facilities (Women's Shelters, Homeless Shelters, and Housing Programs)
Food Banks
Government-Related Care Settings (Military Bases, Veterans Administration)
Health Department and Public Health Agencies
Home Healthcare
Hospice and Palliative Care
Mental Health and Disabilities Offices
Nursing Homes, Continuing Care Retirement Communities, and Residential Care Facilities
Operating Rooms and Other Perioperative Settings
Outpatient Care Centers and Clinics (e.g., Oncology, Dialysis, Cardiac Rehabilitation, Bariatric Care, Pain Clinics, Sports Medicine, Behavioral Health, Occupational Health)
Physician Offices
Preschools and HeadStart Programs
Rehabilitation Centers
Schools
Social Service Agencies
Urgent Care Centers
Wellness Centers

CLINICAL LEARNING IN SPECIALIZED PATIENT CARE SITES

With the diversity of clinical practice sites, there are many examples of clinical learning activities in specialized patient care sites that are often underutilized in clinical education. Several examples are used to illustrate how such sites can be optimized.

Outpatient Clinics

Outpatient settings such as primary care and specialty clinics are often difficult to use effectively for prelicensure clinical learning sites because of the lack of sufficient RN role models and the difficulty placing large numbers of students at one site, which can make clinical teaching by the faculty difficult. This can be addressed through placement of students in a single large clinical facility. Major medical centers may have multiple specialty clinics that allow students to participate in a multidisciplinary approach to patient care focused on specific problems. For example, clinics that focus on pain management, wounds, gastroenterology, women's health, behavioral and mental health, diabetes, rehabilitation and sport medicine, and others may be appropriate for student learning.

Depending on geographic location and availability, faculty can also consider outpatient oncology centers, dialysis centers, rural clinics, or health services for Indigenous populations as possible clinical learning sites. Students will have opportunities to engage in assessment, teaching, and delivery of focused care while interacting with a wide range of healthcare providers in these settings. Nursing staff members provide mentoring of the students while clinical teachers are available and provide regular supervisory visits. Student–teacher conferencing activities allow for an assessment of student learning as well as an opportunity for students to ask questions. Group conferencing with several clinical nursing students can be used to share experiences with other students and enable them to make comparisons and contrasts among the learning settings, the care provided, and the patients seen.

Clinics also provide excellent clinical learning opportunities for graduate nursing students. Working with nursing and interdisciplinary staff in these settings allows students to engage in the practice environment while expanding their care responsibilities and role. The students gain specialized competencies needed for advanced practice roles. Graduate students can refine skills of advanced assessment, develop differential diagnostic abilities, and demonstrate their clinical judgment and decision-making in these settings. Diverse clinics can be used with nurse practitioners and other graduate students and include volunteer free clinics that are faith based, campus based, or community based. These clinics are found in diverse places such as healthcare facilities and in neighborhoods. Some clinics are mobile and deliver care by going to those in need such as the homeless. Other clinics are remote and accessed via telehealth, thus providing care for rural and underserved communities (Bavis et al., 2024; Brommelsiek & Peterson, 2020; Shakoor et al., 2023; Taylor et al., 2022) Regardless of the location or format of these clinics, graduate students providing care in these setting gain valuable population health knowledge, enhance their cultural competence, improve communication skills, and have opportunities to engage in clinical skill development.

Operating Room and Other Perioperative Settings

Most nursing programs eliminated an OR clinical rotation from their undergraduate curricula many years ago, but in doing so, nursing faculty have overlooked rich clinical learning opportunities. Many hospitalized patients for whom acute care nurses provide care pass through the OR at some time during their hospitalization. Knowledge about patients' surgical experiences can greatly enhance the knowledge and skills of the nurse caring for the patients both before and after surgery. Perioperative environments are ideal settings for learning application of the nursing process, and perioperative clinical learning activities can contribute to the achievement of a wide variety of program outcomes. In addition to developing expected skills like aseptic technique, students see the use of the latest technology both in the surgical procedures and in the overall care of surgical patients. Students learn about safety, effective communication, and working with an interdisciplinary team.

Nursing students can develop a wide array of psychomotor skills in perioperative settings, such as catheter care, maintenance of IV lines, pain management, skin and wound care, positioning, and care of unconscious patients. Additionally, inclusion of perioperative learning activities in undergraduate nursing curricula will increase nurses' knowledge of patients' surgical experiences. An integrative review focused on student nurses in the preoperative environment revealed the importance of the positive interpersonal relationship with staff contributed to student learning in this setting (McNamara et al., 2023). Therefore, educators should carefully assess the staff–student relationship in these settings. An added advantage of the OR clinical learning experiences may also increase the number of nursing students who choose the perioperative specialty after graduation, possibly helping to minimize the predicted shortage of nurses in the perioperative setting.

One way to include more perioperative clinical learning activities is with a practicum or capstone experience with preceptor guidance. Such capstone courses allow students to apply knowledge and nursing principles learned from various courses throughout the program while being guided by an expert OR clinician. Another creative approach used by nursing programs to provide OR learning experiences is through elective clinical courses. These elective courses offer students clinical learning experiences in perioperative, intraoperative, and postanesthesia care units, thus allowing students to experience the continuum of care while simultaneously developing specialized skills (Maneval et al., 2020).

Nursing Homes, Rehabilitation Centers, and Residential Care Facilities

Competency in the care of older adults, including frail individuals, is a desired outcome of all nursing curricula. Given the growing aging population in the United States, almost all graduates will be caring for older adult patients, regardless of their future work setting or level of education. An underused clinical learning setting for gaining knowledge and competencies about care for the older adult is the nursing home, rehabilitation center, or extended care facility.

Nursing homes are frequently used as clinical learning sites for beginning students to practice fundamental nursing skills. Given the complex needs of older adult patients, these settings offer opportunities to develop knowledge and skills beyond basic care. With a wide variety of residents, learning needs can be matched with clinical learning assignments as students provide holistic care while developing their health assessment, communication, leadership, and delegation skills. Additionally, students learn about the complex health issues of this population as they address multiple health problems, polypharmacy concerns, cognitive impairments, and age-related and functional health status changes of this population.

Another benefit of student clinical learning in nursing homes is the opportunity to learn about the nursing role in the improvement of care for the residents of the facility. Clinical teachers can serve as clinical experts and role models, and students have the time needed to implement and support programs that help patients achieve objectives that are hard to meet in today's rapidly changing acute healthcare environment. These settings also provide rich opportunities to learn and practice delegation and leadership skills with an interdisciplinary care team (Kolanowski et al., 2024).

There are some barriers to high-quality clinical learning experiences in these residential facilities, particularly those providing care for older adults. One barrier is the negative attitude some students have toward this population, either a preexisting attitude or because of a previous clinical experience. Providing opportunities for positive experiences and designing activities to engage in attitude exploration can help students build effective relationships and attitudes toward this growing population (Parker et al., 2021; Watson et al., 2020).

Faculty members need to carefully consider the agency selected for this clinical learning experience. Because there can be wide variability in quality of care provided to residents from facility to facility, it is critical for the faculty to assess indicators of quality in nursing homes and select appropriately. One measure that may provide insight into quality of care is the adequacy of staffing and appropriate role models. To provide information about other measures of nursing home quality, the Medicare website on nursing homes (www.medicare.gov/nursinghomecompare/search.html) presents reports about nursing home performance on indicators such as quality measures, staffing, and health inspections. This website supplies regular updates and overall ratings for over 15,000 Medicare- and Medicaid-certified nursing homes nationwide. Another consideration when using these facilities involves the staff. For effective clinical experiences, staff need to be willing to work closely with students and provide appropriate role models (Hyun et al., 2024).

Once the quality of the nursing home is assessed, the teacher assigned to this clinical site should work on developing a partner relationship with the nursing home staff. This reciprocal relationship will help to build alliances and enable all staff members, teachers, and students to work collaboratively in delivering care and addressing patients' healthcare needs while providing relevant learning opportunities. While at the clinical site, faculty who have advanced knowledge of geriatric care need to actively support student learning as they confront care challenges and deal with a variety of social and emotional issues (Kolanowski et al., 2024). Students can use this experience to improve collaboration skills as they work with a wide variety of staff members, including nursing assistants, licensed practical or vocational nurses, RNs, physical therapists, occupational therapists, dieticians, social workers, and administrators. Lastly, clinical teachers should plan structured orientation programs that provide needed information to adequately prepare students, particularly for the social and clinical needs they will encounter.

Long-term care facilities also offer excellent opportunities for graduate nursing students. Nurse practitioner students can engage in assessment and management of both acute and chronic physical and mental health conditions for residents. The students can monitor and address issues such as skin integrity and pressure ulcer management, identify and prevent fall risks, assess and direct pain management initiatives, explore polypharmacy concerns, and ensure maintenance of functional ability (Baker et al., 2021).

Hospice and Palliative Care

Competency in delivering end-of-life care is an expected student outcome of nursing education, yet many students may not have opportunities to develop the skills and feel unprepared to deliver the needed end-of-life care and deal with the associated emotional responses they may feel (Camara et al., 2024). It can be difficult to achieve these competencies in traditional acute care settings where students have limited exposure and opportunity to interact with dying patients and their families. Clinical learning in hospice and palliative care settings is an excellent way to expose students to issues related to end-of-life care and to provide opportunities to develop many skills that are needed in all nursing roles and settings. Educators can work with hospice and palliative care providers to arrange for students to partner with nurses and provide care to families receiving hospice or palliative care services. Clinical teachers and faculty working with students at both the prelicensure and graduate levels can use the recommended end-of-life education consortium resources to guide these clinical educational experiences (AACN, 2021b).

Dias et al. (2024) recommend a comprehensive clinical onboarding approach for faculty, students, and preceptors working in hospice and home health settings. They report on the effectiveness of preparing students for this specialty area with content learning modules and providing staff with a preceptor guide. Furthermore, they report that students participating in hospice and home health experiences exhibited increased knowledge and attitudes. Given the sensitive issues that arise during end-of-life care, it is important for clinical teachers to consider the emotional needs of all involved and ensure that students have opportunities to discuss feelings that may surface. This can be accomplished through written reflective journals and structured clinical conference activities that encourage reflection and debriefing about the experiences.

CLINICAL LEARNING IN COMMUNITY-BASED CLINICAL SITES

Almost all patients cared for by nurses in the acute care setting come from and return to the community. In addition, many issues, particularly those related to health promotion and maintenance and management of chronic disease, are best addressed in community settings. Community settings also offer many learning opportunities for the development of key skills and competencies that are hard to meet in the acute care environment. The literature suggests that clinical experiences in community-based settings help students to appreciate health promotion, facilitate patient and family center care, link social determinants to health and illness, and build empathy and communication skills (Meely, 2021). For these reasons, inclusion of community-based clinical learning activities in nursing curricula is important. Community-based learning activities are often implemented under the umbrella of service learning. In service learning, students work collaboratively with community partners to meet both course and community objectives. Reflection on the experience and development of a sense of civic engagement are essential components of these learning experiences.

Community-based experiences can occur in a wide variety of settings. Traditionally, these include health departments, schools, camps, shelters, day care centers for children or senior citizens, and wellness centers where students complete a wide variety of nursing interventions. Given the shift from acute to community care, nursing programs frequently form partnerships with these community-based clinical sites. Working together they identify and create unique community-based learning opportunities. For example, a food bank offers nursing students a clinical learning opportunity to provide health education and health promotion resources to community food bank patrons as well as food bank workers and to understand population health concerns while meeting the community partners' needs (Jin et al., 2022).

Partnerships for Community Experiences and Service Learning

As clinical nursing experiences move into community settings, academic–practice partnerships are essential for developing quality experiences. These formal partnerships between nursing programs and a community partner establish a formal relationship that demonstrates a shared vision, mutual goal setting and benefits, commitment, reciprocity, and collaboration based on respect, trust, and openness. These partnerships lead to enhanced student learning and delivery of needed care and services (Bavis et al., 2024; Osakwe et al., 2023). Frequently service learning experiences rely on academic–practice partnerships. In service learning experiences students participate in an organized service activity that meets identified community and client needs. Service learning combines teaching, reflection, and community-based projects. Through these activities students can learn about the health disparities in their community, become more aware of social determinants of health, enhance their knowledge and increase confidence with care (Tillman et al., 2020; Zhu et al., 2022). **Exhibit 4.2** provides essential components for successful service learning experiences.

As nursing education programs include more community-based learning activities, opportunities to incorporate service learning increase. Meaningful community-based service learning opportunities are based on relationships between the academic unit and the community to be served. For such partnerships to work effectively, there must be a good fit between the academic unit's mission and goals and the needs of the community.

Like other clinical learning activities, planning for a service learning activity begins with the teacher's decision that these learning activities would help students to achieve one or more course outcomes. The success of service learning depends on embedding this pedagogy in an existing academic course with clearly defined outcomes. Service learning experiences help students to develop teamwork, leadership, and collaboration skills; increase understanding of community needs; enhance knowledge of social issues; and improve communication skills, thus offering an attractive learning experience for nursing students (Gresh et al., 2020; Newberry et al., 2023; Zhu et al., 2022).

EXHIBIT 4.2 Essential Components of Service Learning Experiences

- Identify community and student needs
- Link service activities to course outcomes
- Collaboratively plan activities
- Orient participants to the service learning expectations
- Monitor implementation of service learning activities
- Incorporate reflection opportunities for student learning
- Assess and evaluate the experience for all stakeholders

Schools

Decreased inpatient pediatric hospitalizations and improved preventive care have led to the reduction of clinical learning opportunities for nursing students, particularly in smaller community hospitals. Nontraditional community-based clinical learning sites such as schools are an ideal setting for pediatric clinical experiences, yet few programs use these learning sites (Schultz & Krassa, 2022). Some faculty are devising creative school-based learning activities. For example, Forbush and Fortney (2025) describe an innovative experience enabling nursing student to work with high school students who were exposed to adverse childhood experiences such as violence, substance abuse, and unstable housing. Nursing students offered focused health education to these students.

School-based clinical learning activities provide excellent alternative opportunities for prelicensure nursing students to develop pediatric health assessment and communication skills, offer child and family health education, promote health and wellness, conduct screenings and population assessments, and develop awareness of growth and development issues. Based upon population needs, students can engage in health and safety education for students, families, staff, and teachers. Advanced practice students working in school-based health centers can provide physical screenings for sports participation, administer immunizations, address student mental health concerns, and manage chronic illnesses (Beierwaltes, et al., 2020).

Camps

Another community-based site that can meet many clinical learning objectives, particularly those related to the care of children with acute and chronic illnesses, is a camp. Clinical learning activities in summer camps for children provide a rich learning opportunity for nursing students to learn about growth and development, use physical assessment skills, and manage illnesses and emergencies while also gaining insight about primary care. Camps that focus on specific health problems or chronic illnesses, such as diabetes, asthma, cancer, or developmental delays, allow nursing students to learn about these health problems during this immersion experience at the camp.

Students develop communication skills, deliver clinical care, engage in interpersonal relationship building, demonstrate social problem-solving, and promote health (Hendrickx et al., 2020).

For students to be adequately prepared for the experiences, they may need appropriate clinical clearances and they should also be familiar with campers' typical health problems and common medications administered. Since camp nurse responsibilities occur around the clock, students need to be prepared to deliver nursing care at all hours of the day and night and deal with the camp's living conditions and fatigue that may occur. Clinical teachers who guide these learning activities need to provide opportunities for student reflection on their experiences and appropriate mentoring during the experience.

Wellness Centers

Wellness centers offer another creative alternative to traditional clinical learning sites. These clinical sites allow nurses, alone or in collaboration with other healthcare providers, to manage health services that focus on health promotion, disease prevention, symptom control, health education, and wellness. Typically, wellness centers are located in the community in places such as public housing, community or recreation centers, food pantries, shelters, senior centers or other social agencies, or churches where students deliver care for vulnerable and underserved populations. At wellness centers students have opportunities to address critical public health problems such as food insecurity, mental health concerns, addiction recovery, and other health issues. Students gain valuable experience assessing critical community and neighborhood concerns and provide needed holistic health services while advocating for those in underserved communities. They can design programs and provide needed care for vulnerable populations.

CLINICAL LEARNING AT DISTANT SITES

Distance education has become a respected and effective method of providing higher education in the United States. The U.S. Department of Education, National Center for Education Statistics (n.d.) reported that in 2023, 53.2% of students in postsecondary education were enrolled in online education. The COVID-19 pandemic accelerated the use of distance education as nursing programs needed to quickly modify their educational delivery approaches because of pandemic health concerns. Even after the pandemic, online learning continues for many programs.

Students choose distance education programs for a variety of reasons, including barriers related to on-campus access and the desire for learning opportunities that occur anytime and anyplace. Many distance learning programs operate asynchronously, allowing students to choose what time of the day or week they will participate in class activities. This makes distance learning programs especially attractive to adult learners who may be working, providing care for their own families, or dealing with other social issues while furthering their education.

But what about clinical education for distance education students? Nursing education, regardless of the delivery mode, depends on acquiring not only the didactic knowledge base but also a set of essential clinical competencies. Ultimately, students must be able to demonstrate that they can apply clinical judgment and decision making skills and function as safe, competent practitioners in a clinical environment. This is the segment of their education that cannot be completely taught or learned exclusively using computer technology.

Faculty members in distance education programs need to carefully consider how students will acquire the necessary clinical skills and how these students will be evaluated. Available clinical sites and knowledgeable, skilled preceptors are needed. Typically, those preceptors working with online students are physically located in or near students' own communities, which may be hundreds of miles or more away from the nursing program. Although nurse educators have been able to provide didactic education to students who live almost anywhere using internet technologies, schools traditionally have had affiliations only with clinical sites located geographically close to their campuses. Now that students enroll in distance learning from remote geographic locations, faculty need to develop new clinical sites for distance learners. The process of securing an appropriate clinical placement for students at distant locations involves a series of checks and balances to ensure that students receive the education they need. The specific steps involved in selecting, preparing, evaluating, and rewarding preceptors are discussed in more detail in Chapter 10.

Evaluating students in the clinical setting is an ongoing challenge for preceptors and nursing faculty but can be particularly challenging with distance education. Goals of evaluation include identification of student strengths and problem areas as well as documentation of student progress. Faculty members must carefully screen and orient preceptors while developing and maintaining trusting work relationships with clinical preceptors who are located at a distance. Contact between the nursing education program faculty member and the preceptor during a student's clinical experience needs to be timely and consistent. Preceptors need to know how to reach the designated faculty member with questions and concerns. At the same time, teaching and completing student evaluations can be time-consuming for the preceptor, and the nursing education program needs to avoid imposing unnecessary reporting burdens. When working at a distance, electronic communication using email, or other synchronized audiovisual communication, such as Zoom®, can be helpful to busy preceptors and faculty members alike.

Various methods have been developed by faculty members to assist in the evaluation process. Some programs may require students to visit a campus for evaluation sessions and demonstration of essential clinical skills. Often objective structured clinical examinations (OSCEs) are used for this evaluation, particularly with nurse practitioner students. Online nurse practitioner programs are creatively using virtual OSCEs to assess performance using an online videoconferencing platform (Chan et al., 2023). Regardless of whether in-person or remote, these exams assess student clinical competency with standardized patients portraying typical clinical problems. Students rotate through various stations and demonstrate skills such as history taking, assessments, or clinical procedures while a faculty evaluator uses a checklist or other rating tool to evaluate performance. OSCEs are discussed in more detail in Chapter 12 on clinical evaluation. Other emerging possibilities include telehealth applications, virtual communities, and virtual interactive video conferencing. Regardless of the method used, faculty need to plan for clinical learning at distance sites and carefully consider student guidance and evaluation. Chapter 11 focuses on teaching students in distance-based programs and expands on this discussion, and Chapter 12 has additional discussion on evaluating clinical performance in distant sites.

CLINICAL LEARNING IN INTERNATIONAL SITES

Clinical placements in international sites can provide rich opportunities to expand students' comfort and competence in the care of diverse patient populations, beyond what can be gained in traditional classrooms. International learning experiences may increase cultural awareness and sensitivity while developing a better understanding of global issues and differences (Gower et al., 2023). On a personal level, students may explore values, develop confidence, and learn or refine other skills. Nursing students whose clinical activities take place within other cultures, in both developed and developing countries, are challenged intellectually and emotionally to become more culturally aware.

Clinical experiences at international sites present unique challenges and require adequate preparation for both the student and the faculty member. Various factors must be considered as part of the planning process. The nursing education program may have an international placement office that can assist with arrangements, offer travel suggestions, and facilitate the selection of appropriate sites. Establishing relationships with key personnel at the host location may enhance collaboration and facilitate planning. Once a site has been selected, faculty should engage in preparatory activities. **Exhibit 4.3** provides faculty and student travel considerations. Preparations focus on the practice environment and learning activities but faculty also should consider roles and responsibilities, safety, and emergency needs.

An understanding of the overall culture, customs, politics, economics, traditions, communication patterns, and values of the community and country in which they will be placed is also essential.

EXHIBIT 4.3 International Travel Considerations

Faculty Activities

- Clarify trip purpose (education, provision of services etc.)
- Confirm institutional approvals and obtain needed partner agreements
- Establish purpose and duration of the trip
- Determine student eligibility and qualifications
- Check U.S. Department of State travel warnings
- Review security updates at https://travel.state.gov and embassy websites
- Arrange transportation, accommodations, and translators
- Plan onsite learning activities and schedule
- Identify student roles and responsibilities
- Establish practice guides to ensure compliance with health care practices and legal regulations
- Outline appropriate professional behavior and code of conduct
- Share information about cultural norms and review dress code with students
- Prepare medical supplies and pack needed equipment
- Plan for onsite activities and post trip follow-up

Student Preparation

- Ensure passports are current
- Update immunizations and obtain appropriate preventive medications as needed such as antimalarial drugs
- Plan for emergencies and have contact information for U.S. embassy and consulate
- Enroll in the Smart Traveler Enrollment Program (STEP) at https://mytravel.state.gov.s.step
- Purchase supplemental travel health insurance as appropriate
- Review and follow safety and security protocols
- Pack a travel health kit with needed medications and items such as insect repellent, sunscreen, and hand sanitizer
- Review cultural norms and customs

Opportunities for reflection and sharing of experiences are critical because students may encounter emotional issues that need to be addressed. Even with adequate pretrip planning, students may not be prepared for the health disparities and complex health and cultural issues they encounter, the limited resources available, the stereotypes they may experience, and their ethnocentric thinking (Gosse & Katic-Duffy, 2020). Journaling (traditional or electronic format) helps students reflect upon and process their feeling. They may also wish to share their experiences with classmates who did not participate in these activities.

PRACTICAL ASPECTS OF CLINICAL PLACEMENTS IN DIVERSE SITES

When considering practical aspects of clinical placements in diverse sites, there are two major areas of concern. The first reflects the regulatory and accreditation requirements for clinical learning activities; the second involves preparation of the agency, clinical teachers, and students. All clinical learning activities must meet the requirements of state law and regulations (often set by the board of nursing) as well as the policies and requirements of accreditation agencies, the nursing education program (or its parent institution), and the site at which the clinical activities are to take place. Each nursing education program also has procedures in place that describe how contracts and similar formal communication with an agency are to be managed. While often clear from the school's perspective, this is not always the case from the agency's perspective. This is an important point for agencies that usually do not negotiate such contracts and for which there is no clearly identified contact person. Some agencies that appear to be freestanding may be part of larger agencies. When the agency is part of a larger entity (e.g., a hospital system, local government program, state health department, school district, or federal agency such as the Department of Veterans Affairs), it can be both difficult and time-consuming to get the contract signed by all relevant parties. These agreements can dictate student and faculty requirements needed prior to entering the clinical agency for learning. These agreements are especially important when dealing with smaller agencies that may not have procedures in place related to orientation or placement of students in their facilities.

Adhering to the agency guidelines is important to avoid conflicts, especially when multiple programs (nursing and other health professionals) are seeking placements for the same time period. Even if students are at one of the clinical entity's sites, the policy for the overall entity must be followed. Often, smaller and nontraditional sites (e.g., day care settings, church programs, food kitchens) and even some formal agencies that do not have large numbers of staff (e.g., day treatment programs for substance abusers, assisted living facilities) do not require or have a formal orientation program. The clinical teacher should work with the staff to determine what preparation the students need to optimize their learning as well as to protect and provide the best care for the patients they will encounter. A larger institution (e.g., a major hospital system) may be the parent organization of smaller community-based programs, and students may need to complete the full agency orientation to be placed in even a small or offsite location. If these requirements become too onerous, expensive, or time-consuming, the value of clinical learning activities at these sites may be questioned by the nursing education program faculty and administration. Legal aspects of clinical learning experiences are explored more fully in Chapter 6. A few aspects highly relevant to the use of diverse sites are presented in **Exhibit 4.4**.

As competition for clinical sites continues, clinical teachers seek creative ways to effectively and efficiently secure appropriate student learning opportunities. Clinical agency administrators and educators are also ready to embrace creative approaches that will decrease nursing program competition and rivalry in securing clinical sites. They should also work collaboratively to provide an equitable approach that will meet the agency's, nursing program's, and students' needs. Educational programs and healthcare providers must work together to meet common goals. One approach is the formation of a clinical placement consortium. In this model, school representatives, service agency liaisons, and clinical agency representatives meet to find appropriate learning opportunities for all. The use of web-based programs or course management systems is one way to manage and display clinical placement requests and facilitate open communication and negotiation among consortium members.

Regardless of the type of relationship with the clinical agency or location of the clinical site, there are some basic considerations that will help to ensure a collegial working relationship with agency leaders and nursing staff. Details of the clinical learning activity (when will students be there, what are their learning goals, what are they expected to do, and how can they participate) must be communicated to the staff. Settings that rarely host nursing students, as well as those that often do, can have problems getting this information to the staff members who will have the most contact with the students. Explore if there are methods to electronically share information with staff, such as through email, so that it is disseminated in a convenient and efficient way. Misunderstandings about student activities and objectives do occur and can jeopardize the learning experience. Often, course syllabi, clinical objectives, and guides to the clinical learning activity are provided to administrative staff of a clinical agency but may not be

EXHIBIT 4.4 Areas of Consideration When Placing Students in Diverse Clinical Sites

Legal and Regulatory Issues

Does the placement meet the requirements of relevant state laws and accompanying regulations related to approval, contract, faculty ratios, nature of faculty guidance, and student scope of practice?

Must the clinical teacher be present for clinical learning activities for students to practice direct patient care?

Can preceptors be used in the setting and in the manner planned?

Can the clinical teacher delegate guidance and evaluation of students' learning to an RN on staff at the agency, if the clinical teacher is not physically present?

How and where are students documenting care?

Nursing Education Program Issues

Is a contract or legal agreement required?

If the planned clinical learning activity will occur at times other than the usual hours and day of a traditional clinical activity (e.g., on parts of most days of the week, during school breaks, on weekends), is this reflected in the clinical teacher's workload and compensation?

Are there specific requirements of the education program's accreditation body that affect the planned clinical learning activity?

Agency Issues

What are the agency's rules and policies related to nursing student clinical activities? Can the student deliver care or are they primarily observing care?

Does the agency require a contract with the nursing education program? If so, who manages contracts with education programs?

How are requests for clinical placements from multiple nursing education and other programs handled?

What are the agency rules for student clearance (e.g., criminal background, child or elder abuse records, drug screening)?

If screenings or background checks beyond the requirements of the nursing education program are required, who pays for them?

Does the nursing education program need to document that students have demonstrated CPR or other competencies?

What are the health requirements, such as tuberculosis testing or immunizations?

Are there specific Health Insurance Portability and Accountability Act (HIPAA) or patient privacy statements that must be completed?

Does the agency need to keep a record of students at the clinical site for legal or regulatory purposes? If yes, what is needed from the nursing education program?

Student Issues

What modes of transportation are available? Is there parking?

What measures will help to ensure the safety of students?

What is the required orientation?

shared with the staff members who are directly working with the students and could benefit from access to this information. A meeting with the staff members who will work directly with the students, along with providing easily accessible documents, will facilitate communication and ensure that the right people have the right information.

Including nursing staff in planning clinical learning activities can also prevent potential problems. Seeking input from nurses and understanding their workload demands can help clinical teachers plan effectively for student learning activities. Realizing the existing demands on staff members, such as precepting new nurses or supervising other staff members, will help clinical teachers form realistic expectations of the time available to assist students.

Clinical Teacher Preparation

Clinical teachers may need additional education, mentoring, and support as they implement clinical learning activities in new and diverse settings. A highly skilled clinical teacher who is at ease while teaching students to care for acutely ill patients in a critical care unit may not have the necessary knowledge and skills needed to care for those patients in their homes a week after discharge. Like their students, clinical teachers may find that the fine points of adapting care to the home setting while respecting the family in their home and dealing with the virtual loss of the multiple support systems of the acute care setting will be new to them.

The organization and structure of clinical teaching outside of acute care settings may also be new for faculty members. Some logistical issues will need to be addressed. If the students are not all in the same setting, how will faculty members conduct their clinical teaching activities at multiple sites? How will students and teachers communicate with each other? How will clinical conferences occur? What written assignments will be submitted to the teacher and how and when will it be returned to students? Electronic technology can provide solutions for some of these issues. Learning management systems can be used to create forums for posting clinical updates and news, submission of course assignments, or asynchronous discussion boards. Other electronic communication methods can be used to remain in touch with students during clinical time. These methods include cell phones, although they are not always permitted at clinical sites. Text messaging can be used to provide support and instant access between clinical teachers and students during clinical learning experience activities, allowing instant connectivity in an easy-to-use format. However, ensure that messaging is HIPAA compliant if sharing patient information. Some computer applications such as Remind (www.remind.com) are available and can help teachers to schedule and distribute automatic announcements for students. These programs can also be used to share messages without revealing the clinical teacher's phone number.

SUMMARY

Nursing care occurs anywhere clients need the services of a professional nurse, and nursing students can learn to provide care wherever they have contact with clients. Traditionally, much of clinical nursing education has occurred in acute care settings because of long-held assumptions about how nurses must be prepared to practice. However, decreasing length of inpatient stays, high patient acuity, economic pressures to provide care in outpatient and community settings, and increasing competition with other educational programs for the same clinical sites have limited clinical learning opportunities located in traditional acute care settings. Using diverse sites for clinical learning activities can prepare nursing students for the challenges of contemporary nursing practice as clients, health needs, care locations, and approaches to care change over time.

This chapter discussed options for planning and providing clinical learning opportunities for undergraduate and graduate nursing students in a wide variety of clinical sites. Examples of clinical learning opportunities in four categories were presented. The first category included clinical learning in specialized patient care areas that are not used regularly as clinical learning sites (e.g., outpatient clinics, the OR, nursing homes and residential care facilities, hospice and palliative care settings). These sites offer rich learning opportunities for students. The second category included community-based settings such as camps and wellness centers. The third category was clinical learning at distant sites. The final category was the growing use of international clinical learning opportunities.

Practical aspects of clinical placements in diverse sites were also discussed. Two main areas of concern are the need to meet regulatory and accreditation requirements and the need for adequate preparation of agency staff members, clinical teachers, and students. Examples of methods and tools used for the preparation of agency staff members and clinical teachers making the transition from traditional acute care sites were provided.

CNE®cl EXAMINATION TEST BLUEPRINT CORE COMPETENCIES

1. **Function in the Education and Health Care Environments**
   - **A. Function in the Clinical Nurse Educator Role**
     - 2. Foster professional growth of learners (e.g., coaching, reflection, and debriefing)
   - **B. Operationalize the Curriculum**
     - 1. Assess congruence of the clinical environment to curriculum, course outcomes, and learner needs when evaluating clinical sites
     - 4. Prepare learners for clinical experiences (e.g., facility, clinical expectations, equipment, and technology-based resources)
     - 5. Implement clinical activities to help learners develop interprofessional collaboration and teamwork skills
   - **C. Abide by Legal Requirements, Ethical Guidelines, Agency Policies, and Guiding Framework**
     - 1. Apply ethical and legal principles to create a safe clinical learning environment (e.g., privacy laws, confidentiality, error/near-miss situation reporting, remediation, negligence, liability, scope/standards of practice)
     - 4. Inform others of program and clinical agency policies, procedures, and practices
     - 5. Adhere to program and clinical agency policies, procedures, and practices when implementing clinical experiences (e.g., due process, accommodations, academic integrity)
     - 6. Comply with current program and clinical agency policies, procedures, and practices related to personal protective equipment and other infection control measures for self and learners
2. **Facilitate Learning in the Health Care Environment**
   - A. Implement a variety of clinical teaching strategies appropriate to learner needs, desired learner outcomes, course outcomes, setting, and context (e.g., virtual, telehealth, in-person, simulation)
   - D. Create opportunities for learners to develop critical judgment
   - E. Promote a culture of safety and quality in the delivery of health care
   - G. Develop collegial working relationships with learners, faculty, and clinical environment
3. **Demonstrate Effective Interpersonal Communication and Collaborative Interprofessional Relationships**
   - A. Model collaboration within the healthcare environment
   - B. Foster the development of a collegial learning community
   - C. Facilitate opportunities to collaborate within the healthcare team
   - E. Demonstrate respect for learners, healthcare team, colleagues, clients, families, and others
   - F. Use clear and effective communication in all interactions (e.g., written, electronic, verbal, nonverbal, virtual)
   - L. Communicate performance expectations to learners and clinical staff
5. **Facilitate Learner Development and Socialization**
   - F. Create learning environments that promote socialization to the role of the nurse
6. **Implement Effective Clinical Assessment Evaluation Strategies**
   - H. Evaluate the quality of the clinical learning experiences and environment

LEARNING ACTIVITIES

CourseConnect

To access self-assessment questions and interactive, competency-based learning activities for this chapter, visit www.springerpub.com/courseconnect. See inside front cover and tear-out card for CourseConnect details.

REFERENCES

American Association of Colleges of Nursing. (2021a). *APRN clinical training task force report brief.* https://www.aacnnursing.org/News-Information/APRN-Clinical-Training-Task-Force-Report-Brief

American Association of Colleges of Nursing. (2021b). *End-of-life nursing education consortium (ELNEC) fact sheet.* https://www.aacnnursing.org/Portals/42/ELNEC/PDF/ELNEC-Fact-Sheet.pdf

American Association of Colleges of Nursing. (2023). *Guiding principles for competency-based education and assessment.* https://www.aacnnursing.org/Portals/0/PDFs/Essentials/Guiding-Principles-for-CBE-Assessment.pdf

Baker, N. R., Schipper, L., McCumber, S., & Fay, V. P. (2021). Use of long-term care facilities for primary care nurse practitioner students. *Journal of Nursing Education, 60*(2), 99–102. https://doi.org/10.3928/01484834-20210120-08

Bavis, M., O'Brien, B., Hendel, E., & Moss, A. (2024). Creating a win-win: An academic-practice partnership in nurse practitioner training. *The Journal for Nurse Practitioners, 20*(2024), 1–5. https://doi.org/10.1016/j.nurpra.2024.104943

Beierwaltes, P., Bell, S. E., Cornell, R., Ostrow, L. G., Schmitz, N., Verchota, G., Clisbee, D., Houston, R., & Eggenberger, S. K. (2022). A school-based health centre partnership: Faculty practice, nursing student learning and wellness in youth, families, and community. *Journal of Clinical Nursing, 23*(1–2), 332–345. https://doi.org/10.1111/jocn.16246

Brommelsiek, M., & Peterson, J. A. (2020). Preparing nurse practitioner students to practice in rural primary care. *Journal of Nursing Education, 59*(10), 581–584. https://doi.org/10.3928/01484834-20200921-08

Buron, B., Eng, C. A., & Eagleton, A. (2024). Reimagining the future of clinical nursing education: A cohort partnership model. *Nurse Educator, 49*(6), 321–326. https://doi.org/10.1097/NNE.0000000000001681

Camara, C., Rosengarten, L., & Callum, J. (2024). Experiences of nursing students providing end of life care for children and young people: A focus group study. *Nursing Education Today, 137*(2024), 106147. https://doi.org/10.1016/j.nedt.2024.106147

Chan, S. C. C., Choa, G., Kelly, J., Maru, D., & Rashid, M. A. (2023). Implementation of virtual OSCE in health professions education: A systematic review. *Medical Education, 57*(9), 833–843. https://doi.org/10.1111/medu.15089

Colburn, D. A. (2022). Nursing education and social determinants of health: A content analysis. *Journal of Nursing Education, 61*(9), 516–523. https://doi.org/10.3928/01484834-20220705-06

Dias, N., White, M., Harmuth, S., & Horvick, S. (2024). A structured home health and hospice clinical rotation and onboarding model to address the nursing shortage. *Home Healthcare Now, 42*(2), 78–83. https://doi.org/10.1097/NHH.0000000000001237

Forbush, J., & Fortney, C. A. (2025). Use of experiential learning in undergraduate community health curriculum: Adverse childhood events and trauma-informed care. *Nurse Educator, 50*(3), E186–187. https://doi.org/10.1097/NNE.0000000000001781

Gigli, K. H., & Gonzalez, J. D. (2022). Meeting the need for nurse practitioners clinicals: A survey of practitioners. *Journal of the American Association of Nurse Practitioners, 34*(8), 991–1001. https://doi.org/10.1097/JXX.0000000000000749

Goers, J., Mulkey, D., & Oja, K. (2022). A call to reform undergraduate nursing clinical placements. *Nursing Outlook, 70*(2022), 371–373. https://doi.org/10.1016/j.outlook.2022.01.005

Gosse, N. L., & Katic-Duffy, A. (2020). Nursing student and faculty perceptions of reciprocity during international clinical learning experiences: A qualitative descriptive study. *Nurse Education Today, 84*(2020), 1–6. https://doi.org/10.1016/j.nedt.2019.104242

Gower, S., Duggan, R., & Dantas, J. A. (2023). Preparing students for post-COVID nursing careers: The value of international clinical placements. *Journal of Nursing Education, 62*(4), 207–214. https://doi.org/10.3928/01484834-20230208-03

Gresh, A., LaFave, S., Thamilselvan, V., Batchelder, A., Mermer, J., Jacques, K., Greensfelder, A., Buckley, M., Cohen, Z., Coy, A., & Warren, N. (2020). Service learning in public health nursing education: How COVID-19 accelerated community-academic partnership. *Public Health Nursing, 38*, 248–257. https://doi.org/10.1111/phn.12796

Gubrud-Howe, P. (2024). Teaching in the clinical learning environment. In D. M. Billings & J. A. Halstead (Eds.), *Teaching in nursing: A guide for faculty* (7th ed., pp. 387–421). Elsevier.

Hendrickx, L., Pelzel, H., Burdette, L., & Hartung, N. (2020). Pediatric clinical for nursing students in rural areas: The camp nursing experiences. *Online Journal of Rural Nursing and Health Care, 20*(1), 142–155. https://doi.org/10.14574/ojrnhc.v20i1.603

Hyun, A., Tower, M., Bogossian, F., Seib, C., Ryan, C., & Cooper, S. (2024). Factors influencing nursing student satisfaction in aged-care placement: An Australian cross-sectional study. *Nurse Education in Practice, 79*(2024), 104064. https://doi.org/10.1016/j.nepr.2024.104064

Jin, X., Ezeonwu, M., Ayad, A., & Bowman, K. (2022). Using a food bank as a platform for educating communities during the COVID-19 pandemic. *Journal of Community Health Nursing, 39*(1), 50–57. https://doi.org/10.1080/07370016.2022.2037052

Jones-Schenk, J. (2021). Redesigning clinical learning. *The Journal of Continuing Education in Nursing, 52*(9), 402–403. https://doi.org/10.3928/00220124-20210804-03

Kolanowski, A., Bowers, B., Mueller, C., & Harrington, C. (2024). RN staffing shortages in nursing homes: Nursing is part of the solution. *Journal of Gerontological Nursing, 50*(1), 3–5. https://doi.org/10.3928/00989134-20231121-01

Leighton, K., Kardong-Edgren, S. McNelis, A. M., Foisy-Doll, C., & Sullo, E. (2021). Traditional clinical outcomes in prelicensure nursing education: An empty systematic review. *Journal of Nursing Education, 60*(3), 136–142. https://doi.org/10.3928/01484834-20210222-03

Maneval, R., Hepburn, M., Brooks, C., Tamburi, M., Chin, S. D. N., Prado-Inzerillo, M. Haghenbeck-Nunnink, K. T., & Flaum, S. J. (2020). Enhancing the undergraduate nursing education experience with clinical elective courses. *Journal of Professional Nursing, 37*(2), 366–372. https://doi.org/10.1016/j.profnurs.2020.04.014

McNamara, C., O'Brien, B., & O'Reilly, P. (2023). The learning experiences of student nurses in the perioperative environment: An integrative literature review. *Nursing Education Today, 131*(2023), 105985. https://doi.org/10.1016/j.nedt.2023.105985

Meely, N. G. (2021). Undergraduate student nurses' experiences of their community placements. *Nurse Education Today, 106*(2021), 105054. https://doi.org/10.1016/j.nedt.2021.105054

National Academies of Sciences, Engineering, and Medicine. (2021). *The future of nursing 2020–2030: Charting a path to achieve health equity*. The National Academies Press. https://doi.org/10.17226/25982

Newberry, D. M., Spies, L. A., Jones, J. J., & Perez, P. Y. (2023). Evaluation of social determinants of health in nursing education through service learning. *Creative Nursing, 29*(4), 383–388. https://doi.org/10.1177/10784535231212410

Osakwe, Z. T., Horton, J. R., Ottah, J., Eisner, J., Atairu, M., & Stefancic, A (2023). Academic-clinical collaborations to build undergraduate nursing education in hospice and palliative care. *Journal of Gerontological Nursing, 49*(6), 13–18. https://doi.org/10.3928/00989134-20230515-01

Parker, C. N., Harvey, T., Johnston, S., & MacAndrew, M. (2021). An exploration of knowledge of students and staff at residential aged care facilities and implications for nursing education. *Nurse Education Today, 96*(2021), 104639. https://doi.org/10.1016/j.nedt.2020.104639

Schultz, C. M., & Krassa, T. J. (2022). Use of private, parochial and public schools in baccalaureate nursing programs for pediatric practicum. *Nurse Educator, 47*(5), 298–302. https://doi.org/10.1097/NNE.0000000000001200

Shakoor, K., Boelens, L., & Yingling, C. (2023). Improving nurse practitioner practice readiness in an interprofessional student-run free clinic. *The Journal for Nurse Practitioners, 19*(7), 104647. https://doi/org/10.1016/j.nurpra.2023.104647

Taylor, T. L., Remo, E., Hay, B., Johansson, M., Bricker, C., & Maguire, D. (2022). Innovative opportunities for nurse practitioner education uncovered by the pandemic. *Journal of Nursing Education, 61*(3), 153–155. https://doi.org/10.3928/01484834-20211128-02

Tillman, P., Thomas, M., & Buelow, J. R. (2020). Impact of service learning on student attitudes toward the poor and underserved. *Nurse Educator, 45*(6), 316–320. https://doi.org/10.1097/NNE.0000000000000807

U.S. Department of Education, National Center for Education Statistics. (n.d.). *Integrated Postsecondary Education Data System (IPEDS), Fall Enrollment component final data (2012–2022) and provisional data (2023)*. https://nces.ed.gov/ipeds/TrendGenerator/app/answer/2/42

Watson, J., Horseman, Z., Fawcett, T., Hockley, J., & Rhynas, S. (2020). Care home nursing: Co-creating curricular content with student nurses. *Nurse Education Today, 84*(2020), 104233. https://doi.org/10.1016/j.nedt.2019.104233

Zhu, Z., Xing, W., Liang, Y, Hong, L., & Hu, Y. (2022). Nursing students' experiences with service learning: A qualitative systematic review and meta-synthesis. *Nurse Education Today, 108*(2022), 105206. https://doi.org/10.1016/j.nedt.2021.105206

Preparing Learners in Clinical Settings 5

OBJECTIVES:

1. Describe the roles and responsibilities of those involved in clinical learning experiences for nursing students.
2. Suggest methods of preparing learners for clinical learning activities.
3. Discuss the cognitive, affective, and psychomotor domains that influence student learning in the clinical setting.

Preparing nursing students for clinical learning is a multifaced process that requires careful consideration of various factors. Nurse educators must strike a balance between equipping students for the clinical environment and preparing staff members for the presence of learners, all while ensuring patient needs are met. This chapter describes the roles and responsibilities of faculty members, clinical staff, and other individuals involved in clinical teaching. It also offers practical methods for preparing students for clinical learning activities, and addressing cognitive, affective, and psychomotor domains that influence student learning. This chapter discusses essential criteria for selecting appropriate clinical settings, such as the availability of resources, positive role models, and opportunities to meet learning objectives. Additionally, the challenges of selecting clinical settings in a competitive environment are addressed. Finally, the chapter explores how educators can support students in managing anxiety and stress related to clinical learning through orientation and preparation, ensuring a smoother transition into clinical practice. Clinical teaching methods and crafting clinical learning assignments are discussed in Chapter 7.

UNDERSTANDING THE CONTEXT FOR CLINICAL LEARNING ACTIVITIES

To begin preparations for clinical teaching and learning, nurse educators should reflect on the context in which these activities take place. Teachers and learners use healthcare or community settings for learning environments, thus becoming guests within that setting. What are the implications for clinical teaching and learning effectiveness under these conditions and how to best prepare learners for this experience?

Over the last century, basic preparation for professional nursing has moved from service-based training to academic educational programs in institutions of higher learning. As a result of this service–education separation, the clinical teacher and students who enter a clinical setting for learning activities are often regarded as guests of the healthcare agency or community site. They participate in the activities of the established system and attempt to follow the norms of its culture, but they are not a constant presence. Teachers must rely on relationships they develop within the agency to facilitate their sense of belonging to support student learning (Kan & Stabler-Haas, 2025).

Traditionally, clinical teachers and students in an academic nursing education program comprise a temporary system within the permanent culture of the clinical setting. A temporary system is a set of individuals who work together on a complex task for a limited period of time. Although clinical teachers are professional colleagues to nursing staff members and are viewed as nurses by patients, their primary role is that of an educator. Even if they are employed by the agency as a staff member on a casual or part-time basis in addition to their academic positions, faculty members enact a different role when they are guiding the clinical learning activities of students, and role confusion is often inevitable.

Being a good guest involves knowing and adhering to the established routines, policies, and practices of the clinical setting. Clinical teachers negotiate with staff members for access to learning opportunities and resources while simultaneously protecting students from criticism and preventing errors. When possible, the clinical teacher should point out staff members who demonstrate clinical excellence and professionalism. The clinical teacher juggles the complex responsibilities of supporting student learning, developing trusting relationships with staff, and ensuring the delivery of safe quality care.

At times, a clinical teacher's desire for positive relationships with staff members, reluctance to delay or slow patient care, and concern for patient and student safety may lead to minimizing students' risk taking in an effort to prevent errors. For example, teachers may select assignments for students that allow them to demonstrate previously developed competencies rather than choose learning activities that will challenge students to deepen their understanding and develop higher skill levels. If the teacher expects that a student will not be able to complete patient care activities in a timely manner, the instructor may forego a rich opportunity for the student to learn to prioritize, organize, and complete a complex set of tasks for the patient and to work collaboratively and efficiently with other healthcare team members efficiently. Excessive gatekeeping actions of this kind do not allow students to exhibit clinical problem solving, organize care activities, and learn to take appropriate, calculated risks.

Although clinical teachers and nursing students are seen as guests in the healthcare environment, they also serve as a vital resource. Students represent potential future employees, and the learning environment they encounter during the clinical experience can influence their recruitment and job seeking decisions after graduation. Exposure to and immersion in clinical areas influence nursing student decisions about practice upon graduation. Positive clinical learning experiences may encourage nursing students to consider future employment in that agency, and nursing staff members who nurture the development of students can have a powerful influence on such a choice (Anyango et al., 2024).

Many staff members, however, are unaware of or misinterpret these clinical expectations; they expect nursing students to participate fully in all activities, assume responsibility for patient care, and take the same kinds of patient assignments and complete the same patient care tasks as staff members. They may recall their own clinical education as being more rigorous than the contemporary clinical activities that they witness; communicating those perceptions to nursing students can produce self-doubt, discouragement, and dissatisfaction among the novices. Clinicians working with graduate students may expect students preparing to become advanced practice nurses to have well-developed clinical assessment and diagnostic skills and forget these are learners who are refining their knowledge and skills and care efficiency in this new role. The teacher as culture broker must allow students to experience the real world of clinical nursing and, at the same time, communicate to nursing staff that trends and current issues in nursing education have changed. Keeping clinical staff members, managers, and administrators informed about the nature of contemporary nursing education and keeping students updated on current challenges and priorities in the healthcare environment will help to integrate students more effectively into the real world of clinical nursing.

SELECTING CLINICAL SETTINGS

Clinical teachers may have sole responsibility for selecting the settings in which clinical learning activities occur, or their input may be sought by those who make these decisions. In either case, selection of clinical sites should be based on important criteria such as compatibility of school and agency philosophy, availability of opportunities to meet learning objectives, geographic location, agency licensure or accreditation, availability of positive role models, the complexity of patients, level of student, purpose, type of course, and physical resources (Gubrud-Howe, 2024).

Selection Criteria

Nurse educators should conduct a careful assessment of potential clinical sites before selecting those that will be used for learning activities. Faculty members who are also employed in clinical agencies may provide some of the necessary information, and teachers who have previously instructed students in an agency can provide ongoing input into its continued suitability as a practice site. Prior evaluations of the clinical site completed by students and educators can provide helpful information about the experiences and setting and can be useful for guiding clinical site selection. Consider strengths and concerns that have been previously identified by students or faculty.

Educators will also need to consider accreditation or regulatory requirements before selecting a clinical site. State boards of nursing may have specific reporting requirements or forms that need to be completed as part of the selection and approval process for clinical sites. Nursing education programs may need to provide additional information for a board of nursing review. For an example of an agency data form see https://www.pa.gov/content/dam/copapwp-pagov/en/dos/department-and-offices/bpoa/nursing/agency_data_form.pdf.

Assessment of potential clinical agencies should address the following criteria:

- *Opportunity to achieve learning outcomes:* Are sufficient opportunities available to allow learners to achieve learning objectives? For example, if planning, implementing, and evaluating preoperative teaching is an important course objective, the average preoperative patient census must be sufficient to permit learners to practice these skills. If the objectives require learners to practice direct patient care, does the agency allow this, or will learners only be permitted to observe? Will learners from other educational programs be present in the clinical environment at the same time? If so, how much competition for the same learning opportunities is anticipated? Will client fatigue occur if multiple students provide care over several days? Will there be an adequate patient census to ensure that appropriate learning opportunities are available?

- *Level of the learner:* If the learners are undergraduate students at the beginning level of the curriculum, the agency must provide ample opportunity to practice basic skills. Graduate students need learning activities that will allow them to develop advanced practice skills. Are undergraduate students in a capstone course permitted to participate in clinical learning activities under the guidance of an appropriate staff member as preceptor, without the physical presence of a faculty member?
- *Degree of control by faculty:* Does the agency staff recognize the authority of the clinical teacher to plan appropriate learning activities for students, or do agency policies limit or prescribe the kinds and timing of student activities? Do staff members restrict the types of learning activities available? Do agency personnel view learners as additions to the staff and expect them to provide service to patients, or do they acknowledge the role of students as learners?
- *Availability of experienced role models for students:* As previously discussed, students often imitate the behaviors they observe in nursing staff members. Are the nursing staff positive role models for students? Do they have adequate experience to effectively guide students? If learners are graduate students who are learning advanced practice roles, are experienced, positive role models available to serve as preceptors and mentors? Do they have the educational and experiential qualifications to guide students appropriately? Is staffing adequate to permit staff members to interact with students and participate in their learning, or are they overburdened and have demanding workloads? Are staff dismissive, exclusionary, and rude, or are they cooperative, inclusive, supportive, and welcoming of students?
- *Geographic location:* Although the geographic location of the clinical agency is not usually the most important selection criterion, it can be a crucial factor when a large number of clinical agencies must be used. Travel time between the campus and clinical settings for faculty and students must be considered, especially if learning activities are scheduled in both settings on the same day. Is travel to the agency via public transportation possible and safe, especially if faculty and students need to travel in the evening or at night? Are public transportation schedules convenient? Do they allow students and faculty to arrive at the agency in time for the scheduled start of activities, and do they permit a return trip to campus or home without excessive waiting times? Does the value of available learning opportunities at the agency outweigh the disadvantages of travel time and cost? Students attending online educational programs may participate in clinical experiences at remote locations. For students enrolled in clinical experiences at distant locations there may be different needs that faculty will need to consider, such as communication and supervision needs.
- *Physical facilities:* Are physical facilities such as conference space, locker rooms, cafeteria or other dining facility, library, and parking available for use by clinical teachers and students?
- *Staff relationships with teachers and learners:* Do staff members respond positively to the presence of students, engage in effective communications with faculty and students, and welcome appropriate questions from them? Will the staff members cooperate with teachers in selecting appropriate learning activities, participate in orientation activities for faculty and students, and provide useful guidance and feedback about student performance?
- *Orientation needs:* Some clinical agencies require faculty members to attend scheduled orientation sessions before students can enter the clinical setting. The time required for such orientation must be considered when selecting clinical agencies. If faculty members are also employed in the agency as casual or per diem staff, this orientation requirement may be waived. Can any parts of the orientation be completed without being present in the agency, such as online or via self-study? Are technology initiatives such as electronic health records (EHRs) used and do they require faculty and student orientation, password clearances, and access to computer systems? If so, are there mechanisms in place for timely training and to allow clinical teachers and students to use these systems as part of the clinical learning activities?
- *Opportunity for interdisciplinary activities:* As interprofessional skill development emerges as a critical component of nursing education, consider if there are opportunities for learners to practice as members of an interdisciplinary healthcare team. Will learners have contact with other healthcare practitioners, such as physical therapists, pharmacists, nutritionists, respiratory therapists, social workers, infection control personnel, and physicians?
- *Agency requirements:* Unless the educational program and the clinical facility are parts of the same organization, a legal contract or agreement usually must be negotiated to permit students and faculty to use the agency as a clinical teaching site. Such contracts or agreements typically specify requirements such as school and individual liability insurance; competence in CPR and professional licensure for clinical teachers, graduate students, and RN-to-BSN students; immunization and other health requirements; dress code; use of name tags or identification badges; requirements for student drug testing; and requirements for criminal background checks for students and clinical teachers.

- *Agency licensure and accreditation:* Accreditation or other regulatory requirements for educational programs may specify that clinical learning activities take place in accredited healthcare organizations. If the agency must be licensed to provide certain health services, it is appropriate to verify current licensure before selecting that agency as a clinical site.
- *Costs:* In addition to travel expenses, there may be other costs associated with use of an agency for clinical learning activities. Increasingly, some agencies are charging fees for use of the clinical agency for educational purposes. Any fees charged to schools for use of the agency or other anticipated expenses to the educational program and to individual clinical teachers and students should be assessed.
- *Regulatory board approvals:* State boards of nursing often require review and approval of clinical sites before they can be used for clinical nursing education. Faculty members or administrators may need to provide information about the healthcare institution, including bed capacity and average daily patient census, a list of other nursing education programs using the facility, the number of students who will be using the facility, and specific scheduling information.

Healthcare agencies are mandating requirements to ensure patient safety and comply with various regulations. The Centers for Disease Control and Prevention (CDC) and the Advisory Committee on Immunization Practices (ACIP) of the CDC provides updated recommendations about vaccine schedules. Students working in healthcare settings may need to demonstrate evidence of vaccines such as measles, mumps, rubella, hepatitis B, varicella, influenza, tetanus, diphtheria, and pertussis. Given the changing nature of vaccines, particularly since the COVID-19 pandemic, recommendations are regularly updated. Therefore, teachers need to periodically check these guidelines at https://www.cdc.gov/acip-recs/hcp/vaccine-specific/index.html for new information and consult with healthcare agencies to align with their requirements. Students may need to demonstrate compliance by showing evidence of immunizations or immunity, or they may require booster immunizations. Many healthcare facilities may have additional or site-specific clinical requirements such as mandatory drug testing. Institutions may require testing for a specific panel of drugs or drug classifications. Typically, students have a narrow window of time for completion of the drug testing at the start of a clinical experience and must follow a specific protocol for this testing. Depending upon state regulations, students may also need to complete a variety of background checks to screen for offenses and criminal arrest records. These background checks may include child abuse, elder abuse, and criminal history checks. Some agencies require that students meet the same requirements that their staff members must meet for these checks and clearances. All of these requirements, as well as anticipated costs, should be communicated to students. Early and clear communication with students about these requirements will help to ensure that students understand them and have sufficient time to gather evidence of completion by the specified deadlines.

The list of clinical requirements may be quite lengthy and may require significant time and financial investment for students to comply; however, they must be completed before a student can begin clinical activities at a clinical site and risk violating the nursing education program's contract with the agency and jeopardizing future access to that clinical site. Another concern for the educational institution involves managing these records. When gathering personal information about students, nursing education program personnel need to protect student privacy and prevent inappropriate disclosure of personal information obtained for clinical requirements. Some programs contract with agencies that serve as an electronic repository for the various student health requirements and background checks. These companies review the materials submitted by students and provide reports to the nursing program that can guide decisions about completion of the requirements. Student consent is essential when releasing personally identifiable information to such outside agencies to ensure compliance with the Family Education Rights and Privacy Act (FERPA) (20 U.S.C.§ 1232g; 34 CFR Part 99). Thus, nursing education programs should have guidelines for disclosure and a method of keeping this private information separate from students' academic records.

Sufficient time must be allowed before the anticipated start of clinical activities to negotiate a contractual agreement that specifies rights and responsibilities. Legal counsel may be involved in negotiating these legally binding documents that specify roles and responsibilities. Clinical teachers are typically required to hold current, unencumbered professional nursing licenses for each state in which they instruct, unless the clinical agencies are located in states that have adopted the Nurse Licensure Compact (NLC). Over 40 states permit nurses to practice in NLC states as long as they live in an NLC state and meet the licensing requirements in their home state. Other states have pending nurse licensure compact legislation, which may facilitate teaching across state lines (National Council of State Boards of Nursing, 2025).

PREPARATION OF FACULTY MEMBERS

When selection of the clinical site or sites is complete, the nurse educator must prepare for the teaching and learning activities that will take place there. Areas of preparation that must be addressed include clinical competence, familiarity with the clinical environment, and orientation to the agency or setting.

Clinical Competence

Clinical competence has been documented as an essential characteristic of effective clinical teachers. Clinical competence includes theoretical knowledge, expert clinical skills, and judgment in the practice area in which teaching occurs. Students often identify the ability to demonstrate nursing care in the clinical setting as an essential skill of an effective clinical instructor (Gubrud-Howe, 2024).

Accreditation standards and state approval of nursing education programs may require nurse faculty members to have specific educational preparation or clinical experience in the clinical specialty area in which they are assigned to teach. This is particularly important for faculty members who will provide direct, on-site guidance in the clinical area. The combination of academic preparation and professional work experience supports the teacher's credibility and confidence.

Clinical teachers should maintain current clinical knowledge through ongoing participation in continuing education and practice experience. Nurse educators with a concurrent faculty practice or joint appointment in a clinical agency, or those working part time in a clinical role alongside their academic role, can maintain their clinical competence by this means, especially if they practice in the same specialty and clinical agency in which they teach. Faculty working with advanced practice students should also maintain clinical certification and ensure they have current practice experience in the specialty area.

Familiarity With the Clinical Environment

If the clinical teacher is entering a new clinical area, they may ask to work with the staff for a few days prior to returning to the site with students. This enables the teacher to practice using equipment and technology and to become familiar with the agency environment, policies, and procedures. If this is not possible, the teacher should at least observe activities in the clinical area to discern the characteristics and needs of the patient population, the usual schedule and pace of activities, the types of learning opportunities available, the diversity of healthcare professionals in the agency, and the presence of other learners.

As previously mentioned, a clinical agency may require faculty members whose students use the facility to attend an orientation program. Orientation sessions vary in length, from several hours to a day or more, and typically include introductions to administrators or managers; clarification of policies such as whether students may administer IV medications; review of documentation procedures; and safety procedures. Faculty members may be asked to demonstrate competent operation of equipment, such as infusion pumps, that their students will be using or to submit evidence that they have met the same competency standards that are required of nursing staff members. They may also need computer training so they can access EHRs.

Adjunct and Part-Time Teachers

As nursing programs face increasing enrollments, combined with faculty retirements, fiscal constraints, and changing program needs, adjunct or part-time teachers are often hired for clinical teaching responsibilities. Practicing nurses with their extensive clinical knowledge and expertise in the practice setting may fill these needed vacancies. Drawing upon their knowledge of the clinical setting, they can effectively help students learn nursing care practices; however, these skilled clinicians may lack the necessary educational preparation needed to successfully carry out the clinical teacher role (Ross et al., 2024). Specifically, these clinical teachers may need to understand student policies, curriculum, and evaluation practices that are necessary to help students make the connection between theory and practice and provide safe patient care. It is important that all clinical teachers, particularly those newly hired, be oriented to their role, responsibilities, and expectations. Providing opportunities for support, mentorship, and faculty development opportunities aimed at addressing clinical teaching and learning needs will enhance retention and success in the clinical teacher role.

PREPARATION OF CLINICAL AGENCY STAFF

Preparation of the clinical agency staff usually begins with the nursing education program's initial contact with the agency when negotiating an agreement or contract between the program and the agency. Establishing an effective working relationship with the nursing staff is an important responsibility for the clinical teacher. Ideally, nursing staff members would be eager to work with faculty members to help students meet their learning goals. Indeed, in academic health centers and other teaching institutions, participation in education of learners from many healthcare disciplines is a normal job expectation. Serving as a preceptor or working with students may be used for recertification or rewards through a clinical ladder program (Ulrich, 2024). Regardless of the reasons for working with students, some staff members will enjoy working with students more than others. Because teachers may not be able to choose which staff members will be involved with students, it is important for the teacher to communicate the following information to all staff members.

Clarification of Roles

Staff members often expect the instructor to be responsible for the care of patients with whom students are assigned to work. Many clinical teachers remark that if they have 10 students and each student is assigned two patients, the instructor is responsible for 30 individuals. These role expectations are both unrealistic and unfair to all parties involved.

Although the clinical teacher is ultimately responsible for student learning, students have much to gain from close working relationships with staff members. Staff members can serve as useful role models of nursing practice in the real world; students can observe how staff members must adapt their practice to fit the demands of a complex, ever-changing clinical environment. At the same time, staff members are often stimulated and motivated by students' questions and the current information that they can share. The presence of students in the clinical environment often reinforces staff members' competence and expertise, and many nurses enjoy sharing their knowledge and skill with novices. Students should be encouraged to use selected staff members as resources for their learning, especially when they have questions that relate to specific patients for whom the staff members are responsible.

An important point of role clarification is that the responsibility for patient care remains with the staff members of the clinical agency, as mentioned earlier. If a student is assigned learning activities related to the care of a specific patient, a staff member retains overall responsibility for that patient's care. Students are accountable for their own actions, but the primary nurse and student should collaborate to ensure that patient needs are met. Staff members may report patient status and needs to students assigned to work with those patients. Students should be encouraged to ask staff members questions about specific patient care requirements, share ideas about patient care, and report changes in patient condition, problems, tasks that they are unable to complete, or the need for assistance with tasks. These role expectation guidelines should be discussed with both staff members and managers, as well as with students. The guidelines may be written and posted or distributed to relevant personnel and students.

Level of Learners

Staff members can have reasonable expectations of learner performance if they are informed of the students' levels of education and experience. Beginning students will need more guidance; staff members working with these learners should expect frequent questions and requests for assistance. More experienced learners may need less assistance with tasks but more guidance on problem solving and clinical decision-making. Sharing this information with staff members allows them to plan their time accordingly and to anticipate student needs.

It is especially important for faculty members to clearly communicate to agency personnel which specific tasks or activities learners are permitted and not permitted to perform. This decision may be guided by educational program or agency policy, the curriculum sequence, or the specific focus of the learning activities on any given day. For example, during one scheduled clinical session, an instructor may want students to practice communication and active listening skills during health history data collection without relying on physical care tasks. The instructor should inform the staff of this goal and request that they allow students to engage in these activities, rather than focusing on physical care.

Learning Outcomes

The overall purpose and desired outcomes of the clinical learning activities should be communicated to staff members and students. As demonstrated in the previous example, knowledge of the specific objectives for a clinical session permits staff members to collaborate with the teacher and student in facilitating learning. If students have the specific learning objective of administering intramuscular injections, staff members can be asked to notify the teacher if any patient needs an injection that day so that the student can take advantage of that learning opportunity. Students should also remain alert for these learning opportunities.

Knowledge of the learning objectives allows staff members to suggest appropriate learning activities, even if the teacher is unable to anticipate the need. For example, an older adult patient who is confused may be admitted to the nursing unit; the staff nurse who is aware that students are focusing on nursing interventions to achieve patient safety might suggest that a student be assigned to work with this patient.

Need for Positive Role Modeling

The need for staff members to be positive role models for learners is a sensitive but important issue. Teachers often worry that students will learn bad practice habits from nurses who may take shortcuts when giving care. When discussing this issue with staff members, instructors should avoid implying that the only right way to perform skills is the teacher's way. Instead, the teacher might ask staff members to point out when they are omitting steps from procedures and to discuss with learners the rationale for those actions. In this way, staff nurses can model how to think like a nurse, a valuable learning opportunity for nursing students.

Asking staff nurses to be aware of the behaviors that they model for students and seeking their collaboration in fostering students' professional role development is an important aspect of preparing agency staff to work with learners. To accomplish this goal, instructors need to establish mutually respectful, trusting relationships with staff members and to sustain dialogue about role modeling.

The Role of Staff Members in Student Evaluation

Agency staff members have important roles in assessing and evaluating learner performance. The clinical performance of learners must be evaluated formatively and summatively. Formative evaluation takes the form of feedback to the student during the learning process; its purpose is to provide information to be used by the learner to improve performance. Summative evaluation occurs at the end of the learning process; its outcome is a judgment about the worth or value of the learning outcomes (Oermann et al., 2025). Summative evaluations usually result in final clinical evaluations and assignment of academic grades.

Teachers should carefully explain their expectations to both students and staff about the desired involvement of staff members in evaluating student performance. Agency personnel have an important role in formative evaluation by communicating feedback with teachers and learners about student performance. Because staff members are often in close contact with students during clinical activities, their observations of student performance are valuable, but the teacher should keep in mind that staff members may have different expectations for student performance than the instructor does. Staff members should be encouraged to report to the teacher any concerns that they may have about student performance as well as observations of exemplary performance; clinical instructors should accept this input and then validate the report by their own observations.

Staff members should also feel comfortable praising students, pointing out any errors, or offering suggestions for improvement. Immediate, descriptive feedback is necessary for learners to improve their performance and often staff members may be better able than teachers to provide this information to students. However, it is the teacher's responsibility to make summative evaluation decisions. Staff members should know that they are an important source of data regarding student performance and that their input is valued, but it is the clinical teacher who ultimately certifies competence or assigns a grade.

PREPARING THE LEARNERS

Students need cognitive, psychomotor, and affective preparation for clinical learning activities. It is the clinical teacher's responsibility to assist students with such preparation as well as to assess preparation adequacy before students enter the clinical area.

Cognitive Preparation

General prerequisite knowledge for clinical learning includes information about the learning outcomes; the clinical agency; and the roles of teacher, student, and staff member. Students may be expected to prepare ahead of time for each clinical learning session (Putnam & Knowlton, 2022). This preparation may include one or more of the following tasks: gathering information from patient records; interviewing patients and family members; assessing patient needs; reviewing relevant pathophysiology, nursing, nutrition, and pharmacology textbooks; and completing written assignments such as a patient assessment, plan of care, concept map, or instructor-designed preparation activity. In some programs, students complete these types of learning activities during and following their clinical learning activities.

Teachers should ensure that the expected cognitive preparations for clinical learning do not carry more importance than the clinical learning activities themselves; that is, learning should be expected to occur during the clinical learning activities as well as during preclinical preparation. If students receive their learning assignments in advance of the scheduled clinical activity, they can be expected to review relevant textbook information and to anticipate potential patient problems and needs. Some clinical teachers provide students with a list of frequently encountered patient diagnoses or commonly administered medications relevant to the clinical setting. Students may be expected to review these diagnoses, medications, and associated nursing care prior to the clinical experience. If circumstances permit a planning visit to the clinical site, the student may meet and interview the patient and review the patient's health record.

However, requiring extensive written assignments to be completed before the actual clinical activity implies that learning takes place only before the student enters the clinical area. Students cannot be expected to formulate a realistic plan of care before assessing the patient's physical, psychosocial, and cultural needs; this assessment may begin before the actual clinical activity, but it usually comprises a major part of the student's activity in the clinical setting. Thus, preclinical planning should focus on preparations for the learning that will take place in clinical practice. For example, the teacher may require students to review disease pathophysiology, formulate a tentative plan of care, and identify key focused assessments needed for the patient prior to the clinical day. A more extensive written assignment submitted after the clinical activity may require students to evaluate the appropriateness of the care provided and effectiveness of the nursing interventions.

Additionally, because students often copy information from textbooks or other sources to complete such requirements, written assignments submitted before the clinical learning activity may not show evidence of clinical reasoning and problem solving, let alone comprehension and retention of the information. For example, some teachers require students to prepare for medication administration during the clinical experience. Students often copy published pharmacologic information without attempting to retain this information and to think critically about why the medication was prescribed or how a particular patient might respond to it.

A better approach is to ask students to reflect on the pharmacologic actions of prescribed drugs and be prepared to discuss relevant nursing care implications, either individually with the instructor or in a group conference. If it is not possible for students to determine in advance which drugs are being used to treat patients in whose care they will be participating, the clinical instructor may ask students to study particular drug classifications and their prototype drugs and to be prepared to seek and use appropriate information resources when the student obtains the drug list. For example, if students are studying nursing care of patients who are at risk of a cerebral vascular accident, they should be familiar with several classifications of antihypertensive drugs and understand the common desired, side, and adverse effects. Students can then formulate a tentative plan of care for these patients and then modify and individualize the plan when they are able to assess specific patients.

Nursing students should learn to use a variety of reference materials both to prepare for clinical practice and as resources during clinical learning activities. Electronic mobile devices are popular resources that can be used to access reference materials and save time in the clinical setting. Students can use smartphones, tablets, computer applications, and ebooks to support clinical learning. Faculty members should consider the cost, connectivity issues, training needs, technological support, access, privacy and confidentiality concerns, available software, and student comfort if requiring these devices. Teachers may need to plan technology training sessions, collaborate with campus and clinical site technology support personnel, and develop policies and guidelines for appropriate use during clinical learning. Additional information about teaching with technology can be found in Chapter 9.

EXHIBIT 5.1 Sample Preclinical Conference Questioning

What are your priority nursing assessments?

What is your plan of care for the day? What nursing care will you provide first?

What lab or diagnostic tests were performed recently? What are the results? What are your nursing actions based upon these results?

What medications are prescribed for your patient that will need to be administered? Why is the patient taking each medication? What are the actions, side effects, and nursing implications of these medications?

Students should be expected to complete some cognitive preparation before clinical practice, but extensive, detailed written preparation assignments are unrealistic and often shift focus away from learning *during* clinical activities. Encouraging students' identification and use of appropriate, available information resources during clinical practice facilitates development of clinical reasoning and problem-solving abilities.

Meeting with students during a preclinical conference, either in a group or individually, also allows for assessment of student preparation as well as offers anticipatory guidance. Clinical teachers can use questioning techniques to determine if students have adequate knowledge to care for patients. It also provides an opportunity for clarification about anticipated nursing care and allows for correction of students' misconceptions before patient care is provided. Clinical teachers can assess student preparation and feel assured that students have an appropriate plan for care. **Exhibit 5.1** provides sample questions that clinical teachers might use for preclinical conferences with students.

Psychomotor Preparation

Skill learning is an important outcome of clinical teaching. As students develop into competent care providers, they need to have adequate time to learn psychomotor skills in a practice setting and be given appropriate and informative feedback to enhance performance. When learning complex skills, it is more efficient for students to practice in an environment such as a simulation center or skills laboratory, free from the demands of the actual practice setting. In such a setting, students can investigate and discover alternative ways of performing skills, and they can make errors and learn to correct them without fear of harming patients. Technology, such as virtual or augmented reality, may also enhance student skill development, performance, and clinical judgment development (Reaves et al., 2024).

Additionally, some nurse educators are using creative teaching and learning approaches for psychomotor skill teaching and include strategies such as flipped classrooms, blended learning, peer assisted learning, videotaping skill performance, and the use of standardized patients for skill learning and practice. Regardless of the method used to teach students psychomotor skills, students should have ample supported skill practice time before they enter the clinical area so that they are not expected to perform a skill for the first time in a fast-paced, demanding environment. Educators should allow for deliberate practice involving the use of focused activities followed by frequent practice sessions and immediate expert feedback so that the skills are practiced correctly and retained (Aldridge, 2024).

It is the clinical teacher's responsibility to ensure that students have developed the desired level of skill competence before entering the clinical setting. The use of clinical simulation and technology in a nursing skills lab provides students with realistic learning opportunities to develop psychomotor skills in a controlled environment. Use of clinical simulation activities allows students to practice and refine psychomotor skills and incorporates cognitive and affective learning as well. **Exhibit 5.2** provides additional suggestions for teachers to use for psychomotor skill teaching and learning. Chapter 8 presents a comprehensive discussion of the use of clinical simulation.

EXHIBIT 5.2 Strategies for Enhancing Psychomotor Skill Learning

Focus on commonly used psychomotor skills.
Use technology and a variety of teaching–learning methods (visual, auditory, tactile).
Include demonstration and succinct explanations when teaching skills.
Offer a realistic environment for skill learning.
Physically guide students during early psychomotor skill learning.
Allow students opportunities to test different ways of performing skills but ensure critical elements of the psychomotor skills are performed correctly.
Provide focused practice opportunities over time, not just a single practice session.
Cluster steps of a psychomotor skill to facilitate memory.
Practice psychomotor skills to become proficient, coordinated, and efficient.
Intersperse psychomotor skill practice with other learning activities.
Design learning activities that allow students to observe skill performance of others.
Alternate psychomotor skill practice and observation of others' skills practice.
Use simulation for psychomotor skill practice and follow this with debriefing.
Provide prompt, explicit, descriptive, specific feedback focused on the behavior/performance.
Offer coaching about psychomotor skill performance.
Incorporate prompts or cues to allow students to solve problems during psychomotor skill learning.
Provide formative feedback to correct psychomotor performance errors.
Use summative evaluation to verify skill learning.
Incorporate practice to refresh performance if a psychomotor skill is not used frequently.

Source: Adapted from Aldridge, M. D., & Hummel, F. (2019). Nursing students' perceptions of skills learning: A phenomenological study. *Nurse Educator, 44*(3), 170–174. https://doi.org/10.1097/NNE.0000000000000569; Gromer, A. L., Patel, S. E., & Chestnut, S. R. (2024). Strategies for teaching psychomotor skills to undergraduate nursing students: A scoping review. *Teaching and Learning in Nursing,* 20(1), e98–e105. https://doi.org/10.1016/j.teln.2024.08.013

Affective Preparation

Affective preparation of students includes strategies for managing their anxiety and for fostering confidence and positive attitudes about learning. Most students have some anxiety about clinical learning activities. Students report that their initial clinical experience was associated with fear, anxiety, uncertainty, and concern about being a burden (Marriott et al., 2024). The teacher plays a critical role in mediating anxiety and stress and may employ strategies to identify students' fears and reduce their anxiety to a manageable level. A preclinical conference session might assess learners' specific concerns and assure students of the teacher's confidence in them, desire for their success, and availability for consultation and guidance during the clinical activities. For example, during a preclinical conference on the first day of clinical practice in a course, the instructor may state that it is common for students to feel anxious before a clinical activity, but that anxiety usually decreases during the experience. The teacher may encourage students to identify and name the specific source and nature of their anxieties; once these are identified, the teacher can help students to use a problem-solving approach to identify helpful responses. For instance, if students express concern that something may happen that they will not know how to manage, the teacher may help students to list all the potential adverse events and then brainstorm possible responses to them. Throughout such a discussion, teachers should reassure students of their availability to answer questions and assist them with clinical reasoning and problem solving during the clinical learning activities.

Because students may express concerns about communicating with other healthcare staff, providing role–playing activities that allow student rehearsal of common activities such as reporting off to staff may be helpful in ameliorating the anxiety. Or faculty may develop structured communication tools that students can use to facilitate clear communication about patient care (Neal, 2024). Other strategies, such as orientation, can be used to ensure students are adequately prepared.

Orientation to the Clinical Agency

Like clinical teachers, students also need a thorough orientation to the clinical agency in which learning activities will take place. This orientation may take place before or on the first day of clinical activities. Staff members often assist the teacher in orienting students to the agency and helping them to feel welcome and comfortable in the new environment. **Exhibit 5.3** provides suggested orientation topics.

In addition, students need to have the telephone number of the clinical setting to contact in case of personal emergency. They should also be told what procedures to follow in case of illness or other reasons for absence on a clinical day, understand the uniform or dress requirements, and know what equipment to bring (e.g., stethoscope) and what to leave at home (e.g., personal valuables).

Given the growth of informatics in healthcare settings, faculty must consider technology needs for student orientation. Students will require access codes for the technology used at the clinical site, as well as training for computer use such as bar-coded bedside medication systems and EHRs before they can fully deliver care. Preparing students for use of the EHR may require a special training session for students. Staff development practitioners or information technology staff may need to schedule designated EHR training and arrange access for students. Clinical teachers need to coordinate this technology training with nurse educators and healthcare information technology personnel. Clinical teachers also need to ensure that they are up to date on this training so that they are prepared to guide student learning in the clinical setting. However, some clinical agencies are restricting student access to the EHR by allowing read-only access, limited documentation, and restricted diagnostic results, creating variability in skill development for these students. Educators are encouraged to dialogue with clinical agencies to ensure appropriate access and training. If unsuccessful, they may want to adopt an academic EHR system that students can use and practice in a simulated laboratory setting (Kan & Stabler-Haas, 2025).

Not all of this orientation information needs to be presented on site; some clinical teachers have developed electronic resources that provide a virtual tour of the facility. The nursing program may use bar code scanning equipment in clinical practice labs to simulate medication administration. Learners can be expected to review these resources before coming to the clinical site. Self-directed electronic learning modules and learning management systems can be used to orient and prepare students for the clinical experience ensuring an efficient, flexible, and cost-effective delivery method for training. Mandatory education required by healthcare facilities, such as fire safety, Health Insurance Portability and Accountability Act (HIPAA) training, infection control, or other topics can be delivered electronically. Clinical teachers and students can review the training needed and complete appropriate evaluation materials. Spreadsheets or online tracking within a learning management system can efficiently monitor compliance and completion of learning. Electronic delivery of clinical information can also be used throughout the year to share ongoing updates with clinical teachers and students in an efficient manner.

EXHIBIT 5.3 Orientation Topics

- The geographical location of the agency
- The physical setup of the specific unit where students will be placed
- Names, titles, and roles of personnel
- Location of areas such as restrooms, dining facilities, conference rooms, and locker rooms
- Information about transportation and parking
- Agency and unit policies
- Daily schedules and routines
- Emergency protocols (e.g., fire drills, rapid response codes, cardiac arrest procedures, and equipment)
- Review of relevant standards of practice
- Reminders about confidentiality and privacy of information
- Patient information documentation systems, including establishment of passwords and acquiring computer access to electronic health records (EHRs) and bedside medication administration systems

Student Preparation

When students have clinical learning activities in unfamiliar sites or where the learning opportunities are not immediately clear to them, students may feel confused, insecure, isolated, and unprepared for the experience. Provision of specific objectives, learning activities, preparation expectations, activity guides, and written expectations will greatly facilitate learning and make the expectations clear. This is especially true if the faculty member will not always be present at the site. **Exhibit 5.4** is an example of specific preparation, objectives, activities, and written expectations for a community-based experience. Orientation for the clinical experience is based on agency, site, and student needs. Regardless of the clinical setting, an overall orientation to the course expectations with a review of frequently used skills can be helpful. A discussion about preconceptions and expectations will provide students with essential preparation that will enable them to feel confident and prepared for the experience.

Student safety during the clinical learning experience will also need to be addressed. This is an issue in all clinical activities, but it is especially important in situations where students may be in an unfamiliar area, making home visits, or going alone or in small groups to clinical sites at various times during the day or evening. Teachers must provide explicit guidelines for student safety during learning activities and document them in the course syllabus. Safety guidelines should address proper methods of communication with faculty, agency, and patients. Students should have the following information prior to the start of the clinical experience: clinical teacher and emergency contact information, clear travel directions, a reliable vehicle with adequate fuel, availability of a charged cell phone, and guidelines for appropriate dress and behavior while in a patient's home or at an agency or facility without an instructor present. The students must also be prepared for appropriate actions they may need to take if they find themselves in a dangerous situation, be it at an agency, out in the community, or at a patient's home. The faculty member should provide education for how students can prevent and avoid situations that involve harassment or potential violence. It is important to promote a culture of safety and teach students what to do if they experience an adverse event during the clinical time.

For clinical learning occurring outside of the hospital, regular brief visits by the clinical teacher to the clinical site will help prevent problems and address issues that may arise from staff and students during the experience. Individual and group conferences with students will allow for sharing of experiences and provide additional time to assess learning and growth.

EXHIBIT 5.4 Example of Instructions to Students for Community Clinical Sites

Preparation for All Community Clinical Learning Activities

Review objectives and activities listed for each assignment and complete the assigned reading before arriving at the site.

Review key facts or existing guides (e.g., immunization schedules or classification of hypertension in adults) appropriate for the clinical area.

Be at the site at the time indicated by your instructor.

Wear your clean uniform (including identification) and follow the dress code. Dress appropriately for the weather.

Bring a pen, watch with a second hand, stethoscope, notebook, electronic references, and pocket reference books, as appropriate, for the clinical learning activity.

Check on transportation and directions to the site.

Have contact information for your instructor (cell phone number, etc.) with you.

Share your schedule (where and when you are going) with a class member.

Have the phone number and name of the site contact person.

Specific Preparation Before the Clinical Learning Activity Starts

Read assigned chapters in the course text.

Complete and submit the clinical preparation worksheet to your instructor.

Review information about common diagnoses or medications used in the clinical area.

General Clinical Activity Guidelines

Work with the staff for an optimal learning experience.

Your instructor will visit the site each day and be available by cell phone or text messaging.

You should complete assessments, documentation, and teaching as described in the syllabus.

You may only administer medications under the direct observation of the RN identified by your instructor.

Review any unfamiliar medical diagnoses, medications, and care needed for patients you are seeing.

Ask for help if something is unclear.

Clinical Activities

During this clinical learning activity, students will work with staff members to:

Follow the agency policy for client care, including completion of initial assessments.

Review patients' health records for history, diagnoses, medications, and lab test results.

Implement health teaching after review by the instructor.

Complete the required clinical report and course assignments.

The First Day

Students almost always perceive the first day of clinical learning activities in a new setting as stressful; this is especially true of learners in their initial clinical nursing course. Students' first exposure to the clinical environment can either promote their independence as learners or foster dependence on the instructor due to fear. Clinical teachers should plan specific activities for the first day that will allow learners to become familiar with and comfortable in the clinical environment and at the same time alleviate their anxiety. These activities may include tours, conferences, games, and special assignments. Another creative option involves having experienced nursing students serve as peer mentors for beginning nursing students. The experienced students may help enhance student confidence and reduce situation-specific anxiety felt by beginning students during their first clinical experience (Cupelli & Colalillo, 2025). Another option involves partnering new students for a shared dyad clinical assignment, thereby providing peer support, alleviating anxiety, and enhancing client interactions, collaboration, and skill development (Simmonds et al., 2020).

Even if learners have attended an agency orientation, it is helpful to take them on a tour of the specific areas they will use for learning activities, pointing out locations such as restrooms, drinking fountains, fire alarms and extinguishers, emergency equipment, elevators, stairwells, and emergency exits. The instructor should introduce learners to staff members by name and title. If students need agency-specific identification badges, parking permits, or passwords for use of the computer system, the teacher may make the necessary arrangements ahead of time or accompany students to the appropriate locations where these items can be acquired. If an empty patient room is available, the instructor may demonstrate the use of equipment such as bed controls, call bells, oxygen delivery systems, and lighting controls.

Special assignments may include review and discussion of patient records, practice of computer documentation, and a scavenger hunt to help learners locate typical items needed for patient care. **Exhibit 5.5** is an example of a scavenger hunt activity used in orienting students to a medical–surgical unit of a hospital. Learners may be asked to observe patient care for a specified time, interview a patient or family member, shadow a nurse, or complete a short written assignment focused on documenting an observation.

These activities may be followed by a short group conference, during which students are encouraged to discuss their impressions, experiences, and feelings. The teacher should review the roles of students, teachers, and staff members, emphasizing the importance of clear lines of communication. For example, students need to know who to ask for help and under what circumstances—that is, when to ask staff members questions and when to seek assistance from the teacher. Handouts summarizing these expectations and requirements are useful because students can review them later when their anxiety is lower. If a dining facility is available in the clinical setting, pre- or postclinical conferences may take place in that location to allow students to relax with refreshments away from patient care areas. The conference may conclude by making plans for the next day of clinical practice, including selecting assignments and discussing how learners should prepare for their learning activities.

EXHIBIT 5.5 A Scavenger Hunt Activity

Anywhere General Hospital, Unit 2C

Work in pairs to search for the location of the items or areas listed in the following. Check them off as you find them.

Locker room
Restrooms
Oxygen tank
Fire alarms
Fire extinguishers
Emergency exits
Patient teaching materials
Nurse manager's office
Medication dispensing systems
Linen carts
Kitchen
Utility room
Biohazardous waste containers
Waterless hand sanitizer dispensers
Reference materials
Conference room
Medical supply carts (IV bags, dressing change materials, gloves)
Computer workstations
Pulse oximeter
Wheelchairs
Personal protective equipment

SUMMARY

This chapter described the roles and responsibilities of faculty, staff members, and others involved in preparing for clinical learning and suggested strategies for preparing students and staff members. The teacher and learners comprise a temporary system within the permanent culture of the clinical setting. Negative consequences of this relationship can be avoided by establishing and maintaining regular communication between the instructor and staff members. Clinical teachers function as culture brokers and border spanners to help integrate students more fully into the real world of nursing practice.

Settings for clinical learning should be selected carefully, based on important criteria such as compatibility of school and agency philosophy, licensure and accreditation, availability of opportunities to meet learning objectives, geographic location, availability of positive role models, and physical resources. Selection of appropriate clinical settings may be complicated by competition among several nursing programs for a limited number of agencies. Specific criteria for assessing the suitability of potential clinical settings were discussed.

When clinical sites have been selected, educators must prepare for teaching and learning activities.

Areas of preparation include clinical competence, familiarity with the clinical environment, and orientation to the agency. Clinical competence has been documented as an essential characteristic of effective clinical teachers and includes knowledge and expert skill and judgment in the clinical practice area in which teaching occurs. Teachers may maintain clinical competence through faculty practice, joint appointment in clinical agencies, part-time clinical employment, and continuing nursing education activities. The teacher may become familiar with a new clinical setting by observing the staff for a few days prior to returning to the site with students. The clinical agency may require faculty members to attend an orientation program that includes introductions to agency staff, clarification of policies concerning student activities, and review of skills and procedures. Adjunct and part-time clinical teachers need to ensure they are familiar with the curriculum, course, policies, and procedures.

Preparation of the clinical agency staff usually begins with the teacher's initial contact with the agency. Roles of teachers, students, and staff members should be clarified so that staff members have guidelines for their participation in the instruction of learners. An important point of role clarification is that, although students are accountable for their own actions, the responsibility for patient care remains with staff members of the clinical agency. Staff members also need to be aware of specific learning objectives, the level of the learner, the need for positive role modeling, and expectations concerning their role in evaluating student performance. Although staff members' feedback is valuable in formative evaluation, the teacher is always responsible for summative evaluation of learner performance.

Students need cognitive, psychomotor, and affective preparation for clinical learning activities. Cognitive preparation includes information about the learning objectives; the clinical agency; and the roles of teacher, student, and staff member. Students may be expected to prepare for each clinical learning session through readings, interviewing patients, and completing written assignments. However, requirements for extensive written assignments to be completed before the actual clinical activity may imply that learning takes place only before the student enters the clinical area.

The instructor has a responsibility to assess that students have the desired level of skill development before entering the clinical setting. When learning complex skills, it is more efficient for students to practice the parts first in a simulated setting, such as a skills laboratory, free from the demands of the actual practice setting. Students should have ample skill practice time before they enter the clinical area so that they are not expected to perform a skill for the first time in a fast-paced, demanding environment.

Affective preparation of students includes strategies for managing their anxiety and for fostering confidence and positive attitudes about learning. Most students have some anxiety about clinical learning activities. Mild or moderate anxiety often serves to motivate students to learn, but excessive anxiety hinders concentration and interferes with learning. In preparation for clinical learning activities, teachers may employ strategies such as a structured preclinical conference to identify students' fears and reduce their anxiety to a manageable level.

Students also need a thorough orientation to the clinical agency in which learning activities will take place. This orientation should include information about the location and physical setup of the agency, relevant agency personnel, agency policies such as infection control measures, daily schedules and routines, and procedures for responding to emergencies and for documenting patient information.

Students almost always perceive the first day of clinical learning activities in a new setting as stressful. Clinical teachers should plan specific activities for the first day that will allow learners to become familiar with and comfortable in the clinical environment and at the same time alleviate their anxiety. These activities include tours, conferences, games, and special assignments.

CNE®cl EXAMINATION TEST BLUEPRINT CORE COMPETENCIES

1. Function within the Education and Health Care Environments

A. Function in the Clinical Nurse Educator Role

1. Integrate theory and practice in the clinical setting
2. Foster professional growth of learners (e.g., coaching, reflection, and debriefing)
4. Act as a role model of professional nursing within the clinical learning environment

B. Operationalize the Curriculum

1. Assess the congruence of the clinical environment with curriculum, course outcomes, and learner needs when evaluating clinical sites
2. Identify learner goals and outcomes
3. Facilitate meaningful and relevant clinical learning activities to promote optimal learning
4. Prepare learners for clinical experiences (e.g., facility, clinical expectations, equipment, and technology-based resources)
6. Provide opportunities for learners to develop clinical judgment related to course outcomes

C. Abide by Legal Requirements, Ethical Guidelines, Agency Policies, and Guiding Framework

1. Apply ethical and legal principles to create a safe clinical learning environment (e.g., privacy laws, confidentiality, error/near-miss situation reporting, remediation, negligence, liability, scope/standards of practice)
2. Assess learner readiness prior to clinical learning experiences
4. Inform others of program and clinical agency policies, procedures, and practices
5. Adhere to program and clinical agency policies, procedures and practices when implementing clinical experiences (e.g., due process, accommodations, academic integrity)
6. Comply with current program and clinical agency policies, procedures, and practices related to personal protective equipment and other infection control measures for self and learners

2. Facilitate Learning in the Healthcare Environment

A. Implement a variety of clinical teaching strategies congruent with learner needs, desired learning outcomes, course outcomes, setting, and context (e.g., virtual, telehealth, in-person, simulation)
C. Use academic and client-care technology to support the teaching-learning process
D. Create opportunities for learners to develop clinical judgment
G. Develop collegial working relationships with learners, faculty colleagues, and clinical environment personnel

3. Demonstrate Effective Interpersonal Communication and Collaborative Interprofessional Relationships

A. Model collaboration within the healthcare environment
B. Foster the development of a collegial learning community
C. Facilitate opportunities to collaborate within the healthcare team
E. Demonstrate respect for learners, healthcare team, colleagues, clients, families, and others
F. Use clear and effective communication in all interactions (e.g., written, electronic, verbal, non-verbal, virtual)
G. Respond to learner concerns, needs, or questions in a supportive manner
J. Function as an accessible resource to learners and the healthcare team in the clinical learning environment
L. Communicate performance expectations to learners and clinical staff

5. Facilitate Learner Development and Socialization

A. Mentor learners in professional nursing
F. Create learning environments that promote socialization to the role of the nurse

6. Implement Effective Clinical and Assessment Evaluation Strategies

B. Conduct formative and summative evaluation specific to the learner and learning outcomes
E. Provide timely, specific, objective, and constructive feedback to learners
F. Use situational assessment data to facilitate learning in the clinical environment
G. Document learner clinical performance, feedback, and progression
H. Evaluate the quality of the clinical learning experiences and environment

LEARNING ACTIVITIES

CourseConnect

To access self-assessment questions and interactive, competency-based learning activities for this chapter, visit www.springerpub.com/courseconnect. See inside front cover and tear-out card for CourseConnect details.

REFERENCES

Aldridge, M. D. (2024). Is deliberate practice a feasible method for reinforcing indwelling urinary catheterization skill: A pilot study. *Teaching and Learning in Nursing, 19*(4), 342–346. https://doi.org/10.1016/j.teln.2024.05.011

Aldridge, M. D., & Hummel, F. (2019). Nursing students' perceptions of skills learning: A phenomenological study. *Nurse Educator, 44*(3), 170–174. https://doi.org/10.1097/NNE.0000000000000569

Anyango, E., Ngune, I., Brown, J., & Adama, E. (2024). "I changed my mind after my placement": The influence of clinical placement environment on career choices of final-year pre-registration nurses. *Collegian, 31*(2), 69–76. http://doi.org/10.1016/j.colegn.2023.11.004

Cupelli, L. M., & Colalillo, G. C. (2025). Implementing peer learning to enhance academic performance in first-year nursing students. *Teaching and Learning in Nursing, 20*(1), e150–e158. https://doi.org/10.1016/j.teln.2024.09.008

Gromer, A. L., Patel, S. E., & Chestnut, S. R. (2024). Strategies for teaching psychomotor skills to undergraduate nursing students: A scoping review. *Teaching and Learning in Nursing, 20*(1), e98–e105. https://doi.org/10.1016/j.teln.2024.08.013

Gubrud-Howe, P. (2024). Teaching in the clinical learning environment. In D. M. Billings & J. A. Halstead (Eds.), *Teaching in nursing: A guide for faculty* (7th ed., pp. 387–421). Elsevier.

Kan, E. Z., & Stabler-Haas, S. (2025). *Fast facts for the clinical nursing instructor* (4th ed.). Springer Publishing Company.

Marriott, P. H., Weller-Newton, J. M., & Reid, K. J. (2024). Preparedness for a first clinical placement in nursing:

A descriptive qualitative study. *BMC Nursing, 23*(1), 345. https://doi.org/10.1186/s12912-024-01916-x

National Council of State Boards of Nursing. (2025). *Nurse licensure compact*. https://nursecompact.com/index.page#map

Neal, A. R. (2024), Optimizing clinical and work environments through structured communication. *Journal of Nursing Education, 63*(2), 134. https://doi.org/10.3928/01484834-20231205-08

Oermann, M. H., Gaberson, K. B., & De Gagne, J. C. (2025). *Evaluation and testing in nursing education* (7th ed.). Springer Publishing Company.

Putnam, A., & Knowlton, M. C. (2022). Undergraduate supervised clinical practicum activities: An enlightening exploration. *Journal of Nursing Education, 61*(10), 591–593. https://doi.org/10.3928/01484834-20220803-04

Reaves, C., Martel, M., & Rose, K. (2024). Teaching psychomotor skills in undergraduate nursing education: An integrative review. *Journal of Nursing Education, 63*(7), 421–426. https://doi.org/10.3928/01484834-20240505-01

Ross, J. G., Dunker, K. S., Morrell, M., Duprey, M., Parson, T., & Kim, L. (2024). Clinical faculty orientation practices in the United States: A descriptive study. *Nurse Educator, 49*(5), 278–283. https://doi.org/10.1097/NNE.0000000000001625

Simmonds, A., Nunn, A., Gray, M., Hardie, C., Mayo, S., Peter, E., & Richards, J. (2020). Pedagogical practices that influence professional identity formation in baccalaureate nursing education: A scoping review. *Nurse Education Today, 93*, 104516. https://doi.org/10.1016/j.nedt.2020.104516

Ulrich, B. (2024). *Mastering precepting: A nurse's handbook for success* (3rd ed.). Sigma Theta Tau.

Ethical and Legal Issues in Clinical Teaching

6

OBJECTIVES:

1. Analyze how moral reasoning and accountability shape the ethical landscape of clinical teaching.
2. Examine practical guidance for faculty on reinforcing ethical standards and legal awareness in clinical settings, with consideration of how equity and inclusivity influence ethical decision-making and responsibilities.

Clinical teaching and learning occur within a dynamic and multifaceted environment in which interactions among educators, students, staff, and patients frequently present complex ethical and legal challenges. These challenges demand decisions that are not only clinically sound but also ethically and legally informed. Professional values, accountability, and evolving societal expectations further complicate these dilemmas, requiring thoughtful and deliberate navigation.

As nursing education adapts to the digital age, the proliferation of social media and digital communication tools adds new layers of complexity. Although these technologies enhance connectivity and learning opportunities, they also raise significant concerns about privacy, professionalism, and boundary maintenance. Addressing these challenges requires a deep understanding of ethical principles and adherence to professional standards in both online and in-person interactions. Simultaneously, the principles of equity and inclusivity have become indispensable components of ethical and effective education. These principles not only foster environments that support sound decision-making and respect for diverse perspectives, but also enhance the overall quality and outcomes of nursing education. This chapter examines the ethical and legal dimensions of clinical teaching, emphasizing the interconnected roles of moral reasoning, accountability, and inclusivity in addressing dilemmas. It explores the influence of digital professionalism in contemporary nursing education and provides practical guidance for faculty on reinforcing ethical standards and legal awareness. By equipping educators and students with the tools to navigate such complexities thoughtfully, this chapter aims to cultivate a culture of integrity, respect, and ethical excellence in clinical education.

ETHICAL BEHAVIOR IN CLINICAL SETTINGS

Ethical conduct is the foundation of clinical teaching because it shapes the interactions among educators, students, staff, and patients. Conflicts can arise when academic policies and ethical standards diverge, disrupting these relationships—particularly when stakeholders' interests are at odds (Smith Glasgow et al., 2020). Navigating such challenges requires healthcare professionals to recognize and thoughtfully resolve ethical dilemmas by grounding their decisions in established ethical principles. Leaders in nursing education play a crucial role in cultivating a moral mindset, which is essential for delivering high-quality patient care and fostering reflective learning environments.

Educational institutions are tasked with creating cultures rooted in civility, responsibility, safety, and ethical practice. These values underpin both academic integrity and patient care. Nursing faculty hold a shared responsibility to uphold the health, safety, and dignity of patients, which includes addressing bias, respecting autonomy, safeguarding confidentiality, and maintaining professional boundaries (American Nurses Association [ANA], 2025). Such responsibilities demand that healthcare professionals prioritize patient needs, engage in ongoing personal and professional growth, and embody ethical integrity. In increasingly complex clinical teaching environments, moral reasoning and accountability serve as guiding principles that enable educators and students to navigate ethical dilemmas and professional challenges. Together, these principles establish a foundation for fostering integrity, respect, and thoughtful decision-making in nursing education and practice.

Moral Reasoning and Accountability in Clinical Teaching

Moral reasoning is central to ethical decision-making in clinical education, guiding both nursing faculty and students as they navigate complex care scenarios and academic responsibilities (Nunthawong & Ketkomg, 2024). Grounded in ethical theory and professional standards, moral reasoning enables educators to critically evaluate their actions to prioritize patient welfare, student development, and institutional integrity (Masudi, 2024). Beyond compliance with professional standards, moral reasoning fosters a reflective environment in which principles such as beneficence, nonmaleficence, autonomy, and justice are actively examined and integrated into practice (ANA, 2025).

Evidence highlights the value of exposing nursing students to ethical dilemmas through applied learning models, such as simulation-based problem-solving exercises. These strategies enhance moral sensitivity, critical thinking, and the ability to apply ethical frameworks in real-world scenarios, bridging the gap between theory and practice (Qu et al., 2024). Structured discussions and case studies incorporated into curricula further cultivate reflective decision-making and help establish ethical clinical learning environments (Hansen et al., 2024; Tierney et al., 2023). Educators play a pivotal role in fostering these environments by facilitating open discussions that emphasize core values, ethical principles, and behaviors that prioritize patient safety, dignity, and respect.

Accountability complements moral reasoning by upholding ethical standards through transparency and responsible conduct. Educators model ethical behavior, maintain instructional excellence, and foster a culture of continuous improvement among students (Hussein & Hashish, 2023). Accountability extends to guiding students in evidence-based practices, ensuring accurate documentation, promoting clear communication, and safeguarding confidentiality and professional boundaries. At the institutional level, mechanisms such as performance evaluations, adherence to professional codes, and structured feedback loops establish a foundation for ethical vigilance. Policies and procedures informed by the ANA's *Code of Ethics* and other regulatory frameworks reinforce consistent ethical behavior, while case studies and simulations prepare students to navigate the complexities of professional practice (Tierney et al., 2023). Nursing faculty serve as critical role models, demonstrating precision in documentation, compliance with privacy regulations, and the application of best practices in clinical settings.

The synergy between moral reasoning and accountability is transformative, shaping an ethical and professional culture within clinical teaching. Educators who model ethical decision-making inspire students to thoughtfully navigate dilemmas, thus fostering their integrity, compassion, and commitment to ethical practice. Concurrently, accountability frameworks translate ethical principles into actionable practices, enhancing patient safety, strengthening professional relationships, and cultivating moral courage among students (Hussein & Hashish, 2023). This iterative process of developing ethical competence is driven by continuous reflection and learning (Hansen et al., 2024; Nunthawong & Ketkomg, 2024). By embedding moral reasoning and accountability into educational practices, nursing programs prepare graduates who are not only clinically proficient but also ethically grounded and accountable to their profession and communities (Hansen et al., 2024; Hussein & Hashish, 2023). Together, these principles form the cornerstone of ethical nursing education, empowering educators and students to navigate the complexities of clinical environments with integrity, professionalism, and responsibility.

Ethical and Legal Considerations in Digital Communications

The increasing integration of digital communication tools into clinical education presents complex ethical and legal challenges. These tools are indispensable for modern communication and collaboration, but they introduce significant concerns regarding privacy, professionalism, and boundary maintenance. To mitigate potential repercussions, meticulous adherence to ethical and legal standards is essential.

Social media platforms such as Facebook, Instagram, TikTok, Snapchat, X (formerly Twitter), and YouTube provide nursing students with unprecedented opportunities for connectivity. However, these platforms blur the boundaries between personal and professional identities, particularly for "digital natives" from younger generations (Gum et al., 2024). Students may struggle to fully understand their responsibilities on these platforms, which can place them at risk for committing ethical and legal violations (Daigle, 2020; De Gagne et al., 2018). Violations often arise from unintentional oversharing or inappropriate interactions. For example, seemingly innocuous posts may inadvertently disclose identifiable patient information, breaching the Health Insurance Portability and Accountability Act (HIPAA). Such violations compromise patient confidentiality, jeopardize institutional reputations, and expose students and programs to significant legal and professional risks.

The ANA's *Code of Ethics* underscores the importance of maintaining professional boundaries and adhering to ethical guidelines to uphold trust in the nursing profession (ANA, 2025; De Gagne et al., 2018). Misuse of social media can result in disciplinary actions, including dismissal or course failure, and may lead clinical agencies to sever partnerships with offending programs. Additionally, healthcare facilities face reputational damage and legal liability, while patients retain the right to pursue legal recourse for privacy violations. These risks highlight the urgency of integrating comprehensive training on digital professionalism into nursing education curricula (Daigle, 2020; Gum et al., 2024).

Nursing education programs play a pivotal role in promoting ethical digital conduct through robust institutional policies and educational initiatives. Policies should align with established guidelines, such as the ANA's *Principles for Social Networking and the Nurse* (2011) and the National Council of State Boards of Nursing's (NCSBN's) *A Nurse's Guide to the Use of Social Media* (2018), and outline clear expectations and consequences for violations. Students may be required to sign agreements affirming their understanding of these policies and their commitment to compliance (Daigle, 2020; De Gagne et al., 2018).

Educators are instrumental in fostering digital professionalism. Regular discussions, case studies, and simulations help students distinguish between personal and professional online behaviors and understand the potential ramifications of ethical lapses. Key principles to emphasize include

- *Adherence to Conduct Standards:* Nursing students must uphold the same ethical and legal standards as licensed professionals in all clinical settings.
- *Patient Privacy:* Confidential information must remain protected, and patient details should never be shared outside authorized contexts.
- *Maintaining Boundaries:* Online interactions with current or former patients should be avoided to prevent conflicts of interest.
- *Awareness of Visibility:* Digital content may be recoverable and accessible to a broad audience, even after deletion.
- *Separation of Personal and Professional Personas:* Students should carefully curate their online presence, recognizing that privacy settings are not infallible.
- *Responding to Questionable Content:* Inappropriate peer behavior should be addressed privately and escalated if necessary to protect patient interests.
- *Policy Development:* Students should contribute to institutional policies to ensure that they remain relevant and effective.
- *Respect for Colleagues and Employers:* Public discussions that could damage professional relationships or patient care should be avoided (ANA, 2011; De Gagne et al., 2018; NCSBN, 2018).

The concept of digital professionalism, as articulated by Gum et al. (2024), encompasses the competencies required to navigate digital platforms responsibly. It involves balancing technical proficiency, respect for privacy, and adherence to ethical boundaries. These principles enable nursing students and professionals to engage confidently in digital communications while safeguarding their professional integrity and prioritizing patient safety. Cultivating ethical and legal competence in digital communication is integral to preparing nursing students for contemporary practice. By addressing these challenges through education, clear policies, and role modeling, nursing programs empower students to effectively leverage digital tools while upholding the profession's ethical and legal standards. In doing so, they ensure that graduates are well-prepared to navigate the complexities of modern healthcare environments with professionalism, accountability, and respect.

Learners in a Service Setting

Clinical education is founded on the principle that learning occurs most effectively in real-world environments, where direct patient care experiences deepen understanding and develop practical skills. Traditionally, nursing students have been placed in healthcare settings such as acute care hospitals and long-term care facilities. However, the increasing emphasis on cost-effective healthcare and preventive care has expanded clinical learning opportunities to include homes, schools, and community-based environments. In these settings, patients seek care, staff focus on delivering optimal healthcare services, and students are present to learn. Balancing these intersecting purposes often presents ethical and practical challenges. Although learners are supervised by clinical instructors, their developing skills may lead to care that is less efficient or effective compared to that provided by experienced practitioners. Patients, however, expect high-quality, efficient care, and this expectation may conflict with the primary educational goal of student learning (Hussein & Hashish, 2023). This tension raises critical ethical questions, particularly in relation to the principle of beneficence, which emphasizes the duty to help and avoid harm (ANA, 2025).

Patients may experience apprehension about their care being used for educational purposes, citing concerns over privacy and quality of care. At the same time, healthcare staff are often tasked with guiding and supervising students, which can shift their attention away from direct patient care and increase their workload, leading to additional stress. These dynamics underscore the need for ethical and transparent practices when integrating learners into service settings. To address these challenges, clinical educators must take proactive steps to align learning activities with the rights and needs of patients, staff, and students. Clear communication of learning objectives and roles is essential to minimize misunderstandings and conflicts. Patients must be fully informed about the presence of learners and provide consent before participating in teaching activities. Additionally, educators must ensure that students are adequately prepared for their clinical roles, possess the requisite skills, and operate under direct supervision to maintain safety and ethical standards (Hansen et al., 2024).

Educators play a pivotal role in fostering respectful and ethical clinical environments, including engaging healthcare staff in collaborative discussions about integrating students into clinical workflows and addressing potential concerns. Ethical simulations and case studies can help prepare students for real-world dilemmas, and institutional policies should clearly outline expectations for patient care and student learning in clinical settings (Tierney et al., 2023). By carefully balancing the educational needs of students with the service goals of healthcare settings, clinical educators can create environments that are mutually beneficial: Students can develop the skills and ethical foundations necessary for professional practice, while patients continue to receive compassionate, high-quality care. These strategies ensure that clinical education not only supports student development but also contributes positively to the broader goals of healthcare delivery and professional growth. Through thoughtful integration of learners into service settings, nursing education programs can uphold ethical standards while preparing students to meet the complexities of modern healthcare environments.

STUDENT–FACULTY RELATIONSHIPS

The Challenge of Incivility

Incivility is a pervasive issue in higher education that poses significant threats to the integrity of the teaching–learning environment. This disruptive behavior can take various forms, including unpreparedness, side conversations, disrespectful comments, intimidation, and overt aggression (Abedini et al., 2024). Both students and faculty increasingly recognize academic incivility as a pressing concern within nursing education, citing its harmful effects on mental well-being, professional identity, and institutional culture (Abedini et al., 2024; Hudgins et al., 2023).

In clinical settings, uncivil behaviors are particularly concerning because they hinder educational processes and compromise patient safety by disrupting teamwork and clear communication (Small et al., 2023). Contributing factors include high levels of academic stress, financial pressures, competing demands, and mental health challenges, all of which can diminish students' coping mechanisms and lead to frustration and impulsive behaviors. On the other hand, faculty behaviors, such as vague expectations, favoritism, and public criticism, can exacerbate tensions, thus perpetuating cycles of conflict and stress (Abedini et al., 2024; Hudgins et al., 2023).

Respect for Persons

A productive and respectful relationship between clinical teachers and students requires a foundation of mutual trust. Although both parties share responsibility, clinical teachers play a pivotal role by modeling professionalism, discretion, and respectful communication. These practices not only uphold ethical principles such as human dignity and autonomy but also reinforce the professional ethos of nursing education (Hudgins et al., 2023). Teachers foster respectful learning environments by exemplifying civil behavior in interactions with students, colleagues, patients, and healthcare staff (Small et al., 2023).

Managing incivility effectively requires proactive and structured approaches, including prevention, role modeling, and consistent communication. Faculty should establish clear policies that define acceptable and unacceptable behaviors, outline consequences for violations, and articulate performance expectations. These standards should be included in course syllabi, discussed at the beginning of each term, and consistently enforced to foster accountability and fairness (Hudgins et al., 2023; Small et al., 2023). Educational interventions, such as workshops and reflective discussions, help raise awareness about the impact of incivility while providing strategies to promote respectful conduct. Role modeling professional and respectful behavior remains one of the most effective methods for instilling these values in students (Abedini et al., 2024).

Fairness and Justice

The ethical principle of justice demands fairness and equity in evaluating student performance and fostering professional relationships (Oermann et al., 2024). Faculty must consistently apply the same standards to all students to avoid perceptions of favoritism or bias. This is especially significant in clinical education, where unequal treatment can erode trust and hinder learning. A fair and equitable approach creates an environment in which students feel valued, respected, and supported; this is essential for their academic and professional growth (Hudgins et al., 2023).

Maintaining professional boundaries is integral to upholding justice in nursing education. Faculty should clearly differentiate between their professional and personal roles, particularly concerning social media use (ANA, 2011; De Gagne et al., 2018). Social networking can enhance communication and engagement; however, blending personal and professional interactions risks undermining the instructor's authority and mentorship role (De Gagne et al., 2018). Establishing distinct personal and professional accounts preserves faculty integrity while fostering an inclusive and supportive educational environment (Hudgins et al., 2023; Small et al., 2023).

Justice requires the establishment of a transparent and inclusive culture to promote equity and fairness (Charania & Patel, 2022). Collaborative efforts between faculty and students to create and uphold clear guidelines for behavior, evaluation criteria, and penalties for incivility enhance mutual accountability and encourage all stakeholders to contribute to a respectful educational environment. Tools such as the Equity and Inclusivity Checklist (Craig et al., 2022) provide actionable strategies for integrating these principles into clinical education. By revising simulation scenarios to reflect diverse patient populations and challenge implicit biases, such tools foster equity-minded learning environments that prepare students for ethical decision-making in diverse clinical settings (Craig et al., 2022).

Addressing systemic inequities, such as financial barriers and discriminatory practices, is crucial for creating equitable learning environments (Abedini et al., 2024). Integrating equity and justice into clinical education not only enhances inclusivity but also equips students to advocate for fairness in their future roles. This intentional focus fosters empathy, accountability, and a sense of belonging—qualities that are essential for ethical and effective clinical practice. By prioritizing fairness, transparency, and the dismantling of systemic barriers, nursing educators model the ethical responsibilities necessary to navigate complex clinical environments. Such a culture of inclusivity and accountability enriches the learning experience for all students and prepares future nurses to provide equitable and compassionate care.

ACADEMIC DISHONESTY

Academic dishonesty is a significant challenge in higher education, particularly in nursing programs, where integrity is essential to ensuring safe and effective patient care. Defined as intentional engagement in deceptive practices related to academic work, academic dishonesty includes behaviors such as lying, cheating, plagiarizing, and falsifying records (He et al., 2024). The increasing prevalence of online learning, coupled with the rise of generative artificial intelligence (GenAI) tools like ChatGPT, has added complexity to maintaining academic integrity (Kleib et al., 2024) Research highlights a concerning link between academic dishonesty and unethical behavior in clinical practice, revealing that students who engage in dishonesty during their studies are more likely to replicate these behaviors in professional settings (He et al., 2024). This connection raises serious ethical concerns with implications for patient safety, professional trust, and the reputation of nursing graduates.

In clinical environments, academic dishonesty can be manifested in various ways, including by submitting inaccurate clinical logs, fabricating patient data or assessments, misrepresenting skills, claiming collaborative work as individual efforts, and failing to report errors such as medication mistakes. Such actions undermine the educational process, compromise patient safety, and erode public trust in healthcare professionals (He et al., 2024).

Factors Contributing to Academic Dishonesty

The literature identifies several factors that contribute to academic dishonesty among nursing students, which can be grouped into three primary categories (He et al., 2024):

- *Intrapersonal Factors:* Individual traits, such as knowledge gaps, stress, and external pressures, often drive students toward dishonest behaviors. The demanding nature of nursing education can overwhelm students, leading some to resort to unethical shortcuts.
- *Interpersonal Factors:* Peer dynamics, including the influence of classmates and the presence of a competitive academic environment, can normalize dishonest practices. Students may feel pressured to cheat if it is perceived as a common strategy for success among their peers.
- *External Factors:* Institutional culture, high-stakes testing, and the easy availability of online resources that facilitate cheating further complicate the maintenance of academic integrity. GenAI tools exacerbate this challenge by enabling students to bypass traditional learning processes (Kleib et al., 2024).

Implications and Strategies for Addressing Academic Dishonesty

The consequences of academic dishonesty extend beyond risks to individual students; they pose threats to the integrity of nursing education and the safety of patients. Institutions must adopt proactive strategies to mitigate dishonest behaviors and emphasize the serious ramifications of such actions. Clear and comprehensive policies regarding academic and clinical misconduct are essential. These policies should outline specific expectations and consequences for violations in order to foster a culture of accountability in which students understand the ethical standards expected of them (De Gagne et al., 2018).

Creating a supportive learning environment is equally critical. Rather than relying solely on punitive measures, institutions should encourage students to learn from their mistakes in a constructive, non threatening setting. Facilitating discussions around ethical dilemmas and promoting openness about challenges can nurture a culture of integrity and ethical reflection. Faculty members play a pivotal role in this process by modeling ethical behavior, mentoring students, and guiding them through academic and professional pressures. By demonstrating the value of honesty and professionalism, faculty help students to develop a strong sense of responsibility toward their learning and future practice. Similarly, by prioritizing academic integrity, nursing education programs uphold the ethical standards of the profession while preparing students to deliver safe, competent care. An environment that discourages dishonesty prepares nursing graduates to emerge as ethical leaders, equipped to navigate the complexities of modern healthcare with integrity and compassion. A commitment to fostering academic integrity serves to safeguard the trust and safety of the patients and communities nursing graduates will serve (De Gagne et al., 2018).

LEGAL ISSUES

This chapter does not aim to provide an exhaustive discussion of all federal, state, and local laws relevant to clinical teaching and evaluation, nor does it offer legal advice on specific issues. Clinical teachers are encouraged to consult their institution's legal counsel for guidance on policies and procedures. For personal legal concerns, individuals should seek advice from their attorney. This section addresses common legal issues frequently encountered in clinical teaching practice, with a focus on practical implications and compliance with legal standards.

Students' Privacy Rights

The privacy of students' academic and personal information is a cornerstone of ethical and legal standards in education. Sharing information about a student's performance allows clinical instructors to anticipate learning needs and plan appropriate activities, thus ensuring continuity in teaching and learning. However, under the Family Educational Rights and Privacy Act (FERPA) of 1974, the disclosure of students' academic information is restricted to those with a legitimate educational interest; such sharing requires an explicit need-to-know status or the student's written consent.

Baker et al., (2020) emphasize the importance of maintaining confidentiality when addressing necessary disclosures under FERPA. Clinical instructors should focus on sharing specific, factual observations about student performance rather than personal judgments or characterizations. For instance, highlighting a student's need for practice with a specific skill is appropriate, but offering subjective opinions about or labeling a student is unacceptable. This approach upholds FERPA guidelines while reinforcing ethical standards of respect and privacy.

Clinical instructors often face dual responsibilities as educators and supporters when students disclose personal health concerns. Although the desire to provide therapeutic support is natural, an instructor's primary obligation within a teacher–student relationship is to maintain an educational focus. FERPA requires that personal information about a student's health remains confidential unless disclosure is necessary to protect the safety of the student or others. In such cases, the disclosure should be limited to the minimum information required, as emphasized in privacy guidance for public health emergencies (Baker et al., 2020).

Evaluative statements about student performance should be shared only with individuals directly involved in the student's education and must remain objective. When health-related information must be disclosed—whether during routine educational interactions or in extraordinary situations such as public health emergencies—clinical instructors must comply with institutional policies and privacy laws. Aligning communication practices with FERPA and HIPAA requirements protects student trust while maintaining legal compliance (Baker et al., 2020). By adhering to these principles, clinical instructors can establish a professional and legally sound framework for handling sensitive information. Protecting students' privacy while enabling effective teaching and learning ensures that clinical education remains ethical, equitable, and respectful of all stakeholders. These practices not only uphold legal standards but also foster an environment of trust, fairness, and professionalism that benefits both educators and students.

Students With Disabilities

Two federal laws establish the foundation for the education of learners with disabilities in the United States. Section 504 of the Rehabilitation Act of 1973 prohibits federally funded postsecondary institutions from denying access or participation to individuals with disabilities. The Americans with Disabilities Act (ADA) of 1990 and its amendments in 2008 guarantee equal access to educational opportunities for qualified individuals with disabilities. A qualified individual is defined as someone who has a physical or mental impairment that substantially limits one or more major life activities, or has a history of such an impairment, or is perceived to have such an impairment (Smith Glasgow et al., 2020; Southern Regional Education Board [SREB], 2020). The ADA amendments broaden the interpretation of disability to include conditions in remission or episodic conditions that, when active, substantially affect major life activities. This expanded definition ensures protections for a wider range of individuals. Importantly, reasonable accommodations under the ADA do not lower academic standards or eliminate essential technical requirements but are designed to create equitable access for all students (Smith Glasgow et al., 2020).

To support individuals with disabilities, nursing programs must clearly define core performance standards—cognitive, sensory, affective, and psychomotor competencies—necessary for participation in clinical education (SREB, 2020). These standards should be published in institutional materials to help students and applicants determine their need for accommodations. Examples of reasonable accommodations include:

- allowing additional time for assignments or program completion;
- providing assistive devices, such as amplified stethoscopes or interpreters; and
- modifying clinical placements to accessible settings (Smith Glasgow et al., 2020; SREB, 2020).

Accommodations may also involve the use of service animals trained to perform specific tasks for individuals with disabilities (Silbert-Flagg et al., 2020). Although some areas within healthcare facilities may restrict service animals (e.g., operating rooms or sterile environments), clinical placements can be modified to accommodate both the student and their service animal. Effective planning and collaboration among faculty, students, and clinical site personnel are essential to address concerns and ensure compliance with legal protections. Proactive solutions include proper grooming of the animal, identifying designated areas for the animal during clinical activities, and providing personal protective equipment for individuals with allergies (Silbert-Flagg et al., 2020).

Ensuring effective accommodations requires collaboration among students, disability services staff, and clinical educators. Clinical teachers bring a realistic understanding of essential nursing practice, while students are best positioned to articulate their needs and strategies for accommodations. Bridging gaps between disability resource centers and clinical programs is essential, and appointing accessibility coordinators has been suggested as a strategy to enhance support for clinical accommodations (Jamal-Eddine et al., 2024).

Persons with disabilities often encounter structural barriers and stigmatization; therefore, faculty must actively dismantle ableist attitudes that may undervalue their contributions. Creating an inclusive culture not only supports persons with disabilities but also enriches the broader healthcare workforce by integrating diverse perspectives and addressing systemic inequities (Jamal-Eddine et al., 2024). Viewing persons with disabilities as assets rather than liabilities promotes systemic equity and justice but necessitates a reevaluation of traditional norms and the adoption of inclusive policies that prioritize fairness and foster an environment of belonging.

Students requiring accommodations for health concerns should follow the institution's formal disability services process rather than relying on individual faculty decisions. Instructors should encourage students to work with the designated disability services officer to request accommodations. Once the needed accommodations have been approved, clinical instructors should collaborate with students to determine how they can best be implemented in the clinical setting. This structured approach ensures equity, minimizes liability, and maintains the integrity of the educational environment.

Consistent documentation of accommodations offered and their implementation ensures fairness and accountability (SREB, 2020). The American Association of Colleges of Nursing (AACN, 2024) offers a toolkit for accommodating students with disabilities, providing resources to help educators create inclusive learning environments. After accommodations have been implemented and documented, individuals with disabilities must be evaluated using the same criteria as other students to maintain fairness and provided with constructive feedback if they are at risk of clinical failure (Smith Glasgow et al., 2020).

Due Process

The right of students to due process is a critical legal issue in clinical teaching. The 14th Amendment of the U.S. Constitution specifies that the state cannot deprive a person of life, liberty, or property without due process of law, a protection that primarily applies to students in public institutions. In private institutions, due process is governed by contract law, where institutional policies—such as those outlined in student handbooks—may be considered binding agreements. Failure to follow these stated procedures for grievances or disciplinary actions may subject private institutions to legal challenges, including claims of breach of contract (Smith Glasgow et al., 2020).

ACADEMIC DUE PROCESS

Courts distinguish between academic and disciplinary decisions when evaluating due process claims. Academic decisions relate to issues such as assigning a failing grade, delaying a student's progress, or dismissing a student from a program for failure to maintain acceptable academic standing. Academic due process encompasses two critical components:

- *Procedural Due Process*: This refers to the fairness of the methods and processes used to inform students of their academic standing and make decisions regarding their performance.

- *Substantive Due Process:* This pertains to ensuring that the validity and fairness of the actual decision are based on consistent application of academic standards (Smith Glasgow et al., 2020).

A student appealing an academic decision may allege a violation of either type of due process. However, courts typically avoid intervening in faculty evaluations of student performance, whether didactic or clinical, as these decisions rely on the professional judgment of educators (Smith Glasgow et al., 2020). To ensure compliance with substantive due process:

- students must be informed in advance of the academic standards used to evaluate their performance; and
- faculty must apply these standards consistently, using the same criteria for all students and avoiding arbitrary or capricious decisions.

Procedural due process safeguards fairness in the decision-making process. Faculty should notify students of academic deficiencies early, both orally and in writing, and provide specific feedback, suggested improvements, and timelines for progress. The NCSBN Model Rules (2021) emphasize that transparent and consistent evaluation processes are essential for maintaining accountability and minimizing disputes. Students who believe that an academic decision is unjust must follow the institution's stated appeal process, which typically begins with the faculty involved and progresses through higher administrative levels. Courts defer to the academic institution's expertise unless there is clear evidence of due process violations (Smith Glasgow et al., 2020).

DISCIPLINARY DUE PROCESS

Disciplinary decisions, such as dismissal for misconduct, require a higher standard of due process than academic actions. Unlike academic decisions, which rely on faculty's professional judgment, disciplinary actions are often fact-based and subject to judicial review (Smith Glasgow et al., 2020). The NCSBN Model Rules (2021) emphasize the importance of clear and transparent expectations for student conduct, as well as adherence to established institutional procedures for addressing violations. Nursing programs must publish specific codes of conduct, including professional standards unique to the nursing profession, and outline the consequences of noncompliance. Key components of disciplinary due process include:

- *Written Notification:* Students must receive a detailed, written notice of the alleged misconduct and the specific violation of policies or codes of conduct. For example, a student dismissed for repeated absences from required clinical activities should be notified of the specific incidents, the violated policy, and the rationale for dismissal.
- *Fair Hearing:* Students are entitled to a fair and impartial hearing to respond to the charges. They must have the opportunity to speak on their own behalf, present evidence, and question other participants in the case. Although legal counsel may advise students or faculty, attorneys are typically restricted from questioning witnesses during internal proceedings so as to maintain the educational focus of the process.
- *Appeal Rights:* Institutions must provide a clear and transparent process for appealing disciplinary decisions. Appeals generally progress through levels of authority, starting with a faculty hearing panel or administrative review and culminating with senior administrators, such as a dean or university president. This process ensures that students have multiple opportunities to present evidence or address procedural concerns (Smith Glasgow et al., 2020).

If a dismissal decision is upheld, students retain the right to seek remedy through the court system; however, the burden of proof lies with the student to demonstrate that procedural or substantive due process was denied. Courts generally defer to institutional expertise unless there is clear evidence of procedural unfairness or bias (Smith Glasgow et al., 2020).

To reduce disputes and mitigate liability, nursing programs must ensure that disciplinary processes are consistently applied, thoroughly documented, and aligned with published policies. Early intervention, transparent communication, and adherence to due process requirements are essential to maintaining fairness and accountability. Adherence to the NCSBN Model Rules (2021) ensures that disciplinary actions are legally sound and uphold the integrity of nursing education and practice.

Negligence, Liability, and Unsafe Clinical Practice

Determination of whether a given action meets the criteria for professional negligence is based on the standard of care, which is defined as what an ordinary, reasonable, and prudent person would have done in the same context. Importantly, the standard of care for nursing students is not based on what another nursing student would have done; instead, students are held to the same standards of care as RNs. According to the NCSBN Model Nurse Practice Act (2021), nursing students are permitted to practice without licensure provided that they are actively enrolled in and progressing through an approved prelicensure or graduate nursing education program. This practice must occur under faculty supervision and comply with board-established criteria to ensure that students perform safely within the program's oversight.

The NCSBN Model Nurse Practice Act (2021) further emphasizes that unsafe or unprofessional practice and substandard care constitute grounds for disciplinary action. Nurses, including students, must practice with reasonable skill and safety, taking accountability for decisions based on their education and level of experience. For nursing students, this involves adhering to the standard of care appropriate to their educational preparation, seeking guidance when uncertain, and following established protocols. Contrary to a common misconception, nursing students do not practice under the license of their faculty supervisors; rather, personal liability applies to each individual's actions in clinical practice.

Faculty members are generally not liable for negligent acts performed by students if the following specific criteria have been met:

- Learning activities must be appropriately assigned based on clear and defined objectives.
- Faculty must verify that students possess the prerequisite knowledge, skills, and attitudes for assigned tasks.
- Competent guidance must be provided during clinical activities.

However, the NCSBN Model Rules (2021) highlight that RNs may face disciplinary action if they fail to competently oversee student clinical learning activities. Faculty negligence includes assigning tasks that exceed a student's demonstrated capabilities or failing to provide adequate supervision. Even when faculty fulfill their responsibilities, they may still be named as defendants in lawsuits arising from student negligence, a possibility that underscores the importance of clinical faculty carrying individual professional liability insurance to cover potential legal expenses, even when institutional coverage is available. Such precautions allow faculty to protect themselves while continuing to fulfill their vital role in nursing education.

If a student demonstrates unsafe clinical performance resulting in harm, liability may extend to both the student and the faculty member who assigned the task. The NCSBN Model Nurse Practice Act (2021) emphasizes the responsibility of faculty to act promptly when safety concerns arise. Removing a student from clinical activities due to unsafe practice is not an academic decision but rather a disciplinary action focused on protecting patient safety; such an action must adhere to institutional policies and respect the student's right to due process. Rather than denying students access to all learning opportunities, faculty should implement substitute activities to address identified deficiencies. For example, students may be assigned focused library research to strengthen their theoretical understanding or scheduled for additional skills lab sessions to improve psychomotor competencies. These remediation strategies align with the NCSBN Model Rules (2021), which stress the importance of structured frameworks for addressing deficiencies while maintaining public safety.

Nursing education programs should clearly define and enforce standards for safe clinical practice by incorporating them into student handbooks, course syllabi, and clinical policies. Transparency fosters accountability and ensures consistency. Faculty must also meticulously document student progress and any interventions implemented to address performance issues; such documentation is crucial for defending against liability claims and demonstrating adherence to both legal and professional standards. By integrating these provisions, nursing programs can balance their dual responsibilities of safeguarding patients and supporting student learning. Ensuring clarity in expectations, effective faculty oversight, and structured remediation processes fosters a culture of accountability and upholds the integrity of nursing education. Refer to **Exhibit 6.1** for an example of safe clinical practice standards and **Exhibit 6.2** for a policy framework that enforces these standards.

Documentation and Record Keeping

Accurate and thorough documentation is a cornerstone of clinical teaching, serving to evaluate student performance and provide evidence of progress. Faculty should maintain records such as notes about student's performance, summaries of faculty–student conferences, progress reports, and summative clinical evaluations. These records document the feedback provided to students, identify areas of concern, and track progress toward resolving deficiencies.

NOTES ABOUT PERFORMANCE

Notes about students' performance, often referred to as anecdotal notes, are narrative descriptions of observed student behaviors in relation to specific competencies or learning objectives. They may include the faculty member's interpretation of the behavior, although such interpretations should be documented separately to maintain clarity. Limiting notes to observed behaviors linked to clinical competencies, or objectives depending on the format used in the nursing program, avoids extraneous information and ensures that documentation remains focused and time efficient. To present a balanced view of student performance and prevent perceptions of bias, performance notes should capture both positive and negative behaviors. Students

EXHIBIT 6.1 Standards of Safe Clinical Practice

XXXXXX UNIVERSITY
SCHOOL OF NURSING
BSN PROGRAM
STANDARDS OF SAFE CLINICAL PRACTICE

In clinical practice, students are expected to demonstrate responsibility and accountability as professional nurses with the goal of health promotion and prevention of harm to self and others. The School of Nursing faculty believes that this goal will be attained if each student's clinical practice adheres to the Standards of Safe Clinical Practice. Safe clinical performance always includes, but is not limited to, the following behaviors:

1. practicing within boundaries of the nursing student role and the scope of practice of the RN;
2. complying with instructional policies and procedures for implementing nursing care;
3. preparing for clinical learning assignments according to course requirements and as determined for the specific clinical setting;
4. demostrating the application of previously learned skills and principles in providing nursing care; and
5. promptly reporting significant client information in a clear, accurate, and complete oral or written manner to the appropriate person or persons.

ACKNOWLEDGMENT

I have read the XXXXXX University School of Nursing Standards of Safe Clinical Practice, and I agree to adhere to them. I understand that these standards are expectations for my clinical practice and will be incorporated into the evaluation of my clinical performance in all clinical courses. Failure to meet these standards may result in my removal from the clinical area, which may result in clinical failure due to my inability to achieve the required learning outcomes.

Signature: _____________ Date: __________

should have the opportunity to review and comment on these notes. When used effectively, the educator's notes about performance serve as a formative evaluation tool, guiding student improvement (Oermann et al., 2024). In some cases, both the teacher and student may sign the notes to acknowledge their content.

FACULTY–STUDENT CONFERENCES

Faculty–student conferences are essential for addressing performance concerns, creating plans for improvement, and monitoring progress. Summaries of these conferences should include the following details:

- the date, time, and location of the meeting;
- the names and roles of participants; and
- a concise summary of the discussion, including recommendations and action plans.

These meetings should occur in private to maintain confidentiality and professionalism. Conferences offer

EXHIBIT 6.2 Policy on Safe Clinical Practice

XXXXXX UNIVERSITY
SCHOOL OF NURSING
BSN PROGRAM
SAFE CLINICAL PRACTICE POLICY

POLICY

During enrollment in the XXXXXX University School of Nursing BSN program, all students, in all clinical activities, are expected to adhere to the Standards of Safe Clinical Practice. Failure to abide by these standards will result in disciplinary action, which may include dismissal from the nursing program.

PROCEDURES

1. Students will receive a copy of the Standards of Safe Clinical Practice, and they will be reviewed during the Annual Nursing Assembly at the beginning of each academic year. At that time, students will be required to sign an agreement to adhere to the standards. Each student will retain one copy of the agreement, and one copy will be retained in the student's file.
2. Violation of these standards will result in the following disciplinary action:
   a. First violation
      1) Students will be given an immediate oral warning by the faculty member. The incident will be documented by the faculty member on the Violation of Standards of Safe Clinical Practice form. One copy of this form will be given to the student, and one copy will be kept in the student's record.
      2) At the discretion of the faculty member, the student may be required to leave the clinical setting for the remainder of that day. The student may be given an alternative assignment.
      3) If this violation is of a serious nature, it may be referred to the associate dean and the dean of nursing for further disciplinary action as in b and c (see the following).
   b. Second violation
      1) The faculty member will document the incident on the Violation of Safe Clinical Practice form. Following discussion of the incident with the student, the faculty member will forward a copy of the form to the associate dean for review and recommendation regarding further action.
      2) The recommendation of the associate dean will be forwarded to the dean of nursing for review and decision regarding reprimand or dismissal. This disciplinary action process will be documented and placed in the student's record.
   c. If the student has not been dismissed and remains in the program following the disciplinary action, any additional violation will be documented and referred to the associate dean and the dean of nursing for disciplinary action as already stated, which may include dismissal from the program.
   d. The rights of students will be safeguarded as set forth in the XXXXXX University Code of Student Rights, Responsibilities, and Conduct published in the current XXXXXX University Student Handbook.

students the opportunity to clarify and respond to feedback. When necessary, an objective third party, such as a department chair or program director, may participate to ensure mutual understanding and impartial documentation. Depending on institutional policies, the conference documentation may include signatures from all participants. Learning (or action plans) are discussed further in Chapter 12 with an example of a template that can be used.

RETENTION OF RECORDS

Notes about performance and conference records are primarily tools for formative evaluation and should not be included in students' permanent academic files. Faculty should retain these documents in secure private files until there is no reasonable expectation of their being needed. Typically, these records can be discarded once a student completes the program or withdraws in good academic standing. However, if there is potential for an appeal regarding a grade or academic decision, retaining the records until the statute of limitations expires is prudent. Faculty should consult institutional legal counsel to ensure compliance with applicable record retention policies.

Patient Privacy Laws

Enacted in 1996, HIPAA establishes the fundamental right of patients to privacy regarding their personal health information. HIPAA regulations apply to healthcare entities such as hospitals, clinics, and rehabilitation centers. Nursing education programs that place students in these facilities are typically classified as "business associates," obligating them to adhere to the same rigorous privacy standards. Nursing students are bound by HIPAA rules during their clinical activities and must understand that these responsibilities extend beyond the clinical setting to their private conduct.

HIPAA ORIENTATION AND COMPLIANCE

Healthcare facilities often require nursing programs to document that students have been oriented to HIPAA regulations, and this essential requirement can become cumbersome if each facility mandates its own specific orientation process. Nursing education administrators should collaborate with clinical agencies to standardize orientation content, thereby reducing redundancy while ensuring comprehensive training. Students typically sign a verification form acknowledging that they have received HIPAA training and agreeing to comply with its standards. Regularly renewing this verification at the start of each academic year or clinical rotation helps to maintain compliance and awareness.

In addition to HIPAA compliance, healthcare facilities often require nursing programs to verify that students meet specific health requirements, such as immunizations or physical examinations. Because managing individually identifiable health information for these purposes introduces the risk for HIPAA violations, many programs adopt strategies that minimize the collection and transmission of sensitive health data. For example, students may provide verification directly from a licensed healthcare provider that they meet the necessary clinical health standards. Alternatively, student health services at the parent institution can oversee the process and retain the raw data while notifying the nursing program of compliance. These approaches safeguard both student privacy and institutional accountability.

BROADER ETHICAL CONSIDERATIONS

Patient privacy laws protect patient rights but also raise broad ethical considerations in clinical teaching environments. As nursing education programs navigate HIPAA compliance, they must prioritize equity and inclusivity. Ensuring fair access to clinical placements and learning opportunities for all students, regardless of background or identity, is critical to fostering an inclusive educational environment. For instance, international students or those from underrepresented backgrounds may face unique challenges, such as unfamiliarity with U.S. healthcare privacy laws or cultural hesitations about disclosing personal health information. Nursing programs must implement culturally sensitive approaches to HIPAA training and health verification processes to ensure that all students feel supported and respected. Clear communication, inclusive policies, and accessible resources are essential for enabling students to meet legal and ethical requirements confidently.

Nursing education programs must collaborate with institutional legal counsel to develop clear and comprehensive policies for verifying student health information and ensuring HIPAA compliance; these policies must balance the privacy rights of students and patients with the operational needs of clinical agencies. Collaborative efforts between nursing programs and healthcare facilities can streamline compliance processes, reduce administrative burdens, and uphold the highest ethical and legal standards. By integrating these practices, nursing education programs can create a supportive and equitable environment that prepares students to navigate the complexities of privacy laws, clinical responsibilities, and ethical decision-making. This approach fulfills legal obligations, reinforces the profession's commitment to equity, and fosters an inclusive and accountable nursing workforce.

SUMMARY

This chapter explored the ethical and legal complexities inherent in clinical teaching, emphasizing the critical role of moral reasoning, accountability, and adherence to professional standards in fostering an inclusive and equitable learning environment. It highlighted the importance of guiding nursing students through ethical dilemmas and professional challenges while ensuring their accountability for safe and competent patient care. Key topics included the significance of ethical behavior in clinical settings, the integration of moral reasoning and accountability in decision-making, and the transformative role of equity and inclusivity in addressing systemic barriers to learning. The chapter also examined the challenges posed by digital communication tools such as social media and underscored the importance of digital professionalism in safeguarding patient confidentiality and maintaining professional boundaries.

This chapter also discussed learners in service settings and issues related to balancing the educational needs of students with the rights and expectations of patients and staff. Faculty responsibilities were addressed, including practices related to providing fair evaluation, fostering respectful student-faculty relationships, mitigating incivility, and promoting a culture of respect and professionalism.

Finally, the chapter delved into multifaceted legal issues such as due process, negligence, liability, and compliance with patient privacy laws, and underscored the importance of creating clear policies for HIPAA compliance, verifying student health requirements, and safeguarding the privacy of both students and patients. It provided educators with practical tools to navigate the complexities of clinical teaching, create an environment that upholds ethical and legal standards, and prepare nursing students to meet the challenges of contemporary healthcare with integrity, compassion, and professionalism.

CNE®cl EXAMINATION TEST BLUEPRINT CORE COMPETENCIES

1. Function within the Education and Health Care Environment

A. Function in the Clinical Educator Role

4. Act as a role model of professional nursing within the clinical learning environment
5. Create a diverse, equitable, and inclusive learning environment

C. Abide by Legal Requirements, Ethical Guidelines, Agency Policies, and Guiding Framework

1. Apply ethical and legal principles to create a safe clinical learning environment (e.g., privacy laws, confidentiality, error/near-miss situation reporting, remediation, negligence, liability, scope/standards of practice)
4. Inform others of program and clinical agency policies, procedures, and practices
5. Adhere to program and clinical agency policies, procedures and practices when implementing clinical experiences (e.g., due process, accommodations, academic integrity
6. Comply with current program and clinical agency policies, procedures, and practices related to personal protective equipment and other infection control measures for self and learners
7. Demonstrate ethical and legal behaviors in the clinical nurse educator role

2. Facilitate Learning in the Healthcare Environment

E. Promote a culture of safety and quality in the delivery of health care
F. Create a positive and caring learning environment
G. Demonstrate enthusiasm for teaching, learning, and nursing to help inspire and motivate learners

3. Apply Clinical Expertise in the Healthcare Environment

D. Support an environment of frequent, respectful, and civil communication within the healthcare team
E. Demonstrate respect for learners, healthcare team, colleagues, clients, families, and others
F. Use clear and effective communication in all interactions (e.g., written, electronic, verbal, non-verbal, virtual)
G. Respond to learner concerns, needs, or questions in a supportive manner
H. Display a calm, empathetic, approachable, and non-judgemental demeanor in communications
J. Function as an accessible resource to learners and the healthcare team in the clinical learning environment
K. Demonstrate culturally sensitive communication in clinical learning environments
M. Communicate performance expectations to learners and clinical staff

5. Facilitate Learner Development and Socialization

A. Mentor learners in professional nursing behaviors
B. Promote professional integrity and accountability
C. Model professional boundaries with all participants in learning environment
E. Assist learners to use self-assessment, self-reflection, and goal setting for ongoing professional development
F. Create learning environments that promote socialization to the role of the nurse
G. Facilitate learner participation in constructive peer feedback practices

LEARNING ACTIVITIES

CourseConnect

To access self-assessment questions and interactive, competency-based learning activities for this chapter, visit www.springerpub.com/courseconnect. See inside front cover and tear-out card for CourseConnect details.

REFERENCES

Abedini, Z., Hashemi, S., Tehrani, F. J., Eskandari, N., & Saeedi, M. (2024). Incivility in nursing education: A concept analysis. *Iranian Journal of Nursing & Midwifery Research, 29*(5), 542–548. https://doi.org/10.4103/ijnmr.ijnmr_223_21

American Association of Colleges of Nursing. (2024). *Accommodating students with disabilities*. https://www.aacnnursing.org/our-initiatives/education-practice/faculty-tool-kits/accommodating-students-with-disabilities

American Nurses Association. (2011). *ANA's principles for social networking and the nurse: Guidance for registered nurses*. https://www.nursingworld.org/~4af4f2/globalassets/docs/ana/ethics/social-networking.pdf

American Nurses Association. (2025). *Code of ethics for nurses*. https://codeofethics.ana.org

Americans With Disabilities Act of 1990, 42 U.S.C. § 12101 et seq. (1990).

Baker, C., Galemore, C. A., & Lowrey, K. M. (2020). Information sharing in the school setting during a public health emergency. *NASN school nurse (Print), 35*(4), 198–202. https://doi.org/10.1177/1942602x20925031

Charania, N. A. M. A., & Patel, R. (2022). Diversity, equity, and inclusion in nursing education: Strategies and processes to support inclusive teaching. *Journal of Professional Nursing, 42*, 67–72. https://doi.org/10.1016/j.profnurs.2022.05.013

Craig, S., Whitlow, M. L., Quatrara, B., Kastello, J., Ackard, R., Mitchell, E. M., & Kools, S. (2022). A focused checklist for constructing equitable, diverse, and inclusive simulation experiences. *Clinical Simulation in Nursing, 71*, 87–91. https://doi.org/10.1016/j.ecns.2022.05.004

Daigle, A. (2020). Social media and professional boundaries in undergraduate nursing students. *Journal of Professional Nursing, 36*(2), 20–23. https://doi.org/10.1016/j.profnurs.2019.08.007

De Gagne, J. C., Yamane, S. S., Conklin, J. L., Chang, J., & Kang, H. S. (2018). Social media use and cybercivility guidelines in U.S. nursing schools: A review of websites. *Journal of Professional Nursing, 34*(1), 35–41. https://doi.org/10.1016/j.profnurs.2017.07.006

Family Educational Rights and Privacy Act, 20 U.S.C. § 1232g; 34 CFR Part 99 (1974).

Gum, L., Brown, A., Royals, R., Matricciani, L., & Kelly, M. A. (2024). Digital professionalism in preregistration nursing and midwifery students: A scoping review to explore perceptions of professionalism when using social media. *Nurse Education in Practice, 80*, 104128. https://doi.org/10.1016/j.nepr.2024.104128

Hansen, S., Hessevaagbakke, E., Lindeflaten, K., Elvan, K., & Lillekroken, D. (2024). Nurturing ethical insight: Exploring nursing students' journey to ethical competence. *BMC Nursing, 23*(1), 568. https://doi.org/10.1186/s12912-024-02243-x

He, F. X., Fanaian, M., Zhang, N. M., Lea, X., Geale, S. K., Gielis, L., Razaghi, K., & Evans, A. (2024). Academic dishonesty in university nursing students: A scoping review. *International Journal of Nursing Studies, 154*, 104752. https://doi.org/10.1016/j.ijnurstu.2024.104752

Health Insurance Portability and Accountability Act (HIPAA) of 1996. Public Law 104–191.

Hudgins, T., Layne, D., Kusch, C. E., & Lounsbury, K. (2023). An analysis of the perceptions of incivility in higher education. *Journal of Academic Ethics, 21*(2), 177–191. https://doi.org/10.1007/s10805-022-09448-2

Hussein, A. H. M., & Abou Hashish, E. A. (2023). Relationship between nurses' ethical ideology, professional values, and clinical accountability. *Nursing Ethics, 30*(7–8), 1171–1189. https://doi.org/10.1177/09697330231172282

Jamal-Eddine, S., Savage, T., & Gill, C. (2024). Assets, not burdens: Disabled students in nursing education. *International Journal of Nursing Studies, 154*, 104775. https://doi.org/10.1016/j.ijnurstu.2024.104775

Kleib, M., Darko, E. M., Akingbade, O., Kennedy, M., Majekodunmi, P., Nickel, E., & Vogelsang, L. (2024). Current trends and future implications in the utilization of ChatGPT in nursing: A rapid review. *International Journal of Nursing Studies Advances, 7*, 100252. https://doi.org/10.1016/j.ijnsa.2024.100252

Masudi, K. A. (2024). Ethics in education: Teaching moral and ethical decision-making. *Eurasian Experiment Journal of Arts & Management, 5*(3), 45–49. https://www.eejournals.org/public/uploads/1725020108_d3404b7c7f86d3037137.pdf

National Council of State Boards of Nursing. (2018). *A nurse's guide to the use of social media*. https://www.ncsbn.org/NCSBN_SocialMedia.pdf

National Council of State Boards of Nursing. (2021). *NCSBN model act*. https://www.ncsbn.org/public-files/21_Model_Act.pdf

Nunthawong, J., & Ketkomg, T. (2024). An integrative moral development of nursing students. *Global Interactive Journal of World Religions and Cultures, 4*(1), 78–86. https://so18.tci-thaijo.org/index.php/gjwrc_2521/article/view/100/263

Oermann, M. H., Gaberson, K. B., & De Gagne, J. C. (2024). *Evaluation and testing in nursing education* (7th ed.). Springer Publishing Company.

Qu, Z., Sun, J., Li, L., Zhao, L., Jiang, N., Fan, J., Zhang, J., & Liang, B. (2024). The effect of simulated problem learning in nursing ethics on moral sensitivity, empathy and critical thinking of nursing students: A quasi-experimental study. *Nurse Education in Practice, 80*, 104119. https://doi.org/10.1016/j.nepr.2024.104119

Silbert-Flagg, J., Shilling, S. D., Lucas, L., Nolan, M. T., Lin, L., Bellefeuille, P., Foley, M., Mallareddy, D., Baker. D., & D'Aoust, R. (2020). Preparing for a student with a service animal. *Journal of Professional Nursing, 36*(6), 458–461. https://doi.org/10.1016/j.profnurs.2020.03.001

Small, S. P., Cashin, G., English, D., & Moran, G. (2023). "It is essentially about treating each other well": Insights from faculty on incivility in nursing education. *Canadian Journal of Nursing Research, 56*(1), 81–94. https://doi.org/10.1177/08445621231204985

Smith Glasgow, M. E., Dreher, H. M., Dahnke, M. D., & Gyllenhammer, J. (2020). *Legal and ethical issues in nursing education: An essential guide.* Springer Publishing Company.

Southern Regional Education Board. (2020). *The Americans with disabilities act: Implications for nursing education.* http://www.sreb.org/publication/americans-disabilities-act

Tierney, O., Vasilevski, V., Kinsman, L., & Sweet, L. (2023). Advocacy, accountability and autonomy: The learning intention of the midwifery student continuity of care experience. *Nurse Education in Practice, 72,* 103772. https://doi.org/10.1016/j.nepr.2023.103772

II

Strategies for Effective Clinical Teaching

Clinical Teaching Methods and Learning Activities

7

OBJECTIVES:

1. Identify clinical teaching methods and their alignment with learning outcomes, competencies, and student skill levels.
2. Examine diverse clinical assignments and learning activities, including patient care, management activities, observation, and service learning, tailored to different clinical scenarios.
3. Compare types of cases for clinical teaching and their differences to foster critical thinking, clinical judgment, and reflective practice.

One of the most important responsibilities of the clinical educator is selecting teaching methods and planning clinical assignments and other learning activities that are related to the competencies to be developed, appropriate to students' levels of knowledge and skill, but challenging enough to motivate learning. Although having students provide comprehensive nursing care to one or more patients is a typical clinical assignment, it is only one of many possible assignments and not always the most appropriate choice. Alternate options for patient assignments are explored in the chapter. This chapter also describes other clinical teaching methods—discussions with students in the clinical setting, clinical conferences (pre- and postclinical conferences), and written assignments (concept map, short written assignment, nursing care plan, reflective journal, and electronic portfolio). Examples are provided of these clinical teaching methods in the chapter.

Students can analyze various types of case scenarios in a written assignment, clinical group activity, or postclinical conference. Cases describe a clinical situation, based on an actual or a hypothetical patient, for students to apply concepts to clinical situations, solve problems, arrive at carefully thought out decisions, and develop their clinical reasoning and judgment skills. Cases provide a simulated scenario for student review and critique. The case provided for analysis can be short and specific, can be a longer case study with extensive background information, or can be an unfolding case that changes over time. These are discussed in the chapter with examples of each type.

FACTORS AFFECTING SELECTION OF LEARNING ACTIVITIES

Clinical assignments and other learning activities help students apply knowledge to practice, develop competencies, cultivate professional values, and begin to function in the role of the professional nurse. Some of these activities may be assignments in which students provide complete care to one or more patients. However, other assignments may involve specific learning activities such as interviews of patients because these are the best strategies to help students achieve the specific competencies and apply the concepts being examined in class to practice, or because they will meet students' individual learning needs. Clinical teaching methods and learning activities are selected based on the competencies to be developed, individual learner needs, evidence of the effectiveness of the teaching methods and learning activities being considered, and availability of the clinical educator, preceptor, or other clinician to guide learners. Educators also should consider if the patient's nursing care presents enough of a challenge for learners, or if it might be too complex for the student, and if there is concern from patients, family members, or other caregivers about care from a nursing student.

Because one of the purposes of clinical practice is to foster application of theory, clinical learning activities should be related to what is being taught in the classroom. By knowing the concepts that students are learning, the educator can identify learning activities to help students apply exemplars of those concepts in patient care. For example, if beginning students are learning about wound healing, students could have learning activities involving patients with postoperative wounds, pressure ulcers, traumatic wounds, or chronic leg ulcers. It is not necessary for every student to have this learning opportunity. In a postclinical conference, students can report on their care of various patients with wounds with group discussion of commonalities and differences in patients' care, how they provide examples of tissue integrity as a concept, and strategies to maintain tissue integrity.

Many competencies do not need to be met in an acute care, hospital setting. For example, if the competency relates to health teaching, students can develop these skills in a wide range of clinical settings, in simulation, and through other learning activities. Because of the difficulties many schools experience in securing clinical placements for students, scheduling learning activities during evening or night shifts or in the community may offer students better opportunities to develop specific competencies. Segura (2024) described benefits of integrating night shift clinical placements for nursing students to address the competition for day shift opportunities in many hospital settings and provide students with diverse learning experiences.

CLINICAL ASSIGNMENTS

When planning clinical assignments, educators and preceptors typically think about patients for whom students will provide care. The primary role of the student in the clinical setting, however, is that of learner, not nurse. Although students need contact with patients to apply concepts to clinical practice and develop their clinical competencies, caring for patients is not synonymous with learning. Safe, competent nursing practice requires students to integrate theory with practice and develop their clinical reasoning and judgment skills (Nielsen et al., 2021).

Patient Care

The traditional clinical assignment for prelicensure and advanced practice registered nursing (APRN) students whether in acute care, a clinic, or a community setting is to provide complete care for one or more patients. However, many competencies do not require students to provide this care. For example, if the competency is to assess preparation for discharge and home care, students could develop this competency by interviewing a patient or family member in an acute care setting, observing a case manager's assessment of the patient's and family's readiness for discharge, reviewing a physical therapist's assessment of the patient's ability to perform activities at home, interviewing a newly discharged patient in the home or clinic, or participating in a simulation.

All students do not need to have the same learning activities at the same time. Depending on their individual learning needs, some students might focus on activities that allow them to develop a specific competency such as those related to assessment or interviewing, while others could be practicing more integrative activities such as providing complete patient care. One advantage to assigning some students to learning activities that do not involve complete patient care is the educator is more available for closer guidance of students who are caring for patients.

STUDENT–PATIENT RATIO OPTIONS

Although the traditional clinical assignment takes the form of one student to one patient, there are other assignment options. These options include:

- *One student to one patient or multiple patients:* One student is responsible for certain aspects of care (e.g., medication administration) or for comprehensive care for one or more patients. The student works alone to plan and care for the patient. This type of assignment is advantageous when the outcome is to integrate multiple aspects of care.
- *Multiple students to one patient:* Two or more students are assigned to care for one patient. Each learner has a defined role, and all collaborate to provide care. This assignment strategy is particularly useful when patients have complex needs that are beyond the capability of one student, although it can be used in any setting with a large number of students and a low patient census. Other advantages include reducing student anxiety and promoting teamwork and collaborative learning.
- *Multiple students–patient aggregate:* A group of students is assigned to complete activities related to a community or population at risk for certain health problems. For example, a small group of students might be assigned to conduct a community assessment. Clinical activities would include interviewing community residents, identifying environmental health hazards, and documenting the availability of social and healthcare services. The student group would then analyze the data and prepare a report on their findings.
- *Management activities:* Some clinical assignments are chosen to enable learners to meet competencies related to leadership, management of care for groups of patients and staff, and quality improvement.

MAKING A PATIENT ASSIGNMENT

An integrative review by Mella (2021) identified factors for the clinical educator to consider in making a patient assignment for nursing students. These included the needs of patients and families, the students' learning needs and characteristics, course objectives, knowledge of the educator about clinical teaching, and the learning environment. Considering these can make the selection of patient assignments more thoughtful and intentional (Mella, 2021). Three methods of making assignments were identified from the literature review: (a) faculty-led, (b) student directed, and (c) shared by the educator and student. **Exhibit 7.1** lists factors that should be considered when making a patient assignment for prelicensure and APRN students.

EXHIBIT 7.1 Making a Patient Assignment

Consider:

Needs of patients, families, and other caregivers
Current knowledge and competencies of students to care for a particular patient
Competencies to be developed or assessed
Learning needs of students
Course outcomes/objectives
Characteristics of clinical setting, learning environment
Input of staff
Model of clinical teaching used in the setting (e.g., traditional with one educator for group of students, preceptor- or clinician -based, dedicated education unit, other models)
Numbers of students in the clinical setting
Knowledge of educator about clinical teaching

Observation

Observation is an important competency in nursing practice, and teachers should provide opportunities for learners to develop this skill systematically. Observing patients to collect data is a prerequisite to clinical judgment. To make accurate and useful observations, however, the student should have knowledge of the patient's condition or a related concept. As a clinical learning assignment, observation should not be combined with an assignment to provide care. The focus should be on observing purposefully to develop this skill.

Observation also provides opportunities for students to learn through modeling. By observing another person interacting with and caring for patients and others in the clinical setting or community, the learner forms an image of the role of that individual and how interventions are to be performed. Written observation guidelines can be developed to guide learners' attention to important data during the observation.

Service Learning

Another option for clinical learning assignments is service learning. Service learning differs from volunteer work, community service, fieldwork, and internships. Volunteer and community service focus primarily on the service that is provided to the recipients, and fieldwork and internships primarily focus on benefits to student learning. Service learning integrates community service with academic learning, promoting students' understanding of course content, societal issues, and social determinants of health, among other areas, through their direct participation in the community in response to identified community needs (Kuehn, 2024; Marcilla-Toribio et al., 2022; Mayer, 2022; Yoong et al., 2022). In service learning not only do students learn and develop competencies, but the community also benefits.

Some service learning is focused on specific competencies to be developed by students. For example, Bowling et al. (2022) described an intergenerational service-learning experience in a course with the aim of improving the attitudes of nursing students toward older adults. All students completed a minimum of five visits with an independent community-dwelling older adult for their clinical experience. Significant improvements in student attitudes were documented after the service-learning experience (Bowling et al., 2022). Service learning also prepares APRNs for civic engagement and a better understanding of community needs (Wilkinson et al., 2023).

DISCUSSIONS

Discussions between teacher and student, and between preceptor and learner, occur frequently but may not always promote learning. These discussions sometimes involve the teacher telling the learner what to do or not to do for a patient. Discussions, though, should be an exchange of ideas through which the teacher, by asking open-ended questions and supporting learner responses, encourages students to arrive at their own decisions or to engage in self-assessment about clinical practice. Discussions are not intended to be an exchange of the teacher's ideas to the students. In a discussion, both teacher and student actively participate in sharing ideas and considering alternative perspectives. To be effective, discussions should be carried out in an atmosphere in which learners feel comfortable expressing their own opinions and ideas and questioning others' assumptions. With this safe environment, learners have an opportunity to interact with each other and with the educator and to critique and share ideas.

Guidelines for Clinical Discussions

Discussions can be carried out individually with learners or in a small group. The size of the group for a discussion can range from 2 to 10 people. A larger group makes it difficult for each person to participate. An effective teacher keeps the discussion focused, avoids talking too much with students in a passive role, and avoids side-tracking. While the teacher may initiate the discussion, the interaction needs to revolve around the students, not the teacher. Rephrasing students' questions for them to answer suggests that the teacher has confidence in students' ability to arrive at answers and provides opportunities for students to think aloud and share their reasoning. Open-ended questions without one specific answer encourage higher-level thinking. **Exhibit 7.2** summarizes the roles of the teacher and students in clinical discussions.

EXHIBIT 7.2 Roles of Teacher and Student in Discussions

1. *Teacher*
   Plans discussion
   Presents problem, issue, case for analysis, or asks students to do this
   Develops questions for discussion
   Facilitates discussion with students as active participants
   Develops and maintains atmosphere for open discussion of ideas and issues
   Monitors time
   Avoids side-tracking
   Provides feedback
2. *Student*
   Prepares for discussion
   Participates actively in discussion
   Works collaboratively with group members to arrive at solutions and decisions
   Examines different points of view
   Is willing to modify own view and perspective to reach group consensus
   Reflects on clinical experiences and simulation
3. *Teacher and Student*
   Summarize outcomes of discussion and learning

Purposes of Discussions

Discussions promote several types of learning depending on the goals and structure:

- development of problem solving, higher-level thinking, and clinical judgment skills;
- debriefing of clinical experiences;
- development of cooperative learning and group process skills;
- assessment of own learning; and
- development of oral communication skills.

Every discussion will not necessarily promote each of these learning outcomes. The teacher should be clear about the intent of the discussion so it may be geared to the particular outcomes to be achieved. For instance, discussions for critical thinking require carefully selected questions that examine alternative possibilities and "what if" types of questions. This same type of questioning, however, may not be necessary if the goal is to develop cooperative learning or group process skills.

An important purpose of discussions is to promote development of problem solving, higher-level thinking, and clinical judgment skills. Not all discussions, though, lead to these higher levels of thinking. The key is the type of questions asked by the teacher or discussed among students—questions need to encourage students to examine alternative perspectives and points of view in a given situation and to provide a rationale for their thinking. **Exhibit 7.3** presents strategies for directing discussions toward development of higher-level cognitive skills.

EXHIBIT 7.3 Discussions for Development of Higher-Level Cognitive Skills

Ask students to:

Identify problems in a real or hypothetical clinical situation.
Identify possible alternative problems.
Assess the problem and clinical situation further.
Differentiate relevant and irrelevant information for the problem or issue being discussed.
Discuss their own point of view and others' points of view.
Examine their own assumptions and those of other students.
Identify different solutions and interventions that might be used and why.
Compare possible alternatives and defend the choice of one particular action over another.
Take a position about an issue and provide a rationale both for and against that position.
Reflect on own biases, values, and beliefs that influence thinking.
Evaluate the effectiveness of interventions and approaches to solving problems.

Discussions are valuable to help students think through clinical situations and develop their clinical judgment. Questions in a discussion can be used as prompts to lead students through this process. Prompts are planned questions about clinical judgment to make the students' thinking and decision making visible (Billings, 2019; Hensel & Billings, 2020). The questions in **Table 7.1** are examples of prompts for the development of clinical judgment.

Based on their integrative review of teaching strategies for clinical judgment development in clinical education, Gonzalez and Nielsen (2024) recommended clinical educators deliberately make time for discussion with students during the clinical day, in addition to pre- and postconferences. This dedicated time for discussion allows the educator and students to explore the clinical reasoning related to specific patients and nursing care activities.

Discussions also allow students to reflect on their clinical experience and receive feedback from the educator and also from peers about their decisions and other possible approaches they could use. These discussions are valuable in helping students analyze ethical dilemmas, consider different points of view, and explore their own values and beliefs. Discussions also can promote cooperative learning skills where students work in small groups to review a patient's care and propose alternate hypotheses and interventions, and present the results of their discussions to the rest of the students. These can easily be implemented in a postclinical conference.

Discussions provide a means for students to assess their own learning, identify gaps in their understanding, and learn from others in a nonthreatening environment. Students can ask questions of the group and use the teacher and peers as resources for their learning. If

TABLE 7.1 PROMPTS TO TEACH CLINICAL JUDGMENT

Steps of Clinical Judgment	Possible Prompts
Recognizing Cues	What cues did you recognize? What are the most significant findings? What information was less important or distracting?
Analyzing Cues	What findings did you expect based on the client's diagnosis/concern? Are there any findings that seem contradictory? What other information can you gather to help you determine the significance of the cues? What set of cues are most concerning?
Generating Hypothesis	What is most likely occurring? What makes you say that? What will happen if this is not treated? What else could be going on? Which hypothesis is the most important and should be managed first? What are the risks for ignoring other hypotheses?
Generating Solutions	What are the desired outcomes related to your hypothesis? (Give at least two.) What interventions are indicated? What interventions should be avoided?
Taking Action	What intervention(s) are needed immediately? What interventions can you delegate and to whom? What are the mechanisms of actions of any medications, and what are their major nursing considerations? What specific items will you teach the client? What information would you include in a SBAR report for handoff and any referrals?
Evaluating Outcomes	What follow up data are needed? What findings would show an intervention is working? What findings show an intervention is not effective? Are there any critical values to monitor?

SBAR, situation, background, assessment, recommendation.

Source: Hensel, D., & Billings, D. M. (2020). Strategies to teach the National Council of State Boards of Nursing clinical judgment model. *Nurse Educator, 45*(3), 130. https://doi.org/10.1097/nne.0000000000000773. Reprinted by permission Wolters Kluwer Health, January 4, 2025.

the teacher is effective in developing a safe atmosphere for open discussion, students, in turn, will share their feelings, concerns, and questions as a beginning to their continued development.

The ability to present ideas orally, as well as in written form, is an important competency to be achieved by students in clinical courses. Discussions provide opportunities for students to present ideas to a group, explain concepts clearly, and handle questions raised by others. Participation in a discussion requires formulating ideas and presenting them logically to the group.

CLINICAL CONFERENCES

Clinical conferences are planned discussions in which students share information about their clinical experiences, reflect on them, lead others in discussions, and give formal presentations to the group. Clinical conferences can be face-to-face in the clinical or academic setting, or they can be conducted online. Petrovic et al. (2020) examined the literature on meaningful learning in online clinical postconferences. These conferences allow students to connect theory to practice, reflect on current and future practice, gain support from peers and the educator, provide and receive feedback, obtain mentoring, develop critical thinking and leadership skills, and participate actively in learning. With an online discussion following the clinical experience, students have time for reflection about the care they provided and their interactions with patients and others in the clinical setting.

There are many types of clinical conferences. *Preclinical conferences* are small group or one-to-one discussions with the clinical educator, preceptor, or another clinician that precede clinical learning activities. In preclinical conferences, students can ask questions about their patients or other aspects of clinical practice. An important role of the teacher in preclinical conferences is to ensure that students have the essential knowledge and competencies to complete their clinical activities. In many instances, the teacher needs to instruct students further and fill in the gaps in students' learning.

Postclinical conferences are held at the conclusion of clinical learning activities. Postclinical conferences provide a forum for analyzing patient care and exploring other options, thereby facilitating critical thinking. Postclinical conferences may be used for peer review and critiquing each other's work. They are not intended as substitutes for classroom instruction with the teacher lecturing and presenting new content to students. A similar problem often occurs with guest speakers who treat the conference as a class, lecturing to students about their area of expertise rather than encouraging group discussion and student reflection.

Clinical conferences can also focus on ethical and professional issues associated with clinical practice. Conferences of this type encourage critical thinking about issues that students have or may encounter in the future. In these conferences, students can analyze events that occurred in the clinical setting, ones in which they were personally involved or learned about through their clinical experience. A student can present the situation to the group for analysis and discussion. The discussion should focus on varied approaches that might be used and how to decide on the best strategy.

WRITTEN ASSIGNMENTS

Written assignments for clinical learning have three main purposes: (a) assist students in understanding concepts, theories, and other content that relate to care of patients; (b) develop higher-level thinking skills; and (c) examine feelings, beliefs, and values generated from students' clinical experiences. In choosing written assignments for clinical courses, the teacher should first consider the outcomes to be met through the assignments and the competencies that students need to develop in the course and nursing program. Writing assignments should build on one another to progressively develop students' skills. Another consideration is the number of assignments to be completed. How many assignments are needed to demonstrate mastery? It may be that one well-done assignment is sufficient for meeting the outcomes, and students may then progress to other learning activities. Teachers should avoid using the same written assignments repeatedly throughout a clinical practicum and should instead choose assignments to meet specific learning outcomes or competencies.

Promote Understanding

In written assignments, students can describe concepts and other information relevant to the care of their patients and can explain how that knowledge guided their clinical decisions and judgments. Assignments for this purpose need a clear focus to prevent students from merely summarizing and reporting what they read. Shorter assignments that direct students to apply particular concepts to clinical practice may be of greater value in developing higher-level thinking skills than longer assignments for which students summarize readings without any analysis of them.

Examples of written assignments to promote understanding of concepts and other information related to clinical practice are:

- Compare, in no more than three pages, two interventions appropriate for your patient in terms of their rationale and evidence. How will you evaluate their effectiveness?
- Read a research article related to care of one of your patients, critique the article, report on the analysis, and explain why the research findings are or are not applicable to the patient's care.
- Compare data collected from your patient with the description of that condition in your textbook or other readings. What are similarities and differences? Why?
- Develop a concept map (a graphic arrangement of key concepts related to your patient's care) and provide a written description of the relationships among the concepts in your map.
- Investigate the process used in your clinical setting for handoff. Write a summary report. How does the handoff process relate to concepts you learned in your course about communicating patient information between providers?

Develop Higher-Level Thinking Skills

Written assignments provide an opportunity for students to analyze patient and other problems they have encountered in clinical practice, evaluate their interventions, and propose new approaches. In written assignments, students can analyze data and clinical situations, identify additional assessment data needed for decision-making, identify patient needs and problems, propose approaches, compare interventions based on evidence, and evaluate the effectiveness of care. Students can identify assumptions they made about patients' responses that influenced their clinical decisions, critique arguments, take a stand about an issue and develop a rationale to support it, and draw generalizations about patient care from different clinical experiences.

Written assignments for developing higher level thinking skills can be short, ranging from one to two paragraphs to a few pages. In developing these assignments, the teacher should avoid activities in which students merely report on the ideas and thinking of others. Instead, the assignment should ask students to consider an alternative point of view or a different way of approaching an issue. Short assignments also provide an opportunity for teachers to give prompt feedback to students.

Written assignments should have clear directions that relate the assignment to the specific learning outcome and competency. For example, students may be asked to prepare a one-page paper comparing the physiological processes of asthma and bronchitis. Rather than writing on everything they read about asthma and bronchitis, students can focus their papers on the physiology of these two conditions.

Examples of written assignments for developing higher-level cognitive skills are:

- Describe in one paragraph significant information you collected from your patient and why the information was important to your decisions about approaches to use with that patient.
- Select one need or problem you identified for your patient and provide a rationale for it. What is one alternative need or problem you might also consider and why? Complete this assignment in two typed pages.
- Identify a near-miss (close call) or an unsafe practice that you experienced or observed in your clinical setting. Analyze what went wrong and practices that should have been used. Prepare a response integrating the concept of just culture.
- Identify an issue affecting the community. Provide a rationale for actions to be taken and role of the nurse.
- Identify a procedure you performed in your clinical setting. Find the policy. Was your performance consistent with that policy? Why or why not? Are there deviations or workarounds you observed on the unit with that procedure? Write a report about what you learned.
- Identify a patient you cared for in this or a prior course. Briefly describe the patient. What were the most important contributors to that person's health? How do they relate to the social determinants of health?

Examine Feelings, Beliefs, and Values

Written assignments help learners examine feelings generated from caring for patients and reflect on their beliefs and values that might influence that care. Journals, for instance, provide a way for students to record their feelings about a patient or clinical activity and later reflect on these feelings. Assignments may be developed for students to identify their own beliefs and values and analyze how they affect their interactions with patients, families, and staff. Value-based statements may be given to students for written critique, or students may be asked to analyze an ethical issue, propose alternative approaches, and take a stand on the issue.

Examples of writing assignments that help students explore their feelings, beliefs, and values are:

- Identify an issue that affects healthcare. Read about the issue and write an op-ed (opinion piece) that describes how you would address the issue.
- In your journal, write about your feelings about caring for your patient and other patients in this setting. In what way do those feelings influence your care?
- A peer tells you they forgot to reorder a patient's PRN (pro re nata, as needed) medications but is not telling the nurse practitioner who is serving as the preceptor. The patient never asked about these medications. What would you say to your peer? Why did you choose this approach?
- Think about the community in which your patients live. How does that community influence their health?

Types of Written Assignments for Clinical Learning

Many types of written assignments are appropriate for clinical learning: concept map, short written assignment, nursing care plan, reflective journal, and electronic portfolio.

CONCEPT MAP

A concept map is a graphic or pictorial arrangement of key concepts related to a patient's care, which shows the interrelationships of those concepts. By developing a concept map, students can visualize how assessment data, problems, interventions, medications, and other aspects of a patient's care relate to one another.

Concept maps have many uses in clinical learning. First, students may complete a concept map from their readings to assist them in applying new information to their patients. The readings that students complete for clinical practice, and in nursing courses overall, contain vast amounts of facts and specific information. Concept maps help students process this information in a meaningful way, linking new and existing ideas. Second, concept maps help students prepare for clinical practice. They can be developed prior to or at the beginning of a clinical experience as a way of organizing assessment information, relating it to the patient's problems and care. In preclinical conferences, students can present the maps for feedback from the teacher and from peers. Students can modify the maps as they provide care for patients. Third, concept maps may be developed collaboratively by students in clinical conferences. For this purpose, students might present a patient for whom they have cared, and the clinical group then develops a concept map about that patient's care. As another strategy, students can present the concept maps they developed for their patients, and the group can analyze and discuss them. Critiquing each other's concept maps enhances students' thinking, learning from one another, and group process; it also allows for feedback from the teacher and peers.

SHORT WRITTEN ASSIGNMENT

Short written assignments in clinical courses are valuable for promoting higher level thinking and helping students apply what they are learning in class to clinical practice. Short assignments avoid students' reporting on and summarizing what others have written without thinking critically about the content themselves. With a short assignment, students can analyze patient problems, compare interventions with their evidence, explore decisions that might be made in a clinical situation, analyze an issue and approaches, and analyze a case scenario. Sample assignments are found in **Exhibit 7.4**.

EXHIBIT 7.4 Examples of Short Written Assignments for Clinical Courses

The unit clerk is slow about notifying nursing staff when patients use their call bells. It appears that only the assigned staff will answer the call bells; other nurses and staff who happen to be close by the patient's room will not respond. Develop a quality improvement project to address this issue.

Select an intervention or treatment you used in patient care. Search for evidence related to that intervention or treatment. What were your sources of evidence? Summarize the strength of the evidence and discuss what it means for patient care.

Read the article on loneliness. In no more than one page, explain how you would use that concept in an assessment.

Describe patient-centered care and key attributes.

In the handoff, the nurse reports that your patient "had no pain and walked twice around the room." When you assess the patient, he complains of severe pain and says he has not been out of bed for 24 hours. What are two different ways of approaching this situation? What would you do next and why?

The nurse practitioner who is serving as your preceptor makes a decision to admit a patient with heart failure. The patient is agitated, is short of breath, and has swelling of his ankles and legs. What additional data would you collect? Explain why this information is important and would support readmission.

Identify a decision you made in clinical practice involving either patients or staff. Describe the situation and why you responded that way. Propose another approach that could have been used.

Describe the process on your unit for handoff at the end of the shift. What changes would you propose in that process and why?

NURSING CARE PLAN

With care plans, students can record patient data, identify potential problems, select evidence-based interventions, identify outcomes to be measured, and learn about resources for understanding patient conditions and finding evidence to guide practice. Whether the care plan promotes problem solving and higher level thinking is questionable. Often students develop care plans from their textbook or the literature without thinking about the content. Even if the care plan is an appropriate written assignment for the competencies, the question remains as to how many care plans students need to complete in a clinical course. Once these have been achieved, then students can follow whatever type of patient record is used in the healthcare system, clinic, or community agency.

REFLECTIVE JOURNAL

Journal writing assists students in relating theory to clinical practice, linking concepts to care of patients, and reflecting on their clinical learning activities. In a journal assignment, students can reexamine their clinical decisions and propose alternative actions, developing their higher level thinking and clinical judgment skills. Reflective journals also allow students to examine their own values that can affect patient care and interactions with others and reflect on their experiences in clinical practice. Greenleaf Brown et al. (2022) conducted a review of studies on journaling, with most studies indicating that journaling was effective in promoting reflection and developing clinical judgment and emotional competency.

There are different ways of structuring journals, and the decision should be based on the intended outcomes of using the journal in the clinical practicum. The first step for the teacher is to identify the learning outcomes to be met through journal writing, such as reflecting on clinical decisions or describing feelings in caring for a patient, and then how journal entries should be made. Journals are not intended for grading but provide an opportunity for giving feedback to learners and developing a dialogue with them.

ELECTRONIC PORTFOLIO

An electronic portfolio (e-portfolio) provides an opportunity for students to present projects and other materials they developed in their clinical practicum to document the competencies they achieved (Oermann et al., 2025). Portfolios can represent a student's best work for evaluation or can illustrate the growth and development of competencies over a period of time. These can be prepared using commercially available software, or students can upload their e-portfolios in the course management system or at a website for this purpose. Portfolios are effective for competency-based education because they provide a means of collecting evidence and documenting student achievement of clinical competencies (Janssens et al., 2022).

The content of the e-portfolio depends on its purpose. Examples of these materials include documents that students developed for patient care, papers written about clinical practice, selected journal entries, reports of activities in the clinical setting, group work and products, reflections of experiences, self-assessment, and other products (referred to as artifacts) that demonstrate students' competencies. Planning for this type of assignment as part of the evaluation is described in Chapter 12.

CASES

Cases describe a clinical situation, based on an actual or a hypothetical patient, for students to apply concepts to clinical situations, solve problems, arrive at carefully thought-out decisions, and develop their clinical reasoning and judgment skills. Cases provide a simulated scenario for student review and critique. The case provided for analysis can be short and specific, a longer case study with extensive background information, or an unfolding case that changes over time.

Short Cases

Short cases can be used to avoid directing students' thinking in advance. Depending on how the case is written and the questions asked, these cases are effective for applying concepts and other types of knowledge to clinical practice and for promoting development of higher-level thinking skills. With cases, students can analyze patient data, identify potential hypotheses and problems, and decide on the best approaches in that situation after weighing the evidence. Examples of these cases are presented in **Exhibit 7.5**.

Case Study

Case studies are longer and more comprehensive than short cases, providing background data about the patient, family history, and other information for a more complete picture. For this reason, students can analyze case studies in greater depth than with short cases and present a more detailed rationale for their analysis. In their critique of the case study, students can describe the concepts that guided their analysis, how they used them in understanding the case, and the literature they reviewed. Case studies are effective for mirroring clinical practice, providing opportunities for students to develop clinical judgment skills (Silvestri-Elmore & Burton, 2024). Some educators are using artificial

EXHIBIT 7.5 Examples of Short Cases

Your patient has moderate dementia. She lets the nurse practitioner do a pelvic examination because she has a "woman's problem." The examination shows an anterior wall prolapse. While helping the patient get dressed, the nurse practitioner observes that, as soon as the patient stands up, urine begins leaking onto the floor.

1. List and prioritize this patient's problems. Provide a rationale for how the problems are prioritized.
2. Develop a plan of care.

Your patient is admitted from the ED with severe headache, right-sided weakness, and aphasia. His temperature is normal, pulse 120, respirations 16, and blood pressure 180/120.

1. What are possible reasons for these symptoms? Provide an explanation for your answer.
2. What additional data would you collect on admission to your unit? Why is this information important to planning the patient's care?
3. As a group in postclinical conference, develop this case further. Based on the data you added to the case, what information would you include in a report on this patient to the incoming nurse using SBAR (situation, background, assessment, recommendation)?

Your patient is seen for a prenatal checkup. She is in her 24th week of pregnancy. The nurse practitioner notes swelling of the ankles and around the patient's eyes. The patient says she has not been able to wear rings for a week because of swelling. Her blood pressure is 144/96.

1. What are possible problems that might be occurring for this patient? List all problems given the information in the scenario.
2. What additional data should be collected at this time? Why?

You are working in a pediatrician's office. A patient brings in her son for a checkup after a severe asthma attack a month ago that required emergency care. When you ask the mother how her son is doing, she begins to cry softly. She tells you she is worried about his having another asthma attack and this time not recovering from it. When the pediatrician enters the examination room, the mother is still crying. The physician says, "What's wrong? Look at him. He's doing great. There is no reason to worry."

1. What would you say to the mother, if anything, in this situation?
2. What would you say to the pediatrician, if anything?
3. Analyze this case in the context of patient-centered case.

As you record a patient's vital signs in the electronic medical record, the patient asks you to show the computer screen to her husband so he can read about the diagnoses they are ruling out.

1. What would you say to this patient?
2. What principles guide your decision? Provide a rationale for your response.

You have a new patient, 81 years old, with heart failure. The referral to your home health agency indicates that the patient

(continued)

EXHIBIT 7.5 Examples of Short Cases (CONT.)

has difficulty breathing, tires easily, and has edema in both legs, making it difficult for him to get around. He lives alone.

At your first home visit, you find the patient sitting in a chair with his feet on the floor. During your assessment, he gets short of breath talking with you and has to stop periodically to catch his breath.

1. What are problems you anticipate for the patient? Include a rationale for each of these problems.
2. Describe at least three different nursing interventions that could be used in this patient's care.
3. Specify outcome criteria for evaluating the effectiveness of the interventions you selected.
4. What would you teach the patient? How could you use the teach-back method in this situation?
5. Select one of your interventions and review the evidence on its use. What are your conclusions about the effectiveness of the intervention?
6. Identify one published research study that relates to this patient's care. Critique the study and describe whether you could use the findings in caring for him and patients with similar problems.

A grandmother brings her 8-year-old granddaughter to the office for her annual visit. In reviewing the immunization record, the nurse notices that the child never received the second dose of the measles, mumps, rubella (MMR) vaccine. The nurse tells the grandmother not to worry: Her granddaughter can get the second dose when she is 11 or 12 years old.

1. Do you agree or disagree with the nurse's advice? Provide a rationale for your decision.

Read the following statements: One in three adults and one in five adolescents are overweight. Being overweight is prevalent among certain ethnic groups.

1. What additional information do you need before identifying the implications of this statement for your community?
2. Why is this information important?

The heart failure clinic at your hospital has been effective in reducing the number of readmissions, but to save costs the hospital is closing the clinic. As the nurse practitioner in that clinic, write a report about why the clinic should remain open, with data to support your position. To whom would you send that report and why? Then write a report from the perspective of the hospital administration supporting closure of the clinic.

intelligence tools for developing the case data and scenarios (Reed & Dodson, 2024; Silvestri-Elmore & Burton, 2024). An example of a case study is presented in **Exhibit 7.6**.

Unfolding Cases

In an unfolding case, the clinical scenario changes, thereby creating a simulation for students to analyze. New information is added to the case to indicate a change in the patient's condition, clinical situation, or setting similar to what might occur with an actual patient. As the case unfolds, students analyze the new information and make decisions about relevant actions to take. Studies suggest that unfolding cases promote development of critical thinking, clinical decision making, and clinical judgment skills; self-directed learning; and team collaboration (Cheng et al., 2024; Kassabry et al., 2024; Liu, 2024). **Exhibit 7.7** provides an example of an unfolding case.

EXHIBIT 7.6 Example of a Case Study

Your 44-year-old patient is seen in the physician's office with hoarseness and a slight cough. During the assessment, she tells the nurse that she also has shortness of breath, particularly when walking fast and going up the stairs. She has never smoked. Her vital signs are: blood pressure 120/80; heart rate 88 beats per minute; respirations 32 per minute; and temperature 36.6°C (97.8°F).

The patient is married with two teenage daughters. She works part time as a substitute teacher. She has always been health conscious, watching her weight and eating properly. She tells the nurse how worried she is because she has read about women getting lung cancer even if they never smoked.

1. The physician orders a combined PET/CT scan. What is a PET/CT scan, and why was it ordered?
2. What would you teach the patient about the scan so she understands why it was ordered?
3. Identify a potential diagnosis and add data to the case consistent with that diagnosis. What types of problems would you anticipate for her? Describe nursing management for each of those problems.
4. Add data about the patient and her family to the case. Select a family theory and use it to analyze this family. What did you learn about the family, and how will this influence your care?

Using Cases in Clinical Courses

Cases can be integrated in clinical courses throughout the curriculum to assist students in applying concepts they are learning in their courses to clinical situations of increasing complexity. In beginning courses, teachers can develop cases that present problems that are relatively easy to identify and require standard nursing interventions. At this level, students learn how to apply concepts to clinical situations and think through them. Students can work as a group to analyze cases; explore different perspectives of the case, what students noticed about it, and their interpretations; and discuss possible approaches to use.

In the beginning, the teacher should think aloud, guiding students through the analysis, pointing out significant aspects of the case and their own interpretations. By thinking aloud, the teacher can model the clinical judgment process step by step through a

EXHIBIT 7.7 Example of an Unfolding Case

A patient in extended care is seen by the nurse practitioner (NP) for a cough, wheezing, and shortness of breath. The patient's symptoms are worse at night.

1. What additional data would you expect to be collected by the NP in the initial assessment? Why?
2. The NP orders spirometry. Explain this test and why it was ordered.

The following day the patient has increased shortness of breath, more frequent coughing, and fatigue. She seems slightly confused.

1. Does this new information change your impression of her problems? Why or why not?
2. List possible problems for this patient with a brief rationale to support each one.
3. What will you report to the NP?

EXHIBIT 7.8 Examples of Varying Complexity of Cases

Case for Beginning Student

Your patient reports having bad headaches for the last month. The headaches occur about twice weekly usually in the late morning. Initially, the pain began as a throbbing at her right temple. Her headaches now affect either her right or left eye and temple. The pain is so severe that she usually goes to bed. She also describes pain in her neck, and you note tenderness in the posterior neck on palpation.

1. What type or types of headache might this patient be experiencing?
2. Describe additional data that should be collected. Why is this information important to deciding what is wrong with this patient?
3. Select two interventions that might be used. Provide evidence for their use.

More Complex Case

A 55-year-old patient calls for an appointment because he fell yesterday at home. He has a few bruises from his fall and a tingling feeling in his legs. He had been at the eye doctor's office last week because of double vision.

1. What do you think about this patient?
2. What are possible problems this patient might be experiencing?
3. Plan additional data to collect to better understand those problems and explain why that information is important.

case. As students progress through the curriculum, the cases can become more complex with varied problems and approaches that could be used in the situation. **Exhibit 7.8** provides an example of a case for a beginning student in which the problem is described clearly, and sufficient information is included to decide on how to intervene. The exhibit also includes a more complex case for a higher level student. Complexity can be built into a case by making different problems possible, having an incomplete dataset to interpret, or describing a scenario where multiple approaches may be possible.

Students can analyze cases in a postclinical conference, as an independent activity, or online either individually or in small groups. They can share resources they used to better understand the case. If cases are analyzed individually, further discussion about the case can occur with the clinical group as a whole, or students can post their thoughts and responses online for others to reflect and comment on.

SUMMARY

Clinical teachers should select learning activities based on the competencies to be developed or the learning outcomes. These activities need to be appropriate to students' levels of knowledge and skill but challenging enough to motivate learning. Providing complete nursing care to one or more patients is a typical clinical assignment, but it is not always the most appropriate choice. There are different options for clinical assignments (patient care and various options, management activities, observation, and service learning), which were presented in the chapter.

The chapter also described and provided examples of other clinical teaching methods—discussions, clinical conferences, and written assignments. Discussions are an exchange of ideas in a small group format. Discussions promote several types of learning: developing higher-level thinking and clinical judgment skills, reflecting on clinical experiences, assessing one's own learning, and developing oral communication skills. Clinical conferences are discussions in which students analyze patient care and clinical situations, lead others in discussions about clinical practice, present ideas in a group format, and give presentations to the group. Conferences serve the same goals as any discussion.

Written assignments for clinical learning have three main purposes: to learn about concepts, theories, and other content related to clinical practice; develop thinking skills; and examine values and beliefs that may affect patient care. Not all written assignments achieve each of these outcomes. The teacher decides first on the outcomes to be met, then plans the writing assignment with these outcomes in mind. Many types of written assignments such as concept maps, short written assignments, nursing care plans, reflective journals, and e-portfolios, can be used for clinical learning.

Cases describe a clinical situation developed around an actual or a hypothetical patient for student analysis. Case scenarios can be short, can include background information and be more comprehensive such as with case studies, and can unfold with the clinical situation changing to introduce new information for learners to integrate and analyze. With cases, students apply knowledge and concepts to practice situations, identify patient problems, propose varied approaches for solving them considering evidence, decide on actions to take, and evaluate outcomes. As such, cases provide experience for students in thinking through different clinical situations and developing clinical judgment skills.

CNE®cl EXAMINATION TEST BLUEPRINT CORE COMPETENCIES

1. **Function within the Education and Health Care Environment**
   - A. Function in the Clinical Educator Role
     1. Integrate theory and practice in the clinical setting
     2. Foster professional growth of learners (e.g., coaching, reflection, and debriefing)
     4. Act as a role model of professional nursing within the clinical learning environment
   - B. Operationalize the Curriculum
     2. Identify learner goals and outcomes
     3. Facilitate meaningful and relevant clinical learning activities to promote optimal learning
     5. Implement clinical activities to help learners develop interprofessional collaboration and teamwork skills
     6. Provide opportunities for learners to develop clinical judgment related to course outcomes
     7. Implement academic program's assigned models of clinical teaching consistent with course outcomes (e.g., traditional, preceptor, simulation, dedicated education units)
   - C. Abide by Legal Requirements, Ethical Guidelines, Agency Policies, and Guiding Framework
     2. Assess learner abilities and needs prior to clinical learning experiences
     3. Facilitate learning activities that support the mission, goals, and values of the academic institution and the clinical agency
     7. Demonstrate ethical and legal behaviors in the clinical nurse educator role
2. **Facilitate Learning in the Health Care Environment**
   - A. Implement a variety of clinical teaching strategies congruent with learner needs, desired learner outcomes, course outcomes, setting, and context (e.g., virtual telehealth, in-person, simulation)
   - B. Apply teaching strategies from educational theory and evidence-based teaching practices
   - D. Create opportunities for learners to develop clinical judgment
   - G. Develop collegial working relationships with learners, faculty, and clinical environment personnel
   - H. Demonstrate enthusiasm for teaching, learning, and nursing to help inspire and motivate learners
4. **Apply Clinical Expertise in the Healthcare Environment**
   - E. Adjust learner assignments based on client care needs to assure a culture of safety

LEARNING ACTIVITIES

CourseConnect

To access self-assessment questions and interactive, competency-based learning activities for this chapter, visit www.springerpub.com/courseconnect. See inside front cover and tear-out card for CourseConnect details.

REFERENCES

Billings, D. M. (2019). Teaching nurses to make clinical judgments that ensure patient safety. *Journal of Continuing Education in Nursing*, *50*(7), 300–302. https://doi.org/10.3928/00220124-20190612-04

Bowling, H., Murray, L., Eichler, T., Usher, B., & Fennimore, L. (2022). Connecting nursing students and older adults: An intergenerational service-learning experience. *Nurse Educator, 47*(1), 56–61. https://doi.org/10.1097/nne.0000000000001017

Cheng, C. Y., Hung, C. C., Chen, Y. J., Liou, S. R., & Chu, T. P. (2024). Effects of an unfolding case study on clinical reasoning, self-directed learning, and team collaboration of undergraduate nursing students: A mixed methods study. *Nurse Education Today, 137*, 106168. https://doi.org/10.1016/j.nedt.2024.106168

Gonzalez, L., & Nielsen, A. (2024). An integrative review of teaching strategies to support clinical judgment development in clinical education for nurses. *Nurse Education Today, 133*, 106047. https://doi.org/10.1016/j.nedt.2023.106047

Greenleaf Brown, L., Briscoe, G. S., & Grabowsky, A. (2022). The influence of journaling on nursing students: A systematic review. *Journal of Nursing Education, 61*(1), 29–35. https://doi.org/10.3928/01484834-20211203-01

Hensel, D., & Billings, D. M. (2020). Strategies to teach the National Council of State Boards of Nursing clinical judgment model. *Nurse Educator*, *45*(3), 128–132. https://doi.org/10.1097/nne.0000000000000773

Janssens, O., Haerens, L., Valcke, M., Beeckman, D., Pype, P., & Embo, M. (2022). The role of ePortfolios in supporting learning in eight healthcare disciplines: A scoping review. *Nurse Education in Practice, 63*, 103418. https://doi.org/10.1016/j.nepr.2022.103418

Kassabry, M., Al-Kalaldeh, M., Ayed, A., & Abu-Shosha, G. (2024). The impact of applying unfolding case-study learning on critical care nursing students' knowledge, critical thinking, and self-efficacy; A quasi-experimental study. *Nurse Education in Practice, 78*, 104015. https://doi.org/10.1016/j.nepr.2024.104015

Kuehn, J. (2024). Addressing regional social determinants of health through service learning. *Nurse Educator, 49*(6), 341–342. https://doi.org/10.1097/nne.0000000000001727

Liu, W. (2024). Development of clinical decision-making among undergraduate nursing students: The effect of unfolding case-based learning. *International Journal of Nursing Education Scholarship, 21*(1), 20230115. https://doi.org/10.1515/ijnes-2023-0115

Marcilla-Toribio, I., Moratalla-Cebrián, M. L., Bartolomé-Guitierrez, R., Cebada-Sánchez, S., Galán-Moya, E. M., & Martínez-Andrés, M. (2022). Impact of service-learning educational interventions on nursing students: An integrative review. *Nurse Education Today, 116*, 105417. https://doi.org/10.1016/j.nedt.2022.105417

Mayer, K. A. (2022). Facilitators and barriers to critical service-learning goals in a community-academic relationship. *Nurse Educator, 47*(2), E34-E38. https://doi.org/10.1097/nne.0000000000001101

Mella, A. J. (2021). An integrative literature review on selecting patient assignments for undergraduate nursing students in the clinical setting. *Nurse Education Today, 107*, 105103. https://doi.org/10.1016/j.nedt.2021.105103

Nielsen, A., Lanciotti, K., Garner, A., & Brown, L. (2021). Concept-based learning for capstone clinical experiences in hospital and community settings. *Nurse Educator, 46*(6), 381–385. https://doi.org/10.1097/nne.0000000000000964

Oermann, M. H., Gaberson, K. B., & De Gagne, J. C. (2025). *Evaluation and testing in nursing education* (7th ed.). Springer Publishing Company.

Petrovic, K. A., Hack, R., & Perry, B. (2020). Establishing meaningful learning in online nursing postconferences: A literature review. *Nurse Educator, 45*(5), 283–287. https://doi.org/10.1097/nne.0000000000000762

Reed, J. M., & Dodson, T. M. (2024). Generative AI backstories for simulation preparation. *Nurse Educator, 49*(4), 184–188. https://doi.org/10.1097/nne.0000000000001590

Segura, V. (2024). Expanding clinical placement opportunities: Exploring night shift experiences for nursing students. *Journal of Professional Nursing, 55*(2024), 162–166. https://doi.org/10.1016/j.profnurs.2024.10.007

Silvestri-Elmore, A., & Burton, C. (2024). How can nursing faculty create case studies using AI and educational technology? *Nurse Educator, 50*(1), 35–39. https://doi.org/10.1097/nne.0000000000001734

Wilkinson, M. R., Brown, A. B., & Haras, M. S. (2023). Appalachia: Partnering to create a healthy community using service learning. *The Journal for Nurse Practitioners, 19*(10), 104792 https://doi.org/10.1016/j.nurpra.2023.104792

Yoong, S. Q., Liao, A. W. X., Goh, S. H., & Zhang, H. (2022). Educational effects of community service-learning involving older adults in nursing education: An integrative review. *Nurse Education Today, 113*, 105376. https://doi.org/10.1016/j.nedt.2022.105376

Clinical Simulation

8

OBJECTIVES:

1. Discuss how the Healthcare Simulation Standards of Best Practice™ (HSSOBP™) can be used to enhance clinical teaching and simulation.
2. Describe the importance of facilitator training for integration of manikin-based, standardized patient (SP), and computer-based (CB) simulation.
3. Explain how faculty can design, prebrief, debrief, and evaluate simulation.

"Simulation is a technique—not a technology" (Gaba, 2004, i2). This phrase, over two decades old, remains a foundational statement for understanding healthcare simulation where the focus is not on the equipment or high-technology components, but as a pedagogy and teaching strategy rooted in educational research. Healthcare simulation is a technique that uses a situation where learners experience a representation of a real healthcare event for the purposes of practice, learning, evaluation, testing, or gaining understanding of systems or human actions (Lioce, 2024). The science of healthcare simulation is rapidly evolving and plays an important role in clinical nursing education. Nursing programs have long faced competition for limited clinical placement sites and restrictions on what students can do within patient care facilities. When simulation is integrated appropriately, it can involve students in rich dialogue, set high standards, and promote the future healthcare workplace as a place open to psychologically safe conversations and high-quality feedback (Bradley et al., 2020). Evidence continues to support simulation as a useful teaching-learning option to provide students across all levels of nursing education with immersive, experiential learning opportunities outside the patient care environment. However, there is emerging conversation in the simulation community suggesting that untrained educators in simulation pedagogy, even those with the best intentions, may create undesirable experiences for students, leading to student anxiety, incivility, and even abuse (Kardong-Edgren et al., 2024). This chapter discusses how simulation can be used to enhance clinical teaching according to the most recent iteration of Healthcare Simulation Standards of Best Practice™ (HSSOBP™), including a focus on one of the newest standards, preparation and briefing, and other standards/guidelines used in simulation design. Further, this chapter highlights the importance of appropriate facilitator training for integration of manikin-based, standardized patient (SP), and computer-based (CB) simulation. Lastly, the chapter describes how faculty can design, prebrief, debrief, and evaluate simulation for clinical learning according to best practice and recent evidence informing these different modalities of simulation.

BACKGROUND

The term *simulation activity* describes "the entire set of actions and events from initiation to termination of an individual simulation event. This often begins with the briefing (prebriefing) and ends with the debriefing" (Lioce, 2024, p. 59). The principles and practices discussed in this chapter focus specifically on the use of immersive manikin-based, SP, and CB simulation where a scenario is designed, prebriefed, facilitated, debriefed, and evaluated according to the HSSOBP™.

In general, simulations allow students to develop and demonstrate psychomotor skills, clinical reasoning, clinical judgment, problem-solving, and communication skills. Simulation enables teachers to take specific information—such as a patient's personal characteristics; health information; socioeconomic, family, and community components; and their physical, mental, and emotional states—and weave it into a real-life scenario that enhances a student's comprehension of the material because it is meaningful (Jeffries, 2021). In the case of clinical nursing scenarios, simulation provides an opportunity to suspend disbelief, engage in a re-creation of reality, and experience a lower-risk, hands-on opportunity to practice a clinical situation involving patient monitoring, management, communication, and multidisciplinary collaboration.

Simulation is now a standard educational practice in nursing and medical education and is emerging in other health professions education. Borrowing from aviation and the military, simulation has evolved rapidly over the past century moving from the use of life-sized dolls to teach basic nursing skills, to sophisticated, computerized manikins that can mimic human physiology (Karlsaune et al., 2023), and the incorporation and training with SPs. Simulation is now integrated widely across the curriculum providing opportunities for the development and refinement of competencies while helping students to gain self-confidence prior to entering the clinical setting. Nursing education uses simulation in both prelicensure and advanced practice nursing education in diverse courses including specialty clinical courses, leadership, mental health, and interprofessional education. Further, simulation serves as a valuable form of assessment, evaluation, and remediation as nursing education integrates competency-based learning in the nursing curriculum (American Association of Colleges of Nursing [AACN], 2021; Jeffries et al., 2022; National League for Nursing [NLN], 2023).

Various organizations have recognized simulation's value as a teaching technique. The Commission on Collegiate Nursing Education (CCNE) accreditation standards and the NLN Commission for Nursing Education Accreditation (CNEA) encourage the use of innovative teaching methods and simulation (CCNE, 2024; NLN CNEA, 2021). The NLN has also provided long-standing leadership and support for simulation in nursing education, by conducting a national multisite multimethod study investigating the innovative use of simulation to teach nursing care of ill adults and children (Forneris & Fey, 2016) and by publishing a vision statement, in collaboration with the International Nursing Association for Clinical Simulation and Learning (INACSL) for debriefing across the curriculum (NLN, 2015). NLN's leadership continued, in collaboration with Laerdal Medical, with the development of the Simulation Innovation Resource Center (SIRC). SIRC provides education and training about simulation while also allowing participants an opportunity to engage in dialogue with colleagues about simulation and providing resources for the development and integration of simulation in the curriculum (NLN, 2025b). The NLN Leadership Development Program for Simulation Educators offers an opportunity for experienced simulation nurse educators to examine issues related to research in simulation, curricular integration, and the role of simulation in interprofessional education (NLN, 2025a).

Other organizations, such as INACSL and the interdisciplinary Society for Simulation in Healthcare (SSH), are exclusively dedicated to simulation. INACSL publishes a monthly online journal, *Clinical Simulation in Nursing,* and offers an endorsement program. The SSH publishes two journals, *Simulation in Healthcare* and *Simulation Technician Operations Resource Magazine (STORM)*, and provides certification and accreditation opportunities. These organizations offer a wide variety of webinars, scholarships, and other resources to support both beginning and advanced simulationists. In particular, the HSSOBP™ (INACSL Standards Committee, 2021a) and SSH Dictionary (Lioce, 2024) are referenced extensively throughout this chapter. The Association of SP Educators (ASPE) is emerging as the leading organization on integrating simulation with SPs and has released standards of practice; it also provides an opportunity for accreditation.

The National Council of State Boards of Nursing (NCSBN) National Simulation Study provided evidence supporting the use of simulation. The findings from this national study demonstrated that up to 50% of clinical time could be replaced with high-quality simulation with facilitators trained in simulation pedagogy (Hayden et al., 2014). Since the reporting of this landmark study more than 10 years ago, more than half of boards of nursing in the United States have established regulatory guidelines allowing for replacement of clinical time with simulation (Bradley et al., 2019; INACSL Simulation Regulation Committee, 2021). The evidence informing regulation of simulation in nursing education continues to evolve as researchers explore the equivalence of clinical hours and simulation. For example, Sullivan et al. (2019) and Curl et al. (2016) provided evidence to support counting each hour spent in simulation as 2 hours of supervised clinical experiences. While nursing experts agree that time in direct patient care in clinical experiences is important, there remains a lack of evidence linking clinical learning outcomes in traditional clinical experiences (Leighton et al., 2021), leading educators to innovate with clinical nursing education approaches including simulation.

USING SIMULATION AS AN EVIDENCE-BASED TEACHING STRATEGY

Compelling evidence about the benefits and learning outcomes of simulation is encouraging nurse educators to increase their use of simulation as a teaching strategy. Now in the fourth iteration, the NLN Jeffries Simulation Theory has served as a critical framework guiding the design, implementation, and evaluation of simulation in nursing (Jeffries, 2022). One component of this theory focuses on essential simulation design characteristics. Clinical teachers using simulation need to consider the following design characteristics: objectives, fidelity, problem-solving, student support, and debriefing. Another component involves outcomes that include measures of learning (knowledge), skill performance, learner satisfaction, critical thinking, and self-confidence. Finally, clinical teachers using simulation need to consider the facilitator, the participant, and educational practices (Jeffries, 2022). Many of these concepts are explored later in this chapter.

Today's nursing students benefit from pedagogy that is based on hands-on participation and observation. It is common that learners observe a simulation. There is an increasing body of evidence that establishes that the role of the observer in simulation has substantial theoretical support and learning outcomes that are like those in hands-on participant roles (Johnson, 2020; Johnson et al., 2023; Rogers et al., 2020). By engaging learners directly in the simulation and adhering to the HSSOBP™, active learning occurs for those in both participant and observer roles.

INACSL publishes updated standards approximately every 3 years with essential criteria and required elements for simulation. The HSSOBP™ are found in **Table 8.1** and are discussed further in this chapter.

PREPARING FOR SIMULATION

Clinical nurse educators preparing for simulation should carefully plan these activities to ensure optimal learning. This planning should reflect the HSSOBP™ best practices. Teachers must consider the simulation design, create learner outcomes/objectives, determine simulation modality and fidelity, select or design the clinical scenario, and develop prebriefing activities.

Simulation Design and Outcomes/Objectives

Facilitators need to consider many factors and must purposively design clinical scenarios that are based on the HSSOBP™. Beginning with simulation design, educators should conduct a needs assessment and develop measurable objectives for the simulation experience

TABLE 8.1 HEALTHCARE SIMULATION STANDARDS OF BEST PRACTICE™ (HSSOBP™)

Standard	Importance for Planning, Developing, Implementing, and Evaluating Simulations
Professional Integrity (INACSL Standards Committee et al., 2021b)	This standard refers to the Simulationist Code of Ethics (Park et al., 2018) and the ethical behaviors and conduct for facilitators, learners, and participants. Essential behaviors include following HSSOBP™ standards, promoting diversity and inclusivity, and requiring confidentiality.
Professional Development (INACSL Standards Committee et al., 2021e)	This standard challenges simulationists to conduct educational needs assessments for a professional development plan, participate in activities that support those needs, and continually reevaluate professional development needs for lifelong learning.
Simulation Design (INACSL Standards Committee et al., 2021l)	This standard addresses the multiple criteria that are required in designing a simulation that include: involving content and simulation experts, conducting a needs assessment, constructing objectives, and aligning the modality with objectives. Incorporating other HSSOBP™ at this phase, including prebriefing, debriefing, and evaluation plans, as well as piloting the experience prior to implementation, are necessary.
Outcomes and Objectives (INACSL Standards Committee et al., 2021h)	This standard requires that when designing a simulation, learner objectives are developed based on a needs assessment and guided by course, programmatic, and accrediting body outcomes. Objectives should be learner centered and should drive the choice of simulation modality (not vice versa).
Operations (INACSL Standards Committee et al., 2021c)	This standard examines systems and operations level criteria including developing strategic plans, using space and equipment management systems, financial resources, and policies and procedures to support simulation programs.
Prebriefing: Preparation and Briefing (INACSL Standards Committee et al., 2021f)	This standard requires that simulationists develop a prebriefing plan that supports the purpose and objectives of the learning experience based on learner experience and knowledge level. Learners should have material to prepare them for the simulation. A thorough prebriefing is conducted by the facilitator and includes expectations, agenda, logistics, the establishment of a fiction contract, and providing for psychological safety.
Facilitation (INACSL Standards Committee et al., 2021j)	This standard requires that facilitators have knowledge and skills in simulation pedagogy and follow all HSSOBP™ to support learners prior to, during, and after the simulation experience. The standard addresses numerous criteria for successful simulation experiences.
The Debriefing Process (INACSL Standards Committee et al., 2021d)	This standard requires that all simulation experiences include a planned debriefing. Facilitators should be trained and competent in feedback, debriefing, or guided reflection processes that are structured and based on evidence and theoretically derived concepts.
Evaluation of Learning and Performance (INACSL Standards Committee et al., 2021g)	This standard stresses the importance of determining the level of evaluation that is occurring before the simulation experience. Formative, summative, and high-stakes evaluation all have specific elements of evaluation. If this standard is not followed, students may be dissatisfied or the evaluation may not be accurate.
Simulation-Enhanced Interprofessional Education (INACSL Standards Committee et al., 2021k)	This standard supports the integration of simulation with interprofessional education (IPE). Simulations with IPE should be based on theoretical frameworks. The design of a simulation with IPE should begin with all disciplines and be based on an agreed needs assessment with appropriate evaluation.
Glossary (INACSL Standards Committee et al., 2021i)	This standard provides guidance for using consistent terminology related to simulation experiences and should be used with the Healthcare Simulation Dictionary (Lioce, 2024).

(INACSL Standards Committee et al., 2021l). The simulation design standard emphasizes the need to select the simulation modality based on the learning objectives, incorporate an appropriate level of fidelity, include prebriefing and debriefing activities, and consider the assessment of not only the participant, but also the simulation experience, environment, and facilitator. Finally, all simulations should be piloted prior to implementation with learners. Program outcomes and course objectives should direct the type of simulation needed (INACSL Standards Committee et al., 2021h). For example, if a clinical or course objective focuses on client assessment, teachers might decide to create a simulation that has a patient experiencing shortness of breath, decreased oxygen saturation, and abnormal breath sounds. During the simulation, learners could use their problem-solving and critical thinking skills to explore the respiratory status of the patient and complete a respiratory assessment.

Simulation Modalities

Depending on the objectives of the simulation, educators should then select the appropriate modality of simulation aiming to reach a specific level of fidelity. The terms *modality* and *fidelity* are often confused, but what is important is that the modality and fidelity are set *after* the learning objectives are established.

Simulator modality is an overarching term that includes, but is not limited to, manikins, haptic devices, partial task trainers, CB simulation, and SPs (Lioce, 2024). The most common form of simulation is manikin-based, where simulation involves a lifelike manikin that represents a patient with heart and lung sounds, pulses, voice interaction, and other responses that may be controlled by a simulationist using a computer (Lioce, 2024, p. 37). Skill acquisition is often demonstrated on task trainers or partial-task trainers where a simulator is designed for procedural training.

Simulation with SPs, also known as simulated participants or embedded participants, refers to a simulation in which the role of the patient is performed by an individual who is trained to portray a real patient (Lioce, 2024, p. 43). SP simulation must adhere to not only the HSSOBP™, but also to the ASPE Standards of Best Practice (Lewis et al., 2017). This form of simulation incorporates live actors with scripts that portray patients and requires nursing students to engage in nursing care activities with the SP in an environment that simulates patient care areas (Jeffries et al., 2022). Practice with SPs can provide invaluable learning opportunities for students as they refine their communication skills or practice in sensitive or specialized clinical situations. SPs can offer valuable feedback and insight about the patient perspective to the nursing student (Johnson et al., 2020). Involving SPs has also been used for development of competencies such as obtaining a health history, conducting physical health assessments, and demonstrating psychomotor skills. Using an SP can be useful both as a teaching strategy and as an evaluation approach (Costa & Monger, 2024).

Finally, CB simulation is a term that is used to describe activities that involve interactions with simulated systems including virtual patients, screen-based interfaces, and games (Goodwin & Nestel, 2024; Lioce, 2024). Virtual reality, one type of CB simulation, involves a computer-generated 3-D image viewed through a headset. Augmented reality, another type of CB simulation, overlays a computer-generated image, environment, or content to a real-world space (Foronda et al., 2020; Mendez et al., 2020).

While virtual simulation is newer to nursing education, it is increasingly adopted in clinical education. There is substantial evidence through meta-analysis and systematic reviews supporting virtual simulation and its association with positive learning outcomes (Chen et al., 2020; Choi et al., 2022; Foronda et al., 2020). The COVID-19 pandemic provided a catalyst for closer examination of the use of virtual and other CB simulation in healthcare education. Simulated healthcare experiences on one's computer have been used successfully for more than a decade and is an effective teaching method that improves learning outcomes (Foronda et al., 2020; Kononowicz et al., 2019). As nursing shifts toward competency-based education, there is promising evidence supporting CB simulation and the development of increased clinical judgment with the opportunity to provide more realistic learning experiences, resulting in learners feeling more present (Armstrong et al., 2025; Bradley et al., 2024).

Unlike traditional manikin-based and SP-based simulations, CB simulations allow participants to engage with the scenarios at a convenient time and place. Multiple students can complete the simulation and actively participate in the nursing case. Depending on how the CB simulation is designed, the student may receive immediate performance feedback and repeat the simulation. In addition, research has developed best practices for debriefing virtual simulations, and these should be carefully considered when adopting CB simulation pedagogy (Verkuyl et al., 2020). There are opportunities to integrate feedback and redo a simulation, thus making CB simulations ideal for enhanced learning and remediation activities. CB simulations may offer a cost-effective alternative to clinical site visits and performance evaluations, particularly for online or geographically disbursed students. One study comparing manikin-based and CB simulations demonstrated similar learning outcomes between the two types of simulation, but improved cost–utility was associated with the CB simulations (Haerling, 2018). In addition, another study supported that when observing a simulation through virtual telepresence, there were similar learning outcomes compared to learners in active participant simulation roles and traditional observer roles (Dang et al., 2021). As evidence continues to emerge, CB simulation has a bright future for its place in nursing education.

Simulation Fidelity

Clinical nurse educators also should consider simulation fidelity when planning their learning experiences. Fidelity is the "the ability of the simulation to reproduce the reactions, interactions, and responses of the real-world counterpart" (Lioce, 2024, p. 23) and includes conceptual, physical/environmental, and psychological fidelity. Conceptual fidelity reflects the degree to which the case makes sense (INACSL Standards Committee et al., 2021l). For example, do the respiratory rate, blood pressure, and heart rate of the simulator fluctuate in a way that is congruent with the case? All components of the simulation must fit together appropriately. If the simulation scenario involves a patient having a myocardial infarction, then the subjective and objective data provided to the student should be consistent and reflect the typical activities that would normally occur. Physical/environmental fidelity reflects the degree to which the simulation room, props, equipment, and manikin or SP represent the environment being simulated (INACSL Standards Committee et al., 2021l). To support physical fidelity, the teacher should consider the setting, the use of moulage, and realism of the equipment. Finally, psychological fidelity reflects the degree to which the simulated scenario evokes the feelings and thought processes learners would experience if they were involved in a similar scenario in real life (INACSL Standards Committee et al., 2021l).

Increased fidelity and higher technology modalities do not necessarily translate to improved learning outcomes. The objectives of the simulation should dictate the level of fidelity. The type of simulator used in a scenario will affect the level of fidelity. However, it is not the only factor to consider. A task-trainer, such as a disembodied pelvis for catheter insertion simulation or a gel pad for intramuscular injection practice, may offer the appropriate level of fidelity for the learning objective such as demonstrating appropriate technique for a specific skill. Similarly, a simple manikin that produces heart and lung sounds, but does not offer the realism of chest movement, is useful for certain scenarios such as completing an assessment that does not require the interactive features of a more sophisticated simulator. Computerized patient simulators produce the most lifelike scenarios. These full-size manikins react to student manipulations in real time and in realistic ways, such as speaking, coughing, and demonstrating chest movements and pulses.

Scenario Selection/Design

Once some of these preliminary decisions about the simulation have been determined, then clinical nurse educators can create or select the scenario. Scenario development incorporates evidence and professional standards but is also a creative process. The use of a simple storyboard template can provide structure without being overwhelming for teachers who are developing their first scenarios. The template typically includes the specific objectives for the simulation activity, simulator settings and other actions, types of cues that the patient and other team members may provide to the students, expected student actions, and suggested debriefing and reflection topics. The use of a storyboard template by clinical educators as they develop scenarios will increase consistency across a curriculum and encourage them to start with basic information (e.g., identifying three to five simulation objectives and learning outcomes). Further, it is important during the scenario design phase to consider cues that will be delivered that keep learners on track to achieve learning objectives and that are in line with the story and fidelity of the scenario (INACSL Standards Committee et al., 2021j; INACSL Standards Committee et al., 2021l).

Like other learning activities, begin with the objectives and work backward to develop a simulation scenario that will help learners achieve those objectives. If there are specific specialty areas students are not able to access in the clinical environment, these might be areas to first develop for simulation activities. For example, if existing student outcome data reflect deficits in communication, teamwork, medication administration, or other topics, consider simulation as an opportunity for addressing these deficits. The level of the students, specific course objectives, and teacher's clinical expertise all need to be considered when specifying an appropriate learning outcome.

Drawing on common situations seen in clinical practice or relying on past clinical cases will help provide ideas for scenario creation. If using ideas or information from actual patients, make sure case details are generic and that patient privacy is not compromised by revealing too much personal or identifiable information. Sometimes scenarios are a compilation of many patients seen in clinical practice. Scenarios often incorporate unique aspects of care that can be vividly portrayed in simulations. For example, simulations that use a cluttered, dusty, and insect-infested home during a home health simulation; stressed, arguing parents as part of a pediatric simulation; or a patient experiencing homelessness, low literacy skills, comorbidities, and limited support systems can effectively portray challenging situations that nurses face in practice. Regardless of the method used to create scenarios, it is important to ensure that they are student-centered, interactive, related to outcomes, and based on best practices.

Many nursing education programs access or purchase existing scenarios from publishers, simulation manufacturers, other nursing education programs, and professional organizations. These already-developed materials aid teachers by providing well-constructed scenarios with the completed template of essential information and support data needed to implement the simulation. When using prepackaged scenarios, it is important to check alignment with course and program outcomes and needs. Further, when developing scenarios, the use of artificial intelligence (AI) and large language model (e.g., ChatGPT) are also useful for teachers desiring to create realistic patient scenarios. Clinical educators can incorporate local or regional information or patient demographics into the simulation patient's background. AI for simulation creation or support should be used carefully and clinical educators should ensure that information provided is accurate and aligned with objectives. Sometimes tailoring these scenarios to the needs of an individual clinical course may be necessary. Regardless of the origin of the scenario, the scenarios should use lifelike situations that are appropriate for the level of students and clinical course. Fictional characters, popular names, or unrealistic situations should not be incorporated into simulation.

Once the scenario is written, teachers should schedule time with lab staff members (equipment managers and information technology experts for programming the equipment) for a pilot or practice session of the simulation, ideally with students and clinical educators present. Reviewing scenarios for accuracy, current evidence-based practice guidelines, and unnecessary distracters will ensure the quality of the simulation experience for all and help to identify needed resources (e.g., teacher and staff support, props, space, time). Finally, the nurse educator should prepare the manikin or SP with props and include appropriate moulage or a reproduction of special effects so that students are further immersed in a lifelike clinical environment. Further, because electronic health record (EHR) use and its relationship to patient safety and prevention of adverse events has been documented, teachers should consider use of this technology as part of the simulation (Kim et al., 2025). Some nursing programs are using EHRs as a tool to enhance clinical simulation whereas other programs seek to evaluate EHR competency (McBride et al., 2024). Students can use the academic EHR to access simulated patient records and document care provided during a simulation, thus giving students an opportunity to develop these essential informatics skills in a safe environment (Hansbrough et al., 2020). Creating a database of mock patient records as part of the EHR that can be accessed and used during simulation will enhance realism while allowing students to access longitudinal patient data and help ensure that students develop the knowledge and skills needed to function in a technology-rich clinical environment.

Preparation and Prebriefing/Briefing

Learners should be set up for success in simulation and using prebriefing will facilitate the simulation experience. While prebriefing occurs immediately prior to the simulation, there should be thoughtful consideration of prebriefing during the simulation planning and design process. Teachers need to ensure that students participating in simulation experiences see this as a realistic environment and consider various factors when preparing the clinical scenario for simulation. One of the newest HSSOBP™ standards, the Preparation and Briefing standard, suggests that learners have presimulation activities that are thoughtfully scaffolded, enabling them to engage in the simulation and achieve the objectives (Diaz & Anderson, 2021; INACSL Standards Committee et al., 2021f). This required preparation should not just be a reading assignment. Rather, clinical educators and simulation facilitators should consider a variety of activities including videos, websites, and focused readings that will expose learners to content that will directly assist them in achievement of learning outcomes. Often, teachers will use the learning management system, or even email, to provide simulation preparatory material. Teachers may plan learning activities that require students to complete an assignment prior to the simulation, such as reading relevant pathophysiology content, reviewing medications that will be used during the simulation, completing preparation worksheets, practicing technical skills, viewing internet resources, or watching a video or online presentation.

Simulation is not intended to be an activity where learners arrive without any preparation. Evidence supports that while debriefing has a major impact on learning outcomes, prebriefing is essential for a successful debrief (McDermott, 2016). Additionally, learner preparation even for those in the observer role can be designed for optimal learning outcomes (Johnson & Fey, 2023). Learner preparation is only one portion of the preparation and briefing standard.

Other Planning Considerations

There are a variety of factors that the clinical nurse educator should consider when planning for the simulation experience. **Exhibit 8.1** provides questions to consider during the simulation planning. Once these areas have been considered, then further simulation development or selection can occur.

EXHIBIT 8.1 Questions to Consider During Simulation Planning

- What level of student will be participating in the simulation? (e.g., first year prelicensure nursing students versus advanced practice nurses)
- What is the past simulation experience of the students? What is the past clinical experience of the students?
- Will the students need to be oriented to any part of the simulation activities?
- How many students will be participating in the simulation? What are their nursing roles during nursing simulation (nurse, observer, etc.)?
- How does the simulation build upon prior nursing content?
- What new information may be introduced during the simulation?
- What is the reason for the simulation (a clinical day or a make-up activity for a clinical absence)?
- What amount of time is needed for the simulation activities (including introduction to the simulation, prebriefing, and debriefing)?
- Who will be providing simulation operations support?
- Are the needed manikins and resources available?

FACILITATING SIMULATION

Facilitating simulation using the HSSOBP™ best practices requires the clinical nurse educator to prepare prebriefing and briefing activities. Educators will also need to facilitate and implement the simulation scenario.

Preparation and Prebriefing

Prebriefing is an important component of simulation. It involves planning, briefing, and facilitating (McDermott, 2020). Successful prebriefing should establish a psychologically safe learning environment so learners are able to take risks. Psychological safety is one of the most important concepts that can be established in simulation and healthcare environments as it has been directly shown to impact team communication and errors in healthcare (Edmondson, 2019; Rudolph et al., 2014). In simulation, learners need to balance carrying out interventions on a manikin or SP and being watched by their faculty and possibly peers. Learners in simulation, especially those in active participant roles, are at risk of being judged (Brazil & Purdy, 2020).

Often, simulationists hear concerns from faculty and clinical partners that all the preparatory and briefing work is viewed as coddling learners and that establishing psychological safety is "soft" in nature and unrealistic to the "real" world of clinical environments. In a powerful blog, "Safe, Not Soft—Hitting the Sweet Spot for Simulation Based Education," the authors remind faculty that psychological safety is anything but soft; rather, it is a place where learners are held to high expectation and in high regard (Brazil & Purdy, 2020; Rock et al., 2020). It is also where learners feel comfortable taking risks with their thinking, learning from mistakes, and receiving high quality feedback. The authors emphasize that psychological safety is not created all at once; rather, it is created over time (Brazil & Purdy, 2020). The work that facilitators do in the prebriefing helps learners take risks in the simulation environment and is critical for successful debriefing (McDermott, 2016). The Center for Medical Simulation (2024) established The Basic Assumption™, which is a statement read in prebriefing. It encourages risk taking and allows leaders to do their best. Clinical nurse educators may wish to incorporate this or a similar statement into their simulation prebriefing. The Basic Assumption is available at https://harvardmedsim.org/resources/the-basic-assumption/. It is important to note that simply stating beliefs about risk taking prior to simulation does not establish psychological safety. Rather, it is through the actions of the facilitator during prebriefing, simulation, debriefing, and continued experiences in simulation, that will result in learners feeling psychologically safe.

The fiction contract is another component of the prebrief that is important to discuss with learners (INACSL Standards Committee et al., 2021f). The fiction contract is designed as a partnership agreement with facilitators and learners to act as if the events are real even though the experience is taking place in a simulated setting (Rudolph et al., 2014). During the prebrief, facilitators can use statements such as, "I have done everything I can to make this as real as possible, but in the end, it is not reality; I have to depend on you. I ask you to do your best to act as if this is real so that the time we have together is to our best advantage" (Rudolph et al., 2014, p. 342).

Next, provide students with the learning objectives and a brief history of the patient and the diagnosis. This allows students to answer some key questions in preparation for the simulation experience. This part of the prebriefing offers an opportunity for the teacher to assess student preparation for the experience, check on essential student knowledge, review background information about the patient in the simulation, provide instructions, and assign roles for the simulation. Prebriefing is also an opportunity to review expectations about student performance, remind students about confidentiality of the experience, and address the purpose of video recording simulations for continuous quality improvement. Remind students that simulation videos are stored confidentially. Students should be oriented to the simulation room as well as the functions of the manikin, equipment available inside and outside of the room, and how to contact resources (e.g., physician, laboratory, charge nurse.)

during the simulation. Students also should have an idea how long the simulation and overall experience will take as well as logistics of the day including number of breaks and cell phone use, as this indicates the facilitator's care and concerns about learners' needs (Rudolph et al., 2014).

Facilitating the Scenario

Many times, the simulation begins with a report or review of background information about the patient in the form of a handoff or change-of-shift report. It also may include a brief review of the relevant patient health history. Students begin the scenario and enact the assigned roles, which may include primary nurse, charge nurse, medication nurse, or an observer. While often students will engage in the role of a family member, it is important that students of one profession are not portraying roles of another profession. Students should be following the guidelines of their own profession (INACSL Standards Committee et al., 2021b). Instead, SPs can be trained by an expert to act in the role of other health professionals. Or there may be opportunities to collaborate with other disciplines who can serve in their respective roles during the simulation, offering an opportunity for students to engage in interprofessional collaborative practice (INACSL Standards Committee et al., 2021k). The teacher controlling the simulation uses the preplanned scenario to respond to student actions during the simulation. Teachers may use either preprogrammed patient vocal responses or spontaneously respond to student questions and actions on behalf of the simulated patient. Teachers should allow students to make mistakes, solve problems throughout the scenario, and find their own way. Many nursing education programs have video recording capabilities that allow for a recording of all scenario events. These recordings can be used for debriefing after the simulation if there are specific actions the facilitator desires to review.

Finally, as the scenario continues, the facilitator should deliver predetermined cues that were developed during the design phase, or unplanned cues also known as lifesavers, that align with the fidelity of the simulation (INACSL Standards Committee et al., 2021j). Cues can be delivered in a variety of ways. Examples include delivering cues through SPs, laboratory values, comments from the patient or family member, or through equipment alarms (INACSL Standards Committee et al., 2021j).

DEBRIEFING AND GUIDED REFLECTION

Simulation-based educational activities should always include a planned debriefing process. This debriefing process may include activities related to feedback, debriefing, and/or guided reflection (INACSL Standards Committee et al., 2021d). This is not a lecture opportunity. Rather, time immediately following simulation should be guided by the use of established guidelines implemented by formally trained debriefers. Debriefing has been identified as critical for students' learning and satisfaction with their simulation experience; however, it requires adequate time and some preplanning to be effective. Debriefing encourages reflection and self-awareness, and assists in the transfer of knowledge to practice (Alexander et al., 2015; INACSL Standards Committee et al., 2016d). Debriefing allows students to derive meaning from the experience, critique performance while reinforcing learning, and figure out how to apply information to practice.

Because debriefing is critical for learning, teachers need to plan carefully and consider the methods, format, and approach used while also ensuring that they can effectively facilitate this activity. Fey et al. (2022) provided a framework to help teachers identify whether teaching, coaching, or debriefing using the "With Good Judgment" method is appropriate for the learning activity. Similarly, teachers should identify an accepted method for debriefing and receive formal training. It is important to recognize that good lecturing does not equate with high quality debriefing. While these skills in debriefing can inform teaching practice across the curriculum, debriefers should be evaluated regularly and receive coaching feedback about their debriefing (Bradley et al., 2022). Bradley et al. (2022) identified that debriefers may occasionally overestimate their own performance in debriefing and emphasized that regular evaluation of debriefing skills is important. Woda et al. (2023) found that asynchronous training followed by feedback also resulted in improved debriefing.

Clinical educators can select the debriefing approach they want to use. Simulation debriefing methods are listed in **Exhibit 8.2**.

An oral or written format, or a combination of both, may be used to accomplish debriefing. Oral debriefing or discussions about simulation can be done in groups or with individual simulation participants. Group debriefing allows observers, typically other clinical students who observed the simulation, to participate in the debriefing process. Student observers and teachers can provide valuable insight and suggestions after watching the simulation. They may notice actions that the students in the nurse's role may not be aware of and can offer insight from their unique perspective of observer. Sometimes the debriefing process can be sensitive and anxiety-provoking, particularly if the student performance is deficient or problems were encountered. If group debriefing is used, then the teacher should facilitate the use of honest, respectful, and supportive feedback that reinforces elements of The Basic Assumption, or core beliefs about student

EXHIBIT 8.2 Simulation Debriefing Methods

- Debriefing With Good Judgment/Teaching, Coaching, or Debriefing "With Good Judgment"
- Debriefing for Meaningful Learning©
- Diffuse, Discover, Deepen (3D Model)
- Gather-Analyze-Summarize (GAS)
- Promoting Excellence and Reflective Learning in Simulation (PEARLS)

learning in simulation. Often, during prebriefing, facilitators will state that simulation is a place to learn from mistakes. Therefore, how learners are questioned during the debriefing will reinforce whether it is safe to make mistakes in a simulation environment. Thus, it is of utmost importance that debriefers are trained to ask questions in ways that promote psychological safety. It is also important to demonstrate regard for the student and emotional aspect of this experience (INACSL Standards Committee et al., 2016d).

Regardless of the approach used for oral debriefing, teachers should anticipate and plan for adequate time for debriefing. Debriefing typically occurs immediately after the simulation scenario ends. Only during summative and/or high stakes testing environment is feedback not immediate; however, feedback should occur once all testing is complete. This timing for debriefing is helpful in that students can recall recent events and discuss them while they are still current. However, some students may benefit from some additional time to process the simulation events and think about the experience, or they may prefer to privately reflect about the experience in writing rather than orally in a public forum.

Time required for debriefing varies based on several factors including the objectives of the simulation, level of simulation participants, actions of simulation participants within the scenario, and practical time constraints (Dreifuerst et al., 2021). Journaling activities can be assigned to encourage students to personally reflect on the experience, but should not completely replace structured and oral debriefing. Electronic activities such as blogging (in a private rather than public format) or threaded electronic discussions can also be used to engage students who are digital natives and promote reflection after simulation. Either structured or unstructured approaches can be used. For example, students can be asked to compose a reflective journal entry that uses a broad prompt, such as, "Write about what you learned from the simulation." Or they can write more specifically about what went well and what could be improved. Structured prompts could direct students to write about specific examples of actions during the simulation. For example, "What were you thinking when the patient complained of shortness of breath during the simulation? What actions did you take and what else could you have done to address this situation?"

Clinical educators should consider the use of technology for the debriefing, such as whether and how to incorporate video replay of the simulation. It is important to consider the purpose of the video replay in addition to the risks and benefits of creating and using video recordings of simulation activities. Caution should be exercised to prevent inappropriate distribution of the video and potential violation of student confidentiality. Video review can be required as part of the written journaling activities previously discussed. Limited research is available to provide clear guidance about best uses of video replay; however, use of select video snippets of the simulation may help to remind students what happened during the simulation and could lead to rich debriefing discussions.

Once decisions about the method, format, and approach to debriefing are complete, the teacher needs to implement activities that will ensure an appropriate climate for debriefing. The instructor's role during debriefing is that of facilitator, coach, or guide—not lecturer and monopolizer of debriefing conversations. At the beginning of a debriefing session, the teacher should orient students to the debriefing process and code of conduct, review the objectives of the simulation, discuss confidentiality, and articulate teacher expectations for students' participation in evaluating themselves and their peers (INACSL Standards Committee et al., 2016d). Teachers should establish a trusting environment because students may feel vulnerable and anxious, particularly if video playback is used. Sensitive issues need to be openly discussed in a constructive and supportive manner. Once the ground rules of the debriefing session are complete, then discussion about the events and experiences can begin. Most debriefing methods consist of a reaction/description phase, an analysis phase, and a summary phase, and so adequate time is needed to explore each phase of debriefing. As students share their impressions and reflections, teachers should listen, redirect discussion as appropriate, and encourage participation.

The use of probing open-ended questions, particularly during the analysis phase of debriefing, will help to engage students in reflective conversations and explore the thinking and actions that occurred during the simulation. **Exhibit 8.3** provides some sample questions that can be incorporated into simulation debriefing. It is important to not rely solely on planned questions about content; rather, the debriefer should ask questions about specific behaviors observed and why the learner did what they did. Fey and Johnson (2023) encourage debriefers to also remain curious about positive performance and not assume that just because appropriate actions are observed that the thought processes were correct. The debriefing is also a place to reinforce positive actions and positive thinking that healthcare professionals would value seeing in practice (Fey & Johnson, 2023). The teacher should use

EXHIBIT 8.3 Sample Debriefing Questions

Was there anything you missed in the report, or was there other information that you needed so you could act more effectively?
What knowledge do you still need to manage the situation more effectively?
What areas require further practice?
What would you do differently the next time? Why?
Why do you think the patient responded in the manner that they did?
What were you thinking about during the simulation?
Why did you complete the nursing actions in the order that you did?
How could you have acted differently to meet the patient's needs more effectively and efficiently?
What problems did you identify?
What would you do similarly and/or differently if you encountered a similar case?
What If the patient had ___________ (similar pathophysiologic presentation), what would you do similarly and/or differently?

Socratic questions, or questions that the facilitator does not know the answer to, to promote student discussion and higher-level thinking. Not all questions are Socratic, and therefore, training in this type of questioning is recommended (Dinkins & Cangelosi, 2019). During this analysis phase of debriefing, there is a strong focus on assimilation, accommodation, and anticipation. This helps learners see how concepts fit together and differ, and how learning from one situation can be applied to another (Dreifuerst, 2015).

Finally, debriefers should know it is possible to have psychologically safe conversations while asking about unsafe behaviors (Brazil & Purdy, 2020); however, the emphasis on debriefing training, evaluation, and continued training cannot be overstated. Improved debriefing is an element that should be considered in long-term professional development plans for simulation facilitators (INACSL Standards Committee et al., 2021e).

The teacher should conclude the debriefing session with some closing statements about what students identified as effective and efficient, areas they need to work on and takeaway learning messages to summarize the experience. Thanking students for their participation and stating the teacher's appreciation for their attention, efforts in enacting the scenario, and shared reflections provide positive reinforcement and show respect for their efforts.

EVALUATING SIMULATIONS

The final aspect of clinical simulation is evaluation, which involves activity evaluation as well as learner performance evaluation. Activity evaluation is necessary for continuous quality improvement for a simulation program. As simulations occur, teachers can easily identify areas that are working and areas that are problematic. The dynamic process of the simulation allows for some modification during use, but careful note-taking during the scenario and after the debriefing session with students will document changes necessary to enhance the effectiveness of the simulation for the future. Another method commonly used for simulation evaluation involves asking for student feedback or reactions to the experience. This evaluation can occur in a group debriefing session or individually by each student in a written format. This information, while not directly linked to performance, will provide valuable data about the simulation experience, allowing teachers to consider further revisions and improvements. Reviewing student feedback with teachers and simulation specialists who assisted with the technology component of simulation soon after the scenario is completed provides the best opportunities for change and revision. Further, there are numerous resources for facilitators to evaluate elements of the scenario, facilitation, and debriefing using instruments that have demonstrated validity and reliability and provide comprehensive simulation program evaluation, necessary for simulation center accreditation. The website https://www.healthysimulation.com/tools/evaluating-healthcare-simulation/ provides a list of these instruments and how and where to use them for evaluation.

There are also a variety of ways to assess student performance and determine whether the simulation enabled attainment of the learning objectives. The HSSOBP™'s Evaluation of Learning and Performance refers to times when simulation is used to evaluate learner performance (INACSL Standards Committee et al., 2021g). Regardless of the evaluation approach used, clinical educators should select instruments with demonstrated reliability and validity and determine if formative, summative, or high-stakes evaluations will be completed. Student behaviors can be assessed for level of independence, prompting, accuracy, timeliness, and appropriate sequence of activities.

Instruments exist for evaluating multiple aspects of simulation including the facilitator and educational strategies, the participant, simulation design, and simulation outcomes (Haerling, 2021). Two instruments that have been used extensively in the literature to evaluate simulation participant performance are the Creighton Competency Evaluation Instrument (C-CEI) and the Lasater Clinical Judgment Rubric (LCJR). The C-CEI addresses performance in the areas of assessment, communication, clinical judgment, and patient safety (Creighton University, 2025). The developers of the instrument provide extensive resources including access to training and the instrument on their website (https://www.creighton.edu/nursing/academics/competency-evaluation-instrument).

The LCJR is based on Tanner's Model of Clinical Judgment and reflects the four aspects of clinical judgment: noticing, interpreting, responding, and reflecting (Lasater, 2007). Each of the 11 items on the rubric is accompanied by language describing beginning, developing, accomplished, and exemplary performance. This language is useful not only for evaluating performance, but for communicating with simulation participants about their performance and how to improve in the future. Widespread use of both the C-CEI and LCJR contributes valuable evidence about their appropriateness for evaluating student performance.

CLINICAL SIMULATION INTEGRATION INTO THE CURRICULUM

Simulation activities can be integrated into clinical learning in a variety of ways. First, simulation offers opportunities to prepare students for clinical care by offering practice of psychomotor skills, communication, clinical reasoning, and various competencies in a simulated environment. By involving a group of clinical students in simulation activities, students have an opportunity to deliver care, observe performance, reflect on their learning, and critique their practice and that of peers. Simulation also provides a standardized experience for students. It is particularly useful when the clinical teacher would like all students to have practice in a situation that may not be available to everyone due to variability in patient census or setting constraints. Creating a simulation scenario involving a high-risk, life-threatening situation allows all students to experience the same scenario without the potential safety concerns to the patient. Further, creating a simulation scenario around common, everyday situations, such as discharge teaching, allows all students to gain additional experience with patient care clinical activities.

Simulation can also be used as a clinical makeup activity to provide additional clinical learning when a student is absent. Or it can be used for additional review and practice to help remediate at-risk students who are having trouble mastering clinical competencies. Students can participate in repeat practice opportunities with simulation. With video-recording capabilities, simulations can be saved and used for other learning activities such as clinical conferences. Finally, simulation can be used for evaluation purposes as either a way to ensure all students demonstrate satisfactory performance or for competency assessment.

FUTURE IMPLICATIONS

The use of simulation for clinical teaching continues to evolve. Further research is indicated, and some suggestions are provided.

- Simulation research in nursing education needs to move from small-scale, single-site descriptive studies to robust multisite experimental designs using strong methodology, adequate sample sizes, and measurement tools that produce reliable results.
- Nurse educators should continue to work with other related professions to conduct interprofessional simulation activities and evaluate their effectiveness.
- Continued research is needed to demonstrate the efficacy of all types of simulation in nursing education and provide sound, evidence-based support for simulation activities.
- Teacher support, resources, and curricular integration require administrative support, affordable simulation software, and evaluation systems that streamline faculty efforts. As simulation continues to advance, ongoing faculty training on the latest developments is essential to keep nurse educators up-to-date on simulation advances.
- Research regarding the impact of simulation and debriefing on transition to practice and patient outcomes is still needed.

SUMMARY

Clinical simulation plays an increasingly important role in nursing education, and nurse educators will continue to be called on to develop, implement, and evaluate this essential element of clinical nursing education. This chapter discussed the background and evidence related to the use of simulation in clinical nursing education. It provided an overview of some of the most utilized HSSOBP™ standards that inform development of simulations. Simulation design should first involve a needs assessment and learning objectives prior to pursuing modality and fidelity/technology of the simulation. All simulations should be piloted.

Prebriefing is an important component of simulation and was discussed in the chapter. Prebriefing provides an opportunity for the teacher to assess student preparation, check on essential student knowledge, review background information about the patient in the simulation, provide instructions, discuss the fiction contract, and establish a safe container for psychologically safe learning experiences. Perhaps the most important area of clinical simulation involves debriefing and providing an opportunity for guided reflection on the simulation. Debriefing is critical for students' learning and satisfaction with their simulation experience, and it requires adequate time and some preplanning to be effective. The chapter provided a discussion about debriefing with guidelines for implementation.

Simulations should regularly be evaluated to ensure quality and gather ideas for improvement. There are a variety of instruments that are available to inform facilitator competency, debriefing competency, learner engagement in simulation, and other evaluation elements. As the simulation unfolds, teachers can easily identify areas that are working and areas that are problematic. The dynamic process of the simulation allows for some modification during use, but careful note-taking during the scenario and after the debriefing is important to document changes necessary to enhance the effectiveness of the simulation for the future. Simulations also are useful for learner evaluation of performance. As nursing moves toward competency-based education, simulation is an excellent environment for evaluating competencies, but raters must have appropriate training and performance to use evaluation instruments.

Simulation activities can be integrated into clinical learning in a variety of ways, which were described in the chapter. Resources and organizations that can help nurse educators develop and sustain the successful use of simulation were identified throughout the chapter. While research to further develop the science of simulation is ongoing, this chapter and other supportive resources provide guidance for implementing existing best practices.

CNE®cl EXAMINATION TEST BLUEPRINT CORE COMPETENCIES

1. **Function in the Education and Health Care Environment**
   A. **Function in the Clinical Educator Role**
      2. Foster professional growth of learners (e.g., coaching, reflection, debriefing)
      3. Use technologies to enhance clinical teaching and learning
   B. **Operationalize the Curriculum**
      2. Identify learner goals and outcomes
      3. Facilitate meaningful and relevant clinical learning activities to promote optimal learning
      4. Prepare learners for clinical experiences (e.g., facility, clinical expectations, equipment, and technology-based resources)
      5. Implement clinical activities to help learners to develop interprofessional collaboration and teamwork skills
      6. Provide opportunities for learners to develop clinical judgment related to course outcomes
      7. Implement academic program's assigned models of clinical teaching consistent with course outcomes (e.g., traditional, preceptor, simulation, dedicated education units)
2. **Facilitate Learning in the Health Care Environment**
   A. Implement a variety of clinical teaching strategies congruent with learner needs, desired learner outcomes, course outcomes, setting, and context (e.g., virtual, telehealth, in-person, simulation)
   B. Apply teaching strategies from educational theory and evidence-based teaching practices
   C. Use academic and client-care technology to support the teaching–learning process
   D. Create opportunities for learners to develop clinical judgment
   E. Promote a culture of safety and quality in the delivery of healthcare
   F. Create a positive and caring learning environment
5. **Facilitate Learner Development and Socialization**
   A. Mentor learners in professional nursing behaviors
   B. Promote professional integrity and accountability
   E. Assist learners to use self-assessment, self-reflection, and goal setting for ongoing professional development
   F. Create learning environments that promote socialization to the role of the nurse
   G. Facilitate learner participation in constructive peer feedback practices
6. **Implement Effective Clinical Assessment and Evaluation Strategies**
   A. Employ a variety of strategies to determine achievement of learning outcomes
   B. Conduct formative and summative evaluation specific to the learner and learning outcomes
   D. Maintain integrity (e.g., ethical, nonbiased) in the assessment and evaluation of learners
   E. Provide timely, specific, objective, constructive feedback to learners

This chapter was prepared based on work by Katie Ann Haerling in the sixth edition of the book.

REFERENCES

Alexander, M., Durham, C. F., Hooper, J. I., Jeffries, P. R., Goldman, N., Kardong-Edgren, S. S., & Tillman, C. (2015). NCSBN simulation guidelines for prelicensure nursing programs. *Journal of Nursing Regulation, 6*(3), 39–42. https://doi.org/10.1016/s2155-8256(15)30783-3

American Association of Colleges of Nursing. (2021). *The essentials: Core competencies for professional nursing education*. https://www.aacnnursing.org/Portals/0/PDFs/Publications/Essentials-2021.pdf

Armstrong, E., Bradley, C. S., & Flaten, C. (2025). Immersive virtual reality in nursing didactic courses: Bringing the patient to the classroom to foster clinical judgment. *Clinical Simulation in Nursing, 100*, 101689. https://doi.org/10.1016/j.ecns.2025.101689

Bradley, C. S., Aebersold, M., DiClemente, L., Flaten, C., Muehlbauer, M. K., & Loomis, A. (2024). Breaking boundaries: How immersive virtual reality is reshaping nursing education. *Journal of Nursing Regulation, 15*(2), 28–37. https://doi.org/10.1016/S2155-8256(24)00053-X

Bradley, C. S., Dreifuerst, K. T., Johnson, B. K., & Loomis, A. (2022). More than a meme: The Dunning-Kruger effect as an opportunity for positive change in nursing education.

Clinical Simulation in Nursing, 66, 58–65. https://doi.org/10.1016/j.ecns.2022.02.010

Bradley, C. S., Johnson, B. K., & Dreifuerst, K. T. (2020). Debriefing: A place for enthusiastic teaching and learning at a distance. *Clinical Simulation in Nursing, 49*, 16–18. https://doi.org/10.1016/j.ecns.2020.04.001

Bradley, C. S., Johnson, B. K., Dreifuerst, K. T., White, P., Conde, S. K., Meakim, C. H., Curry-Lourenco, K., & Childress, R. M. (2019). Regulation of simulation use in United States prelicensure nursing programs. *Clinical Simulation in Nursing, 33*, 17–25. https://doi.org/10.1016/j.ecns.2019.04.004

Brazil, V., & Purdy, E. (2020). *Safe, not soft—Hitting the sweet spot for simulation-based education*. ICE Blog. https://icenet.blog/2020/11/03/safe-not-soft-hitting-the-sweet-spot-for-simulation-based-education/

Chen, F., Leng, Y., Ge, J., Wang, D., Li, C., Chen, B., & Sun, Z. (2020). Effectiveness of virtual reality in nursing education: Meta-analysis. *Journal of Medical Internet Research, 22*(9), e18290. https://doi.org/10.2196/18290

Choi, J., Thompson, C. E., Choi, J., Waddill, C. B., & Choi, S. (2022). Effectiveness of immersive virtual reality in nursing education: Systematic review. *Nurse Educator, 47*(3), E57–E61. https://doi.org/10.1097/NNE.0000000000001117

Commission on Collegiate Nursing Education. (2024). *Standards for accreditation of baccalaureate and graduate degree nursing programs*. https://www.aacnnursing.org/Portals/0/PDFs/CCNE/CCNE-Education-Standards-2024.pdf

Costa, L. A., & Manger, E. J. (2024). Criteria to evaluate graduate nurse proficiencies in obtaining a health history and perform physical assessment in simulation-based education: A narrative review. *Nurse Education in Practice, 77*, 103984. https://doi.org/10.1016/j.nepr.2024.103984

Creighton University. (2025). *Competency evaluation instrument*. https://nursing.creighton.edu/academics/competency-evaluation-instrument

Curl, E., Smith, S., Chisholm, L., McGee, L., & Das, K. (2016). Effectiveness of integrated simulation and clinical experiences compared to traditional clinical experiences for nursing students. *Nursing Education Perspectives, 37*(2), 72–77.

Dang, B., K., Johnson, B. K., Butzlaff, A., Gilbert, G. E., Schleicher, M., Palicte, J., Wood, A. M., & Kardong-Edgren, S. (2021). A multi-site evaluation of observer roles and telepresence technology in simulation with prelicensure nursing students. *Clinical Simulation in Nursing, 55*, 86–94. https://doi.org/10.1016/j.ecns.2021.03.007

Diaz, D. A., & Anderson, M. (2021). Structuring simulation-based education (SBE): From pre-simulation to debriefing. In P. R. Jeffries & National League for Nursing (Eds.), *Simulation in nursing education: From conceptualization to evaluation* (3rd ed., pp. 69–82). National League for Nursing.

Dinkins, C. S., & Cangelosi, P. R. (2019). Putting Socrates back in Socratic method: Theory-based debriefing in the nursing classroom. *Nursing Philosophy, 20*(2), e12240. https://doi.org/10.1111/nup.12240

Dreifuerst, K. T. (2015). Getting started with debriefing for meaningful learning. *Clinical Simulation in Nursing, 11*(5), 268–275. https://doi.org/10.1016/j.ecns.2015.01.005

Dreifuerst, K. T., Bradley, C. S., & Johnson, B. K. (2021). Debriefing: An essential component for learning in simulation pedagogy. In P. R. Jeffries & National League for Nursing (Eds.), *Simulation in nursing education: From conceptualization to evaluation* (3rd ed., pp. 45–68). National League for Nursing.

Edmondson, A. (2019). *The fearless organization: Creating psychological safety in the workplace for learning, innovation, and growth*. Wiley & Sons.

Fey, M. K., & Johnson, B. K. (2023). 'They didn't do anything wrong! What will I talk about?' Applying the principles of cognitive task analysis to debriefing positive performance. *International Journal of Healthcare Simulation*, 1–6. https://doi.org/10.54531/gevl9221

Fey, M. K., Roussin, C. J., Rudolph, J. W., Morse, K. J., Palaganas, J. C., & Szyld, D. (2022). Teaching, coaching, or debriefing with good judgment: A roadmap for implementing "with good judgment" across the simzones. *Advances in Simulation, 7*, 39. https://doi.org/10.1186/s41077-022-00235-y

Forneris, S. G., & Fey, M. (2016). NLN vision: Teaching with simulation. In P. R. Jeffries (Ed.), *The NLN Jeffries simulation theory* (pp. 43–49). Wolters Kluwer.

Foronda, C. L., Fernandez-Burgos, M., Nadeau, C., Kelley, C. N., & Henry, M. N. (2020). Virtual simulation in nursing education: A systematic review spanning 1996 to 2018. *Simulation in Healthcare, 15*(1), 46–54. https://doi.org/10.1097/SIH.0000000000000411

Gaba, D. M. (2004). The future vision of simulation in health care. *Quality and Safety in Health Care, 13*, i2–i10. https://doi.org/10.1136/qhc.13.suppl_1.i2

Goodwin, B., & Nestel, D. (2024). Demystifying simulators for educators in healthcare. *International Journal of Healthcare Simulation, 1*(8). Advance online publication. https://doi.org/10.54531/MUIF5353

Haerling, K. (2018). Cost-utility analysis of virtual and mannequin-based simulation. *Simulation in Healthcare, 13*(1), 33–40. https://doi.org/10.1097/SIH.0000000000000280

Haerling, K. (2021). Simulation evaluation. In P. R. Jeffries & National League for Nursing (Eds.), *Simulation in nursing education: From conceptualization to evaluation* (3rd ed., pp. 83–99). National League for Nursing.

Hansbrough, W., Dunker, K. S., Ross, J. G., & Ostendorf, M. (2020). Restrictions on nursing students' electronic health information access. *Nurse Educator, 45*(5), 243–247. https://doi.org/10.1097/NNE.0000000000000786

Hayden, J. K., Smiley, R. A., Alexander, M., Kardong-Edgren, S., & Jeffries, P. (2014). The NCSBN national simulation study: A longitudinal, randomized controlled study replacing clinical hours with simulation in prelicensure nursing education. *Journal of Nursing Regulation, 5*(2), S1–S64. https://doi.org/10.1016/S2155-8256(15)30062-4

INACSL Simulation Regulation Committee. (2021, May). *INACSL simulation regulation map*. https://www.inacsl.org/simulation-regulation-map

INACSL Standards Committee. (2021a). Healthcare simulation standards of best practice™. *Clinical Simulation in Nursing, 56*, 66. https://doi.org/10.1016/j.ecns.2021.08.018

INACSL Standards Committee, Bowler, F., Klein, M., & Wilford, A. (2021b). Healthcare simulation standards of best practice™ professional integrity. *Clinical Simulation in Nursing, 58*, 45–48. https://doi.org/10.1016/j.ecns.2021.08.014

INACSL Standards Committee, Charnetski, M., & Jarvill, M. (2021c). Healthcare simulation standards of best practice™ operations. *Clinical Simulation in Nursing, 58*, 33–39. https://doi.org/10.1016/j.ecns.2021.08.012

INACSL Standards Committee, Decker, S., Alinier, G., Crawford, S. B., Gordon, R. M., Jenkins, D., & Wilson, C. (2021d). Healthcare simulation standards of best practice™: The debriefing process. *Clinical Simulation in Nursing, 58*, 27–32. https://doi.org/10.1016/j.ecns.2021.08.011

INACSL Standards Committee, Hallmark, B., Brown, M., Peterson, D., Fey, M., Decker, S., Wells-Beede, E., Britt, T., Hardie, L., Shum, C., Arantes, H., Charnetski, M., & Morse, C. (2021e). Healthcare simulation standards of best practice™ professional development. *Clinical Simulation in Nursing, 58*, 5–8. https://doi.org/10.1016/j.ecns.2021.08.007

INACSL Standards Committee, McDermott, D., Ludlow, J., Horsley, E., & Meakim, C. (2021f). Healthcare simulation standards of best practice ™ prebriefing: Preparation and briefing. *Clinical Simulation in Nursing, 58*, 9–13. https://doi.org/10.1016/j.ecns.2021.08.008

INACSL Standards Committee, McMahon, E., Jimenez, F. A., Lawrence, K., & Victor, J. (2021g). Healthcare simulation standards of best practice™ evaluation of learning and performance. *Clinical Simulation in Nursing, 58*, 54–56. https://doi.org/10.1016/j.ecns.2021.08.016

INACSL Standards Committee, Miller, C., Deckers, C., Jones, M., Wells-Beede, E., & McGee, E. (2021h). Healthcare simulation standards of best practice™ outcomes and objectives. *Clinical Simulation in Nursing, 58*, 40–44. https://doi.org/10.1016/j.ecns.2021.08.013

INACSL Standards Committee, Molloy, M., Holt, J., Charnetski, M., & Rossler, K. (2021i). Healthcare simulation standards of best practice™ simulation glossary. *Clinical Simulation in Nursing, 58*, 57–65. https://doi.org/10.1016/j.ecns.2021.08.017

INACSL Standards Committee, Persico, L., Belle, A., DiGregorio, H., Wilson-Keates, B., & Shelton, C. (2021j). Healthcare simulation standards of best practice™ facilitation. *Clinical Simulation in Nursing, 58*, 22–26. https://doi.org/10.1016/j.ecns.2021.08.010

INACSL Standards Committee, Rossler, K., Molloy, M., Pastva, A., Brown, M., & Xavier, N. (2021k). Healthcare simulation standards of best practice™ simulation-enhanced interprofessional education. *Clinical Simulation in Nursing, 58*, 49–53. https://doi.org/10.1016/j.ecns.2021.08.015

INACSL Standards Committee, Watts, P. I., McDermott, D. S., Alinier, G., Charnetski, M., Ludlow, J., Horsley, E., Meakim, C., & Nawathe, P. (2021l). Healthcare simulation standards of best practice™ simulation design. *Clinical Simulation in Nursing, 58*, 14–21. https://doi.org/10.1016/j.ecns.2021.08.009

Jeffries, P. R. (2021). *Simulation in nursing education: From conceptualization to evaluation* (3rd ed.). Wolters Kluwer.

Jeffries, P. R. (2022). *The NLN Jeffries simulation theory* (2nd ed.). Wolters Kluwer.

Jeffries, P. R., Dreifuerst, K. T., & Haerling, K. A. (2022). Clinical simulations in nursing education: Overview, essentials, and the evidence. In M. H. Oermann, J. C. De Gagne, & B. C. Phillips (Eds.), *Teaching in nursing and role of the educator: The complete guide to best practice in teaching, evaluation, and curriculum development* (3rd ed., pp. 133–158). Springer Publishing Company.

Johnson, B. K. (2020). Observational experiential learning: Theoretical support for observer roles in health care simulation. *Journal of Nursing Education, 59*(1), 7–14. https://doi.org/10.3928/01484834-20191223-03

Johnson, B. K. & Fey, M. (2023). Setting observers up for success in simulation. *Nurse Educator, 48*(6), 321–325. https://doi.org/10.1097/NNE.0000000000001433

Johnson, B. K., Zulkosky, K., & O'Regan, S. (2023). Observer roles: Their purpose, power, and value to health care simulation. In P. R. Jeffries (Ed.), *Clinical simulations in nursing education: Advanced concepts, trends, and opportunities* (2nd ed.). Wolters Kluwer.

Johnson, K. V., Scott, A. S., & Franks, L. (2020). Impact of standardized patients on first semester nursing students self-confidence, satisfaction, and communication in a simulated clinical case. *SAGE Open Nursing, 19*(6), 1–7. https://doi.org/10.1177/2377960820930153

Kardong-Edgren, S., Wells-Beede, E., & Wands, L. M. (2024). Student abuse in simulation: Causes and solutions. *Teaching and Learning in Nursing, 19*(2), 145–149. https://doi.org/10.1016/j.teln.2024.02.007

Karlsaune, H., Antonsen, T., & Haugan, G. (2023). Simulation: A historical and pedagogical perspective. In I. Akselbo and I. Aune (Eds.), *How can we use simulations to improve competencies in nursing?* Springer Publishing Company.

Kim, M. J., Kang, J., Chu, M., Min, H., & Kim, S. (2025). Use of electronic medical records in simulated nursing education and its educational outcomes: A scoping review. *Clinical Simulation in Nursing, 101*, 101703. https://doi.org/10.1016/j.ecns.2025.101703

Kononowicz, A. A., Woodham, L. A., Edelbring, S., Stathakarou, N., Davies, D., Saxena, N., Tudor Car, L., Carlstedt-Duke, J., Car, J., & Zary, N. (2019). Virtual patient simulations in health professions education: Systematic review and meta-analysis by the Digital Health Education Collaboration. *Journal of Medical Internet Research, 21*(7), e14676. https://doi.org/10.2196/14676

Lasater, K. (2007). Clinical judgment development: Using simulation to create an assessment rubric. *Journal of Nursing Education, 46*(11), 496–503. https://doi.org/10.3928/01484834-20071101-04

Lewis, K. L., Bohnert, C. A., Gammon, W. L., Hölzer, H., Lyman, L., Smith, C., Thompson, T., Wallace, A. & Gliva-McConvey, G. (2017). The Association of Standardized Patient Educators (ASPE) standards of best practice

(SOBP). *Advances in Simulation, 2*, 10. https://doi.org/10.1186/s41077-017-0043-4

Leighton, K., Kardong-Edgren, S., McNelis, A. M., Foisy-Doll, C., & Sullo, E. (2021). Traditional clinical outcomes in prelicensure nursing education: An empty systematic review. *Journal of Nursing Education, 60*(3), 136–142. https://doi.org/10.3928/01484834-20210222-03

Lioce, L. (2024). *Healthcare simulation dictionary version 3.0*. Agency for Healthcare Research and Quality. https://www.ahrq.gov/patient-safety/resources/simulation/terms.html

McBride, S., Thomas, L., Decker, S., Pierce, M., Burson, S., Song, H., & Adamson, K. H. (2024). Validation of a tool to evaluate nursing students' electronic health record competency in simulation. *Nursing Education Perspectives, 45*(3), 161–168. https://doi.org/10.1097/01.NEP.0000000000001240

McDermott, D. S. (2016). The prebriefing concept: A delphi study of CHSE experts. *Clinical Simulation in Nursing, 12*(6), 219–227. https://doi.org/10.1016/j.ecns.2016.02.001

McDermott, D. S. (2020). Prebriefing: A historical perspective and evolution of a model and strategy (Know: Do: Teach). *Clinical Simulation in Nursing, 49*, 40–49. https://doi.org/10.1016/j.ecns.2020.05.005

Mendez, K. J., Piasecki, R. J., Hudson, K., Renda, S., Mollenkopf, N., Nettles, B. S., & Han, H-R. (2020). Virtual and augmented reality: Implications for the future of nursing education. *Nurse Education Today, 93*, 104531. https://doi.org/10.1016/j.nedt.2020.104531

National League for Nursing. (2015). *Debriefing across the curriculum* [NLN Vision #9]. https://www.nln.org/news/newsroomnln-position-documents/nln-vision-series

National League for Nursing. (2025a). *Simulation innovation resource center*. https://www.nln.org/education/education/sirc/sirc/sirc

National League for Nursing. (2025b). *Leadership development for simulation educators*. https://www.nln.org/education/leadership-institute/centers-for-nursing-educationnln-center-for-transformational-leadership2b/leadership-development-for-simulation-educators

National League for Nursing. (2023). *Integrating competency-based education in the nursing curriculum* [NLN Vision #21]. https://www.nln.org/news/newsroomnln-position-documents/nln-vision-series

National League for Nursing Commission for Nursing Education Accreditation. (2021). *Accreditation standards for nursing education programs*. https://irp.cdn-website.com/cc12ee87/files/uploaded/CNEA%20Standards%20October%202021-4b271cb2.pdf

Park, C. S., Murphy, T. F., & the Code of Ethics Working Group (2018). *Healthcare simulationist code of ethics*. https://www.ssih.org/healthcare-simulationist-code-ethics

Rock, L. K., Rudolph, J. W., Fey, M. K., Szyld, D., Gardner, R., Minehart, R. D., Shapiro, J., & Roussin, C. (2020). "Circle up": Workflow adaptation and psychological support via briefing, debriefing, and peer support. *NEJM Catalyst, 1*(5). https://catalyst.nejm.org/doi/full/10.1056/CAT.20.0240

Rogers, B., Baker, K. A., & Franklin, A. E. (2020). Learning outcomes of the observer role in nursing simulation: A scoping review. *Clinical Simulation in Nursing, 49*, 81–89. https://doi.org/10.1016/j.ecns.2020.06.003

Rudolph, J. W., Raemer, D. B., & Simon, R. (2014). Establishing a safe container for learning in simulation: The role of the presimulation briefing. *Simulation in Healthcare, 9*(6), 339–349. https://doi.org/10.1097/SIH.0000000000000047

Sullivan, N., Swoboda, S. M., Breymier, T., Rutherford-Hemming, T., Budhathoki, C., & Kardong-Edgren, S. (2019). Emerging evidence toward a 2:1 clinical to simulation ratio: A study comparing the traditional clinical and simulation settings. *Clinical Simulation in Nursing, 30*, 34–41. https://doi.org/10.1016/j.ecns.2019.03.003

Verkuyl, M., Lapum, J. L., St-Amant, O., Hughes, M., Romaniuk, D., & McCulloch, T. (2020). Exploring debriefing combinations after a virtual simulation. *Clinical Simulation in Nursing, 40*, 36–42. https://doi.org/10.1016/j.ecns.2019.12.002

Woda, A., Bradley, C. S., Johnson, B. K., Hansen, J., Loomis, A., Pena, S., Singh, M., & Dreifuerst, K. T. (2023). Testing the impact of an asynchronous online training program with repeated feedback. *Nurse Educator, 48*(5), 254–259. https://doi.org/10.1097/NNE.0000000000001405

Pedagogical Technologies in Clinical Education

9

OBJECTIVES:

1. Analyze the role of technological advancements, including artificial intelligence (AI), in clinical education to prepare nursing students for the evolving demands of healthcare.
2. Examine strategies for integrating pedagogical technologies, such as simulated electronic health records (EHRs), telepresence, telehealth, virtual gamification, and emerging tools, into clinical teaching practices.
3. Reflect on the evolution of virtual clinical learning and the transition to more robust, technology-enhanced learning models in the postpandemic era, offering practical guidance for clinical educators.

Practice experience in the clinical learning environment enables nursing students to apply theoretical knowledge and develop critical clinical skills as well as clinical judgment and reasoning. Technological advancements shape how clinical skills are practiced. New technologies such as simulated electronic health records (EHRs), telehealth, virtual learning platforms, and artificial intelligence (AI) offer new avenues for enhancing skill development and are transforming clinical education. Clinical teaching methods must be regularly reassessed to ensure that nursing students are adequately prepared for the complexities of modern healthcare.

Nursing leaders and educators should strategically integrate pedagogical technologies into clinical education as an ongoing process aligned with best practices. Innovative technologies can connect students to cutting-edge tools that enhance data collection, advance delivery of high-quality healthcare (American Association of Colleges of Nursing [AACN], 2021), and foster development of the complex nursing skills and competencies required in the evolving healthcare landscape.

This chapter examines a range of technologies currently shaping clinical teaching, including simulated EHRs, telepresence, telehealth, virtual gamification, and emerging tools such as AI; reflects on the evolution of virtual clinical learning, underscoring the transition to more robust, technology-enhanced learning models in the postpandemic era; and offers practical guidance for clinical nurse educators to effectively integrate emerging technologies into their teaching practices to ensure continued success in providing cutting-edge healthcare education.

TECHNOLOGY USE IN CLINICAL TEACHING

Clinical skills for nursing students have traditionally been developed through a combination of laboratory activities and direct observation in clinical practice. Over time, students gradually take on more responsibility for patient care under the supervision of nurse educators and clinical staff. Today's students, already immersed in multimedia environments, expect technology tools, ranging from simple supplements to primary methods of instructional delivery and skill practice, to be seamlessly integrated into their clinical courses and learning experiences. In some instances, external pressures—such as the COVID-19 pandemic—have forced educators to rapidly replace traditional (and sometimes outdated) teaching methods with new technologies for teaching and learning. However, although the swift pandemic-era shift helped to maintain educational continuity, it often led to fragmented and less-than-satisfactory learning experiences. Many nurse educators lacked a structured approach to effective adoption and resorted to trial and error.

The current generation of nursing students (often referred to as Generation Z or digital natives) grew up surrounded by digital technologies and anticipate learning experiences that are interactive, engaging, and technologically integrated. Although Generation Z may be proficient with digital devices, the assumption that their familiarity equates to true digital literacy has been challenged. Reid et al. (2023) argue that digital literacy involves more than a fundamental understanding of how to use technology. It requires the ability to critically engage with digital tools, proficiently navigate complex information systems, and thoroughly evaluate digital content for accuracy and relevance. This nuanced understanding of digital literacy underscores the importance of teaching nursing students both the functional use of digital technologies and how to use them with optimal effectiveness in clinical practice.

Technology Stewards and Champions

The successful adoption of technology into clinical teaching can be greatly enhanced by identifying technology stewards or superusers within the learning community who can help learners choose, organize, and apply technology to meet their needs. It is not uncommon for students to take on leadership roles and join the technology champion team to help troubleshoot issues and provide support to peers and instructors who are adopting new technologies.

Technology champions must possess a clear understanding of their learning community's needs—both expressed and implied. Although advanced technological expertise is helpful, even a basic awareness of available tools and possibilities can catalyze the process of selecting and implementing new technologies. During the adoption phase, champions serve leadership functions, managing the direction and pace of change. Once technology has been implemented, these stewards continue to support the ongoing evolution of practices and integration of emerging technologies in response to evolving needs (Tischendorf et al., 2024). Clinical teachers who are open to new ideas often make excellent candidates for technology champion roles; however, a team-based approach is crucial for the successful implementation of more complex systems. The following are some benefits of adopting the technology champion role:

- the satisfaction of advancing initiatives that may lack a designated leader;
- opportunities to improve learning and educational practices;
- a chance to develop leadership, teaching, and technical skills; and
- enhanced reputation and credibility in both academic and practice settings.

To achieve a sustainable integration of digital tools into nursing education, clinical teachers must not only adopt new technologies but also must ensure that nursing professionals actively contribute to their development, testing, and implementation. Technology stewards, such as champions, are integral in creating an inclusive and adaptive learning environment. They bridge the gap between technical knowledge and practical application by fostering collaborative, participatory approaches to technology integration. Digital literacy in nursing must be seen as a core competency at all levels of nursing education, from initial training to ongoing professional development (Reid et al., 2023). Engaging nursing staff in the codevelopment of digital solutions ensures that technologies meet real-world needs and align ethically with healthcare values (Tischendorf et al., 2024).

SELECTING TECHNOLOGY FOR CLINICAL TEACHING

Educational technology plays a pivotal role in enhancing students' learning experiences, but its successful implementation depends on choosing the right tool for a specific teaching purpose. Clinical teachers who wish to integrate pedagogical technologies into their courses must first consider both their course and program outcomes and the learners' characteristics. The most effective approach is often to start small, with simple, easy-to-implement strategies. For example, teachers can introduce a single electronic postclinical conference activity using a technology with which they are already familiar, rather than switching to a completely new system or attempting a drastic overhaul of the entire course structure. A phased approach allows smoother integration and reduces the learning curve associated with new technologies.

After carefully choosing a technology, the clinical teacher should test and practice its use before attempting a full-scale implementation; this will ensure a more seamless experience for both instructors and students. It can be especially useful to have a colleague, student, or faculty member test the technology in a practice scenario before introducing it to the entire class. Additionally, educators should leverage available technology training resources such as those offered by product distributors, online platforms, or campus technology staff. When selecting technologies, educators should prioritize strategies that simultaneously foster engagement, intellectual development, and meaningful rapport among students (Chunta et al., 2021).

Educators can employ evidence-based models to facilitate effective technology integration. One such model is the SECTIONS framework developed by Bates (2022), which provides a systematic approach to selecting appropriate technologies by considering the following elements: **S**tudents, **E**ase of use, **C**ost, **T**eaching functions, **I**nteraction, **O**rganizational issues, **N**etworking, and **S**ecurity and privacy. Although the SECTIONS model was initially designed as a universal framework for integrating technology into curricula, it is particularly valuable in clinical education because it helps educators make informed decisions that align with both educational goals and the specific needs of clinical courses.

The SECTIONS model emphasizes that successful technology integration is not achieved simply by selecting the most advanced or costly tools; rather, faculty must thoughtfully choose technologies that align with their course content, learning objectives, and teaching methods. Additionally, they must consider factors such as accessibility, ease of use, and the potential to engage students to achieve better student outcomes (Bates, 2022). The SECTIONS framework allows clinical educators to identify tools that will best enhance the clinical learning experience and enable nursing students to develop essential skills as they prepare for the dynamic challenges of modern healthcare.

Start Small and Build Confidence

Many technological tools serve multiple functions, and certain learning objectives can be supported by more than one tool. For example, simulation and virtual reality-based learning provide experiential learning opportunities in immersive environments. These platforms allow students to engage with virtual patients to develop critical thinking and clinical decision-making skills and reflect on and refine their understanding of clinical practice (Forneris, 2023). Teachers can choose virtual environments that both replicate real-world best practices and offer opportunities to explore ethical issues and professional boundaries. Such environments prepare students for real-world scenarios in a supportive virtual context, thus serving as a foundation for learning that will extend into future clinical experiences.

FAMILIAR TECHNOLOGY FOR BETTER ENGAGEMENT

Leveraging technology with which students are already familiar can enhance their engagement in clinical learning. For example, a clinical educator can establish a separate account on X (formerly Twitter) to interact with students, adjusting privacy settings to limit visibility to a designated group of students. Through this platform, the educator can share mini-lessons, updates, and relevant resources. Additionally, social media platforms allow clinical teachers to take advantage of teachable moments outside the clinical setting—such as sharing insights from a conference, alerting students to a newly published article, or recommending a documentary related to their current studies. To encourage interaction, the educator could post a weekly question or brainteaser related to the competencies on which students are currently working. For students involved in clinical activities across diverse settings, X can also facilitate postclinical conferences at a set time, for which the educator posts discussion prompts (e.g., Q1, Q2) and invites student responses (labeled R1, R2, etc.). This approach fosters a dynamic exchange of ideas and reflections and promotes collaborative learning even outside scheduled class time.

SECURE AND HEALTH INSURANCE PORTABILITY AND ACCOUNTABILITY–COMMUNICATION

Students and clinical instructors may prefer to engage in electronic discussions without the use of social media. Learning management systems (LMSs) provide a venue for interactive discussions which allows students to reflect and comment upon experiences, pose questions, and dialogue with clinical classmates and the clinical instructor in a secure environment. LMSs work well for clinical conferencing activities that do not require an immediate response from others; however, text messaging services provide an appropriate alternative when a clinical teacher or student requires quick access to support, needs clarification about questions, or seeks dialogue about a clinical situation. It is essential that educators exercise caution while text messaging, in compliance with the Health Insurance Portability and Accountability Act (HIPAA), to ensure that personal patient information remains uncompromised. Secure HIPAA-compliant text messaging services for healthcare providers allow for streamlined, connected, and secure text messaging among clinical students and instructors (Benavente et al., 2023).

SELECTING THE RIGHT TOOLS FOR THE LEARNING OBJECTIVE

It is important to remember that most educational technologies are tools to achieve learning goals, not ends in themselves. The most advanced or expensive technology is not always the best choice for supporting clinical learning. In fact, simpler, less costly tools may be more effective for achieving specific clinical objectives. Educators should avoid overcomplicating the learning process by relying on complex technology for a single task or assignment. Instead, they should focus on selecting tools that align with learning outcomes, ensuring that the technology complements the teaching strategy without overshadowing the core educational objectives.

Proficiency with technologies such as EHRs is essential for students' future careers, but educators must be careful not to prioritize specific tools over broader learning goals. For example, if the learning objective is to develop a patient education pamphlet or an electronic clinical portfolio, design or presentation software will be needed. On the other hand, if the objective is to develop clinical decision-making skills, tools such as human patient simulation, virtual reality environments, or online case studies will likely be more appropriate. Before selecting technology for clinical teaching, educators should carefully consider their learning objectives and the types of interactions that will best support the achievement of their goals. **Table 9.1** provides a guide to selecting technology that aligns with various educational strategies. Clinical educators can refer to this table to identify appropriate technology tools that match specific learning intentions to help them create an effective and targeted learning experience.

TABLE 9.1 SELECTING TECHNOLOGY TO SUPPORT EDUCATIONAL STRATEGIES

Educational Intention	Related Technology
Direct experience	Electronic health records, virtual reality environments, e-learning modules, telepresence, telehealth, multiplayer online role-playing games, electronic escape rooms, virtual case simulations, high-fidelity simulation
Discussion/reflection	Online discussion boards, virtual chat, video conferencing, telepresence, social media sites
Project production	Software or online sites for design and publishing, presentation creation, video recording, posting on discussion forums, blogs, video-sharing platforms, course management systems, commenting sites
Information access	Websites, mobile applications, online newspapers and journals, pre-recorded or real-time presentations
Drill and practice	Quizzing software, electronic response systems, polling software, online/digital flashcards, knowledge-based games

ELECTRONIC HEALTH RECORDS

EHRs are now integral to the healthcare system, serving as vital tools for managing patient information, improving care coordination, and enhancing the quality of healthcare delivery (Okolo et al., 2024). Nursing students must be proficient in using EHRs for documentation, retrieving patient information, and developing essential information technology skills that are expected of graduates. However, despite the widespread use of EHRs, some clinical agencies have policies that limit students' and clinical faculty access and their ability to enter data into these systems (Samadbeik et al., 2020; Whitt et al., 2024). Such restrictions are based on concerns about security, privacy, and the potential for breaches of protected health information (Basil et al., 2022). As EHR systems become more complex and interconnected, it is crucial that students understand these security issues and the importance of data privacy and protection under HIPAA. However, restricted access may hinder their full engagement with the technology and impede their ability to develop the skills required for modern nursing practice.

Developing Partnerships for Electronic Health Record Access

One approach to gaining access to a healthcare facility EHR involves forming partnerships with specific healthcare organizations. Such partnerships can provide students with repeated immersive clinical learning experiences with in-depth training on the use of EHR systems. Orientation to an EHR can sometimes take days of training, but partnerships offer students continued, hands-on exposure to a site-specific EHR system during their clinical rotations. This repeated exposure allows students to develop familiarity with the operations and technology used at the healthcare facility, gain valuable insight into EHR use, and become attractive as potential employees who may require less training once hired (Whitt et al., 2024).

Academic Electronic Health Record Integration

In addition to partnerships, educators have identified several strategies to support nursing students in learning electronic documentation and data review. One solution involves leasing or purchasing simulated EHR systems similar to those used in hospitals and ambulatory health settings; however, such simulated systems can be costly. A more cost-effective solution for academic institutions is to develop their own Academic Electronic Health Record (AEHR). Although this approach offers more customization and affordability, it requires considerable time, technological expertise, and support services (Samadbeik et al., 2020; Whitt et al., 2024). Choosing the right AEHR requires thoughtful consideration to meet the needs of students, faculty, and the curriculum. The AEHR selected should provide realistic scenarios that help students learn how to read health documents and document clinical assessments. Additionally, the AEHR should allow for system upgrades and the integration of program-specific requests, such as bar-code technology to improve patient safety and reduce medication errors (Kan & Stabler-Hass, 2025; Whitt et al., 2024). Faculty should thoroughly review the AEHR before making any purchase decisions.

Successful Integration and Overcoming Barriers

Educators can plan strategies to make implementation of an AEHR successful and meaningful for both faculty and students. An AEHR can be integrated across all curriculum levels, allowing users to complete assignments such as planning care or developing written Situation, Background, Assessment, Recommendation (SBAR) reports. Clinical faculty can also implement EHRs in nursing programs by having students interact with health records developed for simulation patients. This hands-on experience allows students to practice searching for critical information (e.g., allergies, diagnostic test results, medications) while also documenting assessments and interventions performed during simulations.

The use of an AEHR as a teaching strategy across various learning environments (e.g., classrooms, skills labs, simulation labs) exposes students to diverse scenarios that enhance their professional role readiness. Repetitive practice opportunities with AEHRs develop student competence in using such systems in clinical settings. Additionally, integrating simulated AEHR patients across multiple courses within a semester can reinforce key content and enable students to become more familiar with and skilled in electronic documentation.

Addressing Challenges in AEHR Implementation

Despite the advantages of AEHRs, there are several barriers to their use in nursing education, including limited funding for AEHR integration, resistance from faculty, and lack of adequate faculty training. Additionally, technical challenges such as internet connectivity issues, inadequate backup systems, and software incompatibility may hinder AEHR implementation (Mollart et al., 2020). A strategic plan should be in place to address such challenges before AEHR implementation is undertaken. Engaging faculty in the planning process and providing ongoing training and support can often overcome resistance and ensure successful integration. Administrative support and funding are also crucial for overcoming the financial challenges associated with AEHR implementation (Whitt et al., 2024).

Successful implementation of AEHRs often involves the presence of a program champion—someone who is an early adopter of technology and has a positive attitude toward its use. Program champions can serve as change leaders by providing initial training, refresher courses, and ongoing support to faculty and students. Their involvement is critical in ensuring the long-term success of AEHR integration into a nursing education program.

VIRTUAL LEARNING IN CLINICAL EDUCATION

Virtual learning, a modality enhanced by using computers and the internet, presents students with opportunities to gain clinical experience outside the traditional face-to-face clinical setting. Virtual learning experiences range from simple online case studies to more advanced, technologically sophisticated simulations that incorporate video-based, interactive, and simulated environments. A key advantage of virtual learning is that its flexibility enables students to complete clinical activities at their own pace while offering opportunities for repeated practice and mastery.

One approach to virtual learning that clinical educators can adopt involves creating e-learning modules within an LMS. These modules focus on one or two topics and integrate various teaching tools, such as videos, weblinks, narratives, and games. Students engage in self-directed activities and assessments that they complete independently. Clinical teachers can leverage these modules to prepare students for pre- and postconference discussions or other learning experiences. For instance, an e-learning module could be developed to cover cardiovascular disease. Students would complete the module before their clinical day, using embedded resources that reinforce course content, such as weblinks and videos on lifestyle changes, medications, or dietary recommendations. During a virtual discussion, the teacher can pose probing questions to engage students and encourage them to demonstrate clinical judgment and reasoning. This format supports the integration of classroom and clinical education, facilitating the application of theory to practice. Student responses to discussion prompts can serve as a foundation for in-depth dialogue during postconference sessions. E-learning modules are versatile and applicable across all student levels and clinical areas.

Virtual learning addresses some limitations of traditional clinical training, particularly the constraints of clinical learning spaces. For instance, students can participate in virtual activities without the logistical costs of traveling to clinical sites. Furthermore, the virtual environment provides opportunities for experiences that might not be available in real clinical rotations. For example, although students may not gain direct experience in neonatal intensive care units, the creation of virtual reality-based learning activities—such as simulations of high-risk neonatal infections—can enable the repetitive practice of critical clinical and problem-solving skills (Yu & Mann, 2021). The use of simulated patients within a virtual environment ensures that each student has access to a consistent experience at an appropriate level of complexity.

Telepresence

Clinical learning experiences can present challenges when the virtual activity requires students to interact synchronously from different locations. Telepresence is a modality that can extend the nuances and presence of face-to-face clinical interactions to a virtual learning experience (Leoste et al., 2022). Telepresence technology overcomes the barrier of distance and allows remote students to feel as if they are physically present with their peers. Recent studies have reinforced the effectiveness of telepresence in promoting student engagement, satisfaction, and self-confidence when completing clinical learning activities. Specifically, telepresence technology, through its ability to simulate physical presence, has been shown to support enhanced interaction and engagement in learning experiences, which is vital for remote clinical education (Leoste et al., 2022).

Telepresence is most commonly incorporated using a robot in simulated clinical learning experiences in which students are participating both in-person and remotely (Leoste et al., 2022). A telepresence robot is a roaming, remote-controlled wheeled device with a screen that allows for face-to-face real-time interactions among the teacher, in-person students, and remote students. This technology enables remote students to interact within a classroom or clinical simulation as if they were physically present (Li et al., 2024). To participate, remote students use a computer with a webcam and an internet connection to control the robot and actively engage in the clinical activity, thus overcoming the typical limitations of distance learning. **Figure 9.1** demonstrates this technology in operation. The image shows an elegant telepresence robot, featuring a high-definition display, moving through a state-of-the-art simulation lab.

There are many benefits to using telepresence technology as a clinical teaching strategy. Telepresence creates an immersive opportunity that allows remote students to transition from being passive observers to engaged learners. Remote students who participate in simulated activities via telepresence, as opposed to cloud-based audio/video communications, report feeling more present and engaged in the virtual learning activity. Telepresence enhances the social presence of remote learners, allowing them to feel more connected to their peers and instructors (Leoste et al., 2022). Additionally, it provides unique learning opportunities that support the development of effective communication and collaborative problem-solving skills, which are essential for future healthcare professionals.

Telepresence technologies offer the potential to create interprofessional learning opportunities in simulated clinical activities, particularly for undergraduate prelicensure students and nurse practitioner students. By facilitating collaborative learning across disciplines, telepresence prepares students for the interconnected nature of modern healthcare environments. Exposure to such technologies during clinical learning equips students with the knowledge and experience to function effectively in complex healthcare settings and prepares them for future roles in telemedicine and remote patient care (Li et al., 2024).

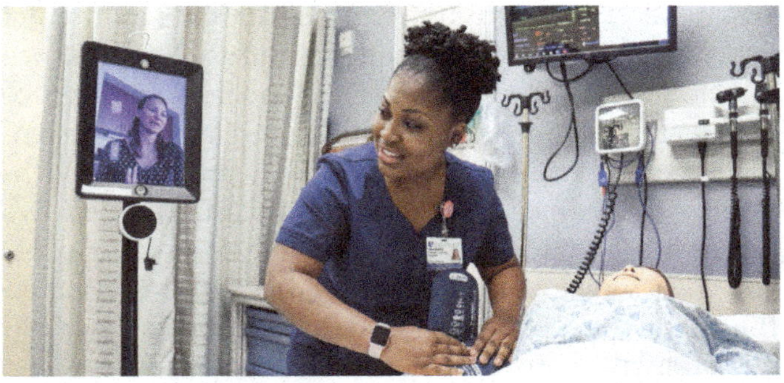

Figure 9.1. Telepresence in action. Source: https://nursing.duke.edu/sites/default/files/2024-07/Duke-Difference-Nursing-Virtual.jpg, Reprinted by permission, Duke University School of Nursing, February 3, 2025.

Telehealth

Telehealth, like telepresence, is an emerging technology that is becoming an integral part of routine healthcare practices. In nursing education, telehealth encompasses a broad range of applications, including remote patient monitoring, the delivery of patient education, and the facilitation of consultations through audio and video communications. This innovative modality holds significant promise for enhancing traditional face-to-face clinical encounters, offering virtual and electronic experiences that provide students with rich opportunities for learning in dynamic, real-world contexts (Koppel et al., 2022). The integration of telehealth into clinical teaching allows students to gain exposure to digital health tools that are essential in preparing them for the future of healthcare delivery. Telehealth technologies, particularly those used in remote monitoring and patient education, play a critical role in equipping nursing students with the skills necessary to navigate the rapidly evolving digital health landscape (Kleib et al., 2024).

A key aspect of telehealth in nursing education is its role in fostering rapport and strong clinician–patient relationships, particularly during videoconferencing visits. Although telehealth can present challenges related to personal connection, it also offers opportunities to develop and refine communication strategies that are essential in maintaining trust and empathy in virtual settings. Techniques such as maintaining eye contact, using empathetic language, and actively listening help nursing students to overcome the limitations of digital communication and establish meaningful connections with patients, even from a distance. The ability to build rapport is especially important in sensitive areas of practice, such as oncology, in which the establishment of trust is fundamental to providing effective care (Koppel et al., 2022).

Telehealth-based interventions, such as continuous glucose monitoring with data sharing, provides a compelling example of how telehealth can be leveraged to improve collaboration between patients with chronic conditions and their care partners. A study by Bristol et al. (2023) illustrates how the use of telehealth in diabetes management encouraged shared responsibility for care, leading to better health outcomes and strengthened relationships between patients and their care partners. The transformative potential of telehealth to support patient-centered care highlights the need for collaborative approaches that can be seamlessly integrated into nursing education. By equipping students with the tools to engage in these virtual care models, educators prepare them to manage complex, real-world healthcare challenges effectively.

Telehealth simulations in nursing education can also substantially improve students' knowledge, confidence, and competency. In a recent study by Wittler et al. (2025), telehealth virtual simulations, integrated across a nurse practitioner curriculum, significantly enhanced students' confidence in using telehealth equipment and conducting virtual consultations. These simulations, embedded into multiple courses throughout the curriculum, provided students with repeated exposure to telehealth scenarios, thereby reinforcing their understanding and technical proficiency. For instance, in an advanced health assessment course, students demonstrated significant improvement in telehealth knowledge after participation in a simulation that involved standardized patients voiced by independent actors. The study reinforces the value of incorporating multiple, evolving telehealth simulations throughout nursing programs to help students develop both the technical and interpersonal skills necessary for providing effective virtual patient care.

Despite their educational value, virtual telehealth experiences often elicit strong emotional responses from students, particularly in relation to sensitive topics. For this reason, Kleib et al. (2024) recommend that instructors carefully prepare for virtual clinical encounters to alleviate students' anxiety and help them focus on learning objectives. Before the experience, structured prebriefing can help set expectations and provide necessary context. Following virtual experiences, reflection and debriefing sessions are needed to reinforce key learning points. These sessions not only ensure that the students are meeting learning objectives but also provide them with opportunities to develop cultural sensitivity and improve communication skills—qualities essential for navigating complex, real-world clinical scenarios. In particular, debriefing allows students to process their emotional reactions, integrate their learning experiences, and better understand their roles in the patient care process, thus fostering a deeper, more holistic approach to nursing practice.

VIRTUAL GAME-BASED LEARNING

Virtual game-based learning engages students by allowing them to make decisions, face consequences, and explore clinical scenarios in a dynamic, risk-free environment. These games often feature evolving narratives that change based on students' actions, providing a rich context for decision making and reflection. As Cant et al. (2023) note, virtual simulations, including games, offer nursing students immersive and controlled settings in which they can practice clinical reasoning, hone psychomotor skills, and experiment with decision-making processes. This pedagogical approach aligns closely with the learning preferences of Generation Z, a cohort that has grown up surrounded by technology and expects interactive, technology-rich learning experiences. Generation Z values educational tools that are engaging, individualized, and enriched by digital technologies—characteristics that make virtual game-based learning an ideal platform for their educational needs (Reid et al., 2023).

In virtual game-based environments, students take on a role (e.g., nurse) and use it to gather information, address clinical challenges, and make decisions that directly affect the outcome of the scenario. This approach fosters critical thinking by requiring students to evaluate the consequences of their choices and consider multiple potential outcomes based on their decisions (Reid et al., 2023). Instead of passively receiving information, students actively shape the scenario, which encourages deeper engagement and promotes reflection on their decision-making processes. This method is particularly beneficial for developing clinical judgment, as it challenges students to consider various perspectives and assess their actions through a dynamic, evolving narrative.

One of the key advantages of virtual game-based learning is its ability to offer repeated practice opportunities, which is not possible in traditional clinical settings. In real-world clinical practice, nursing students cannot revisit a previous patient encounter to explore alternative decisions. However, virtual game-based learning allows students to engage with the same scenario multiple times, make different choices, and learn from the resulting consequences. Flexibility to experiment and make mistakes in a controlled environment fosters reflective practice by presenting errors as opportunities for growth rather than failures. This type of learning environment supports continuous feedback, enabling students to refine their clinical decision-making skills. The opportunity to explore multiple solutions to a clinical problem encourages critical thinking, adaptability, and, ultimately, the development of clinical competence, thus providing students with a strong foundation for future practice (Cant et al., 2023).

Electronic Escape Rooms

Escape rooms have rapidly evolved from recreational activities into powerful educational tools that are gaining popularity, especially in healthcare education (Quek et al., 2024). These immersive, game-based learning experiences engage students in problem-solving tasks, fostering active learning and critical thinking—skills essential to nursing practice. Particularly in their electronic format, escape rooms offer an engaging and effective method for developing critical clinical nursing skills.

In nursing education, escape rooms are traditionally designed as face-to-face activities in which students collaborate to solve clinical challenges rooted in realistic patient scenarios. These activities aim to apply theoretical knowledge, improve clinical reasoning, and encourage teamwork as students unlock a series of puzzles or "locks" (Rushdan et al., 2024). Typically, students follow a clinically based storyline, gathering clues related to patient assessment, medication administration, and specific nursing interventions. In many cases, students use digital devices such as smartphones, tablets, or laptops to access web-based resources that support their decision making, an approach that guides them to apply evidence-based practice in clinical scenarios (Yang et al., 2023).

The primary advantage of escape rooms in education is their capacity to promote teamwork and collaboration—fundamental elements of effective nursing practice (Quek et al., 2024). Designed to simulate real-world clinical situations, escape rooms require students to engage in collaborative problem-solving and critical thinking. These activities not only enhance cognitive and psychomotor skills but also help students develop essential attributes, including communication, leadership, and adaptability—qualities that are crucial for success in clinical environments (Rushdan et al., 2024; Yang et al., 2023). Asynchronous electronic escape rooms offer flexibility, allowing students to work independently at their own pace; synchronous versions, often facilitated through video conferencing tools, provide opportunities for real-time collaboration, simulating clinical team dynamics and reinforcing interpersonal skills (Quek et al., 2024).

Escape rooms are particularly effective in nursing education as formative evaluation tools. Kim et al. (2025) specifically explored how escape rooms serve as an alternative formative assessment method. Their study evaluated first-year nursing students' clinical reasoning, decision making, and teamwork skills and found that escape rooms create an immersive environment in which students participate in collaborative problem-solving tasks that are essential for developing practical clinical competencies. The real-time feedback provided during escape room activities allows educators to assess student progress, identify areas for further instruction, and offer immediate insights into students' understanding and application of nursing concepts. This feedback mechanism aligns with the formative nature of the assessment by supporting student skill development throughout the learning process (Kim et al., 2025; Yang et al., 2023).

By incorporating electronic escape rooms into both asynchronous and synchronous learning formats, educators can effectively reinforce core competencies such as critical thinking, problem-solving, and interprofessional collaboration. Escape rooms not only support immediate learning but also enhance knowledge retention as students engage deeply with clinical scenarios that mirror real-world healthcare situations (Kim et al., 2025). These digital tools serve as both innovative methods for skill development and dynamic ways to engage students; moreover, they make the learning process both enjoyable and impactful (Quek et al., 2024; Rushdan et al., 2024). Such innovative, game-based learning strategies will likely soon become indispensable for preparing students to meet the challenges of modern healthcare and ensuring that they excel academically and thrive in real-world clinical settings.

ARTIFICIAL INTELLIGENCE IN CLINICAL EDUCATION

As healthcare continues to evolve, so must nursing education. Given the increasing integration of AI into clinical settings, it is essential that nursing students be equipped with the knowledge and skills to effectively use these technologies in their practice. AI is no longer a distant concept; it has become a pivotal part of healthcare, with applications ranging from clinical decision support systems to predictive analytics and patient monitoring tools (Cary et al., 2024). To prepare students for the future of healthcare, nursing education must adapt to this technological shift by incorporating AI into clinical teaching.

Artificial Intelligence's Role in Ethical Decision Making

AI technologies offer unique opportunities to enhance nursing students' clinical reasoning and decision making. One key area in which AI can play a transformative role is in promoting health equity. Cary et al. (2024) highlight how AI can assist nursing students in addressing healthcare disparities by providing them with tools to make more informed, equitable decisions as they engage with diverse patient populations. AI can help students to identify and address social determinants of health, ultimately improving patient outcomes.

AI tools are becoming more prevalent in clinical practice, offering clinical educators valuable new opportunities to guide students in the critical skill of ethical decision making. Shin et al. (2024) demonstrated that AI-assisted learning can help nursing students explore complex clinical scenarios and improve their ability to navigate ethical dilemmas, such as balancing patient autonomy with clinical data. AI allows educators to design exercises that not only teach students how to use AI but also challenge them to apply ethical frameworks aligned with nursing values to make ethically sound decisions.

AI-enhanced debriefing in nursing simulations has the potential to boost clinical skills development. Benfatah et al. (2024) found that AI-assisted debriefing provides personalized feedback that increases student engagement, confidence, and critical reflection. AI tools that analyze performance in real-time allow educators to provide objective data to help students identify their strengths and areas for improvement and refine their clinical decision making, thereby enhancing their overall ethical decision-making process. However, it is crucial that AI-driven feedback be integrated with traditional teaching methods to ensure a comprehensive approach to ethical reasoning and clinical practice (Shin et al., 2024).

Personalized Learning Through Artificial Intelligence

Another exciting application of AI in nursing education is its ability to personalize learning. AI-driven systems can adapt to each student's unique learning needs, offering targeted learning opportunities that match their pace and understanding. This personalized approach is crucial for helping students master complex clinical concepts and improve their decision-making skills. Taskiran (2023) emphasizes how AI-driven courses can enhance students' readiness for clinical AI applications by providing real-time feedback and adjusting learning challenges according to their performance. For clinical educators, AI presents an opportunity to create a customized learning environment that offers individualized support. By leveraging AI systems, clinical educators can ensure that students receive tailored instruction that enables them to progress at their own pace, focusing on specific areas for improvement while reinforcing their strengths and clinical decision-making capabilities.

Artificial Intelligence-Integrated Healthcare Workforce

AI must be incorporated into nursing education not only to enhance students' technical skills but to prepare them to competently navigate an increasingly AI-integrated healthcare workforce. As AI tools become more widespread in clinical settings, clinical educators need to integrate AI literacy into their teaching to ensure that nursing students fully understand their use, benefits, limitations, and the ethical considerations surrounding their use. Simms (2025) emphasizes that AI literacy is essential for nursing students as it enables them to navigate the complexities of AI-driven healthcare systems while ensuring patient safety.

AI tools are reshaping nursing education by improving clinical reasoning, and ethical decision making, while ensuring that nursing students are prepared to work effectively in AI-integrated clinical environments. The future of nursing practice will see AI play a significant role in clinical decision making and patient care. Yalcinkaya et al. (2024) found that nursing students' attitudes toward and readiness to adopt AI technologies directly influence how successfully they integrate AI into their practice. Therefore, clinical educators must assess students' preparedness and attitudes toward AI, ensuring that they are comfortable and confident with using these tools in clinical settings.

As AI continues to evolve, clinical educators must ensure that nursing students are equipped with AI literacy, ethical decision-making skills, and the ability to interact with AI systems responsibly and effectively. Incorporating AI-focused curricula that emphasize critical thinking, problem-solving, and ethical considerations will prepare nursing students to meet the evolving demands of modern healthcare. By integrating these elements into nursing education, clinical educators can ensure that students not only excel academically but also thrive in real-world clinical settings. **Exhibit 9.1** summarizes actionable strategies that clinical educators can use to integrate AI into their teaching to enhance student learning and prepare future nurses for the AI-enhanced healthcare environments they will encounter in their clinical practice.

EXHIBIT 9.1 Strategies for Integrating Artificial Intelligence (AI) Into Clinical Teaching

- Integrate AI-assisted case studies and simulations: Use AI-driven simulations to create realistic clinical scenarios that enable students to practice decision making and receive real-time feedback to refine their clinical judgment.
- Promote AI literacy: Develop AI literacy modules to introduce students to AI tools and ensure that they understand AI's role in clinical decision making and patient care.
- Facilitate ethical decision making through AI: Implement AI-powered ethical decision making simulations to help students explore complex clinical scenarios and weigh the ethical implications of their decisions.
- Personalize learning pathways using AI: Use adaptive AI systems that adjust learning challenges based on individual performance to provide targeted support that meets students' unique needs.
- Assess AI readiness: Conduct preassessments to evaluate students' familiarity with AI tools and adjust teaching strategies to support their confidence in using AI in clinical practice.
- Encourage critical evaluation of AI-generated information: Train students and faculty to critically assess AI-generated outputs, recognizing both the potential benefits and limitations of AI in clinical decision making.
- Stay informed on emerging AI advancements: Given the rapid evolution of AI, educators should stay up to date with new developments and best practices to ensure that AI integration in clinical teaching remains relevant and evidence based.

CONSIDERATIONS FOR TECHNOLOGY INTEGRATION

As we move beyond the immediate challenges of the COVID-19 pandemic, the landscape of health professions education continues to evolve, propelled by the rapid pace of technological advancement. The pandemic underscored the pivotal role of technology in reshaping educational practices, driving innovation and adaptation across fields such as medical and nursing education (Sungkono et al., 2024). Virtual learning, enriched by technologies such as telepresence, AI, and virtual reality, has dramatically expanded possibilities in clinical teaching. These tools not only enable immersive learning experiences but also provide students with the chance to refine essential clinical skills in dynamic, simulated environments. However, the integration of these technologies into clinical teaching presents unique challenges. Clinical educators must address issues related to accessibility and digital literacy, ensuring that technology enhances, rather than complicates, the clinical learning experience.

Looking ahead, nursing education programs must continue to prioritize a holistic and thoughtful approach to technology integration that aligns with the core competencies required in modern healthcare (AACN, 2021). The seamless adoption of new technologies necessitates a deep understanding of their ethical, practical, and pedagogical implications within the clinical setting. For instance, as AI and telehealth tools become increasingly embedded in healthcare systems, it is imperative that nursing students are prepared not only to use these tools effectively but also to engage with them critically and competently (Cary et al., 2024; Koppel et al., 2022). These tools have the potential to transform clinical practice, and clinical educators must ensure that students remain focused on patient-centered care while navigating the ethical complexities they may present.

One of the key opportunities arising from the integration of new technologies is the potential for interprofessional learning within the clinical environment. The COVID-19 pandemic forced many healthcare education systems to rapidly adopt remote learning technologies that have now opened doors for more flexible, immersive training. Tools such as telepresence and telehealth platforms enable real-time collaboration between nursing students and professionals from diverse healthcare disciplines, fostering critical communication and teamwork skills. This collaboration is invaluable in preparing students to work effectively within multidisciplinary teams, a critical skill in the complex, interconnected healthcare environments they will soon enter. By fostering these interprofessional learning opportunities, clinical educators can better prepare students to thrive in diverse, team-oriented clinical settings (Elendu et al., 2024).

Equally important to successful technology integration in clinical teaching is the role of technology champions within nursing education programs (Tischendorf et al., 2024). These champions are instrumental in overcoming barriers to adoption, providing continuous support to both faculty and students and advocating for the ongoing evolution of digital learning practices. The integration of these advanced tools into clinical teaching requires leadership that bridges the gap between traditional practices and new technology, ensuring a smooth transition and promoting sustained use. As catalysts for change, technology champions ensure that innovations are adopted and adapted to meet the specific needs of clinical education. Cultivating a culture of innovation that encourages faculty, students, and technology experts to collaborate in shaping and testing new educational tools is crucial for keeping nursing education dynamic, forward-thinking, and responsive to emerging healthcare trends (Tischendorf et al., 2024).

At the heart of these efforts is the overarching goal of preparing nursing students for the future of healthcare. By thoughtfully integrating pedagogical technologies into clinical nursing education, educators can provide students with rich, engaging learning experiences that refine their clinical judgment, strengthen their decision-making abilities, and better prepare them for the evolving demands of patient care. As healthcare becomes increasingly technology-driven, the role of clinical nurse educators will be pivotal in ensuring that students are not only competent in utilizing these tools but also equipped to use them ethically, responsibly, and effectively in clinical practice.

SUMMARY

Clinical practice experiences are essential for ensuring that nursing students can apply theoretical knowledge and develop key clinical skills. As the healthcare landscape evolves, pedagogical technologies are increasingly shaping how these skills are taught, necessitating a shift in clinical teaching strategies. The integration of technologies such as simulated EHRs, telehealth, virtual learning platforms, and AI is transforming clinical education, providing students with new opportunities to refine their abilities in dynamic, real-world contexts.

Pedagogical technologies are essential for preparing nursing students to meet the complex demands of modern healthcare. The ongoing integration of these technologies into clinical education, guided by best practices, connects students with innovative tools that foster the development of critical competencies. These technologies not only support data collection but also play a pivotal role in delivering high-quality healthcare. Nursing leaders and educators must strategically integrate these tools to cultivate advanced clinical skills and ensure that graduates are equipped to excel in today's healthcare environments.

This chapter explored how emerging technologies are reshaping clinical teaching. Practical guidance was provided for clinical educators to effectively integrate these technologies into their teaching practices. Additionally, the chapter reflected on the evolution of virtual clinical learning, underscoring the transition in the postpandemic era to more robust, technology-enhanced learning models that meet the evolving demands of healthcare education.

CNE®cl EXAMINATION TEST BLUEPRINT CORE COMPETENCIES

1. **Function within the Education and Health Care Environments**
   A. Function in the Clinical Nurse Educator Role
      1. Integrate theory and practice in the clinical setting
      2. Foster professional growth of learners (e.g., coaching, reflection, and debriefing)
      3. Use technologies to support clinical teaching and learning
   B. Operationalize the Curriculum
      3. Facilitate meaningful and relevant clinical learning activities to promote optimal learning
      4. Prepare learners for clinical experiences (e.g., facility, clinical expectations, equipment, and technology-based resources)
      5. Implement clinical activities to help learners develop interprofessional collaboration and teamwork skills
      6. Provide opportunities for learners to develop clinical judgement related to course outcomes
2. **Facilitate Learning in the Healthcare Environment**
   A. Implement a variety of clinical teaching strategies congruent with learner needs, desired learner outcomes, course outcomes, setting, and context (e.g., virtual, telehealth, in-person, simulation)
4. **Apply Clinical Expertise in the Healthcare Environment**
   F. Demonstrate competence with technologies available in the clinical learning environment
5. **Facilitate Learner Development and Socialization**
   F. Create learning environments that promote socialization to the role of the nurse
6. **Implement Effective Clinical and Assessment Evaluation Strategies**
   A. Employ a variety of strategies to determine achievement of learning outcomes
   B. Conduct formative and summative evaluation specific to the learner and learning outcomes
   F. Use situational assessment data to facilitate learning in the clinical learning environment
   H. Evaluate the quality of the clinical learning experiences and environment

This chapter was prepared based on work by Meigan Robb in the sixth edition of the book.

LEARNING ACTIVITIES

CourseConnect

To access self-assessment questions and interactive, competency-based learning activities for this chapter, visit www.springerpub.com/courseconnect. See inside front cover and tear-out card for CourseConnect details.

REFERENCES

American Association of Colleges of Nursing. (2021). *The essentials: Core competencies for professional nursing education.* https://www.aacnnursing.org/Portals/42/AcademicNursing/pdf/Essentials-2021.pdf

Basil, N. N., Ambe, S., Ekhator, C., & Fonkem, E. (2022). Health records database and inherent security concerns: A review of the literature. *Cureus, 14*(10), e30168. https://doi.org/10.7759/cureus.30168

Bates, A. W. (2022). Choosing and using media in education: The SECTIONS model. In *Teaching in a digital age* (3rd ed.). https://pressbooks.bccampus.ca/teachinginadigitalagev3/part/9-pedagogical-differences-between-media

Benavente, K., Banaschak, C., & Szotek, P. (2023). Replacing conventional telecommunication with a freeform HIPAA compliant healthcare texting app: A survey of patient preference. *Surgical Endoscopy, 37*, 2182–2188. https://doi.org/10.1007/s00464-023-09869-z

Benfatah, M., Youlyouz-Marfak, I., Saad, E., Hilali, A., Nejjari, C., & Marfak, A. (2024). Impact of artificial intelligence-enhanced debriefing on clinical skills development in nursing students: A comparative study. *Teaching and Learning in Nursing, 19*, e574–e579. https://doi.org/10.1016/j.teln.2024.04.007

Bristol, A. A., Litchman, M., Berg, C., Grigorian, E., Small, D., Glazener, A., Jones, C., & Allen, N. A. (2023). Using continuous glucose monitoring and data sharing to encourage collaboration among older adults with type 1 diabetes and their care partners: Qualitative descriptive study. *JMIR Nursing, 6*, e46627. https://doi.org/10.2196/46627

Cant, R., Ryan, C., & Kelly, M. A. (2023). Use and effectiveness of virtual simulations in nursing student education: An umbrella review. *CIN: Computers, Informatics, Nursing, 41*(1), 31–38. https://doi.org/10.1097/CIN.0000000000000932

Cary, M. P., Jr., De Gagne, J. C., Kauschinger, E. D., & Carter, B. M. (2024). Advancing health equity through artificial intelligence: An educational framework for preparing nurses in clinical practice and research. *Creative Nursing, 30*(2), 154–164. https://doi.org/10.1177/10784535241249193

Chunta, K., Shellenbarger, T., & Chicca, J. (2021). Generation Z students in the online environment: Strategies for nurse educators. *Nurse Educator*, *46*(2), 87–91. https://doi.org/10.1097/NNE.0000000000000872

Elendu, C., Amaechi, D. C., Okatta, A. U., Amaechi, E. C., Elendu, T. C., Ezeh, C. P., & Elendu, I. D. (2024). The impact of simulation-based training in medical education: A review. *Medicine*, *103*(27), e38813. https://doi.org/10.1097/MD.0000000000038813

Forneris, S. (2023). Teaching and learning using simulation. In D. M. Billings & J. A. Halstead (Eds.), *Teaching in nursing: A guide for faculty* (7th ed., pp. 422–448). Elsevier.

Kan, E. Z., & Stabler-Haas, S. (2025). *Fast facts for the clinical nursing instructor* (4th ed.). Springer Publishing Company.

Kim, C., Ke, F., & Brewer, V. (2025). Escape rooms as formative knowledge assessment: A quasi-experimental study. *Nurse Education Today*, *147*, 106572. https://doi.org/10.1016/j.nedt.2025.106572

Kleib, M., Arnaert, A., Nagle, L. M., Ali, S., Idrees, S., Costa, D. D., Kennedy, M., & Darko, E. M. (2024). Digital health education and training for undergraduate and graduate nursing students: Scoping review. *JMIR Nursing*, *7*, e58170. https://doi.org/10.2196/58170

Koppel, P. D., De Gagne, J. C., Docherty, S., Smith, S., Prose, N. S., & Jabaley, T. (2022). Exploring nurse and patient experiences of developing rapport during oncology ambulatory care videoconferencing visits: Qualitative descriptive study. *Journal of Medical Internet Research*, *24*(9), e39920. https://doi.org/10.2196/39920

Leoste, J., Virkus, S., Talisainen, A., Tammemäe, K., Kangur, K., & Petriashvili, I. (2022). Higher education personnel's perceptions about telepresence robots. *Frontiers in Robotics and AI*, *9*, 976836. https://doi.org/10.3389/frobt.2022.976836

Li, Y., Wang, M., Wang, L., Cao, Y., Liu, Y., Zhao, Y., Yuan, R., Yang, M., Lu, S., Sun, Z., Zhou, F., Qian, Z., & Kang H. (2024). Advances in the application of AI robots in critical care: Scoping review. *Journal of Medical Internet Research*, *26*, e54095. https://doi.org/10.2196/54095

Mollart, L., Newell, R., Geale, S. K., Noble, D., Norton, C., & O'Brien, A. P. (2020). Introduction of patient electronic medical records (EMR) into undergraduate nursing education: An integrated literature review. *Nurse Education Today*, *94*, 1–13. https://doi.org/10.1016/j.nedt.2020.104517

Okolo, C. A., Ijeh, S., Arowoogun, J. O., Adeniyi, A. O., & Omotayo, O. (2024). Reviewing the impact of health information technology on healthcare management efficiency. *International Medical Science Research Journal*, *4*(4), 420–440. https://doi.org/10.51594/imsrj.v4i4.1000

Quek, L. H., Tan, A. J. Q., Sim, M. J. J., Ignacio, J., Harder, N., Lamb, A., Chua, W. L., Lau, S. T., & Liaw, S. Y. (2024). Educational escape rooms for healthcare students: A systematic review. *Nurse Education Today*, *132*, 106004. https://doi.org/10.1016/j.nedt.2023.106004

Reid, L., Button, D., & Brommeyer, M. (2023). Challenging the myth of the digital native: A narrative review. *Nursing Reports*, *13*(2), 573–600. https://doi.org/10.3390/nursrep13020052

Rushdan, E. E., El-Sayed Mohamed, M. A., Abdelhalim, G. E., El-Ashry, A. M., & Ali, H. F. M. (2024). Effect of an escape room as a gamification evaluation tool on clinical reasoning and teamwork skills among nursing students: A quasi-experimental study. *Nurse Education in Practice*, *82*, 104188. https://doi.org/10.1016/j.nepr.2024.104188

Samadbeik, M., Fatehi, F., Braunstein, M., Barry, B., Saremian, M., Kalhor, F., & Edirippulige, S. (2020). Education and training on electronic medical records (EMRs) for healthcare professionals and students: A scoping review. *International Journal of Medical Informatics*, *142*(2020), 104238. https://doi.org/10.1016/j.ijmedinf.2020.104238

Shin, H., De Gagne, J. C., Kim, S. S., & Hong, M. (2024). The impact of artificial intelligence-assisted learning on nursing students' ethical decision-making and clinical reasoning in pediatric care. *CIN: Computers, Informatics, Nursing*, *42*(10), 704–711. https://doi.org/10.1097/CIN.0000000000001177

Simms, R. C. (2025). Generative artificial intelligence (AI) literacy in nursing education: A crucial call to action. *Nurse Education Today*, *146*, 106544. https://doi.org/10.1016/j.nedt.2024.106544

Sungkono, Makrufardi, F., Fairuz, A., Azizah, N., Ekaputra, F., & Sungkono, M. (2024). Exploring challenges, innovations, and technological integration in medical education after COVID-19 pandemic: An in-depth analysis. *Journal of Medicine*, *25*(2), 166–172. https://doi.org/10.3329/jom.v25i2.74377

Taskiran, N. (2023). Effect of artificial intelligence course in nursing on students' medical artificial intelligence readiness: A comparative quasi-experimental study. *Nurse Educator*, *48*(5), E147–E152. https://doi.org/10.1097/NNE.0000000000001446

Tischendorf, T., Heitmann-Möller, A., Ruppert, S.-N., Marchwacka, M., Schaffrin, S., Schaal, T., & Hasseler, M. (2024). Sustainable integration of digitalisation in nursing education—An international scoping review. *Frontiers in Health Services*, *4*, 1344021. https://doi.org/10.3389/frhs.2024.1344021

Whitt, K. J., Allen, C. L., Hogg, C. W., Pericak, A., Beebe, S. L., Braungart, C., Knestrick, J., Harrod, T., & McNelis, A. M. (2024). The use of electronic health records in advanced practice nursing education: A scoping review. *Journal of Professional Nursing*, *50*, 83–94. https://doi.org/10.1016/j.profnurs.2023.11.007

Wittler, A., Perez, A., & Griffin, V. (2025). Telehealth virtual simulation across the family nurse practitioner curriculum. *Nursing Education Perspectives*, *46*(1), 52–54. https://doi.org/10.1097/01.NEP.0000000000001262

Yalcinkaya, T., Ergin, E., & Yucel, S. C. (2024). Exploring nursing students' attitudes and readiness for artificial intelligence: A cross-sectional study. *Teaching and Learning in Nursing*, *19*(4), e722–e728. https://doi.org/10.1016/j.teln.2024.07.008

Yang, C.-L., Chang, C.-Y., & Jen, H.-J. (2023). Facilitating undergraduate students' problem-solving and critical thinking competence via online escape room learning. *Nurse Education in Practice*, *73*, 103828. https://doi.org/10.1016/j.nepr.2023.103828

Yu, M., & Mann, J. S. (2021). Development of virtual reality simulation program for high-risk neonatal infection control education. *Clinical Simulation in Nursing*, *50*, 19–26. https://doi.org/10.1016/j.ecns.2020.10.006

Preceptors as Clinical Teachers

10

OBJECTIVES:

1. Appraise the effectiveness of preceptorship experiences for nursing student learning.
2. Examine the advantages and disadvantages of preceptorships in clinical nursing education.
3. Suggest effective approaches for selecting, preparing, implementing, evaluating, and rewarding preceptors who work with nursing students.

Preceptorship experiences are widely used across all educational levels as an alternative to the traditional clinical teaching model. In the preceptor model, an experienced nurse, known as a preceptor, guides student learning in a clinical setting. This approach, drawing upon apprenticeship theory, allows students to be immersed in clinical learning with an expert as the coach and primary teacher. The preceptor directs the student and provides opportunities for the student to gain clinical nursing knowledge and skills, and facilitates opportunities to translate theory into practice. Additionally, the preceptor helps socialize the student in understanding the role of the nurse.

Preceptorships have been used with prelicensure nursing students, graduate students preparing for advanced practice roles, and new staff nurse orientees (Ulrich, 2024). These preceptor experiences may be known by other names such as practicums, internships, immersion experiences, clinical partnerships, coaching models, capstone experiences, or externships (National Advisory Council on Nurse Education and Practice, 2024). Regardless of the name used, this experience allows students an opportunity to work one-to-one in a clinical setting with an expert who facilitates and supervises clinical learning. This chapter discusses the effective use of preceptors as clinical teachers and coaches. The advantages and disadvantages of preceptorships are examined, and suggestions are made for selecting, preparing, implementing, evaluating, and rewarding preceptors.

PRECEPTORSHIP MODEL OF CLINICAL TEACHING

A preceptorship involves a time-limited, one-to-one relationship between a learner and an experienced nurse who is employed in a healthcare setting in which the learning activities take place. Since the academic clinical teacher may not be physically present during the learning activities, the preceptor assumes the teaching responsibilities and guides the learner to develop their clinical competence, confidence and clinical reasoning. Regardless of learners' levels of education and experience, preceptorships provide professional enculturation and opportunities for socialization into professional nursing roles. They also enhance the personal and professional development of the preceptors and allow preceptors to contribute to the growth of the profession through this service (National Center for the Apprenticeship Degree [NCAD], 2024).

The preceptor model is collaborative. The teacher is a faculty member who has overall responsibility for the quality of the clinical teaching and learning. The teacher provides the link between the educational program and the practice setting by selecting and preparing preceptors, assigning students to preceptors, providing guidance for the selection of appropriate learning activities, serving as a resource to the preceptor–student pair, and evaluating student and preceptor performance. The preceptor functions as a role model and provides individualized clinical instruction, coaching, support, and socialization for the learner. The preceptor also serves as protector or advocate for the student and provides input into the evaluation of learner performance.

USE OF PRECEPTORSHIPS IN NURSING EDUCATION

In academic programs that prepare nurses for initial entry into practice, preceptorships are usually used for students in their final year of study. The decision to use preceptors for clinical teaching should be based on the perceived benefits to students, the educational program and focus, student learning needs, clinical sites and staff available, and accreditation and practice requirements.

Apprenticeships are another related emerging area of growth in prelicensure nursing education that involves preceptor experiences. These apprenticeships offer an alternative educational pathway for students to gain real-world training, mentoring, and support while pairing classroom learning with paid, hands-on clinical experiences under the guidance of a nursing clinical supervisor or a preceptor. In states such as Alabama, Kentucky, Nevada, and North Dakota, student apprentices working under state regulations are paid for supervised clinical work in healthcare settings. State or federal funding may also support additional financial incentives for the clinical preceptors who validate student skill mastery and guide clinical performance with nursing skills and activities (Lerman et al., 2024; [NCAD], 2024). As nursing seeks to address workforce development and funding initiatives are created, apprenticeships will offer an alternative educational pathway, allowing students to gain practical supervised experience in the workplace along with payment for their work.

Preceptorships are frequently used in graduate programs that prepare nurses for advanced clinical practice, administration, and education roles. At this level, a preceptorship involves well-defined learning objectives based on the student's education and experience. The student participates in learning activities that demonstrate functional role components, allowing rehearsal of role behaviors in a safe setting before assuming the advanced practice role. Depending upon the focus of the graduate program, these learning experiences can involve 500 or more clinical hours with preceptors. Recently, the National Task Force (NTF) for Quality Nurse Practitioner Education increased the required clinical hours for NP tracks to have a minimum of 750 direct patient care clinical hours (NTF for Quality Nurse Practitioner Education, 2022). The preceptor for graduate students must be an expert practitioner who can model the advanced practice role functions including decision making, problem solving, clinical reasoning and judgment, and leadership. Additionally, the NTF for Quality Nurse Practitioner Education (2022) provides a faculty and preceptor checklist that specifies the role of faculty and preceptors for NP students' clinical experience and outlines expectations for orientation, clinical experiences, communication, and evaluation.

ADVANTAGES AND DISADVANTAGES OF USING PRECEPTORS

The use of preceptors in clinical teaching has both advantages and disadvantages for the parties involved. Effective collaboration and adequate preparation of students and preceptors are required to minimize the drawbacks and achieve advantages for the educational programs, clinical agencies, teachers, preceptors, and students.

Preceptorships hold many potential advantages for preceptors and the clinical agencies that employ them. Nurses serving in preceptor roles report this experience helps to keep them current, remain stimulated in the profession, and contribute to the profession (Gholizadeh et al., 2022). While preceptors enjoy sharing their clinical knowledge and skill, they also appreciate the stimulation of working with students who challenge the status quo and raise questions about clinical practice. Preceptors also report increased job and career satisfaction (Ciocco, 2021). The interest and enthusiasm of students are often rewarding to nurses who take on the additional responsibilities of the preceptor role. In agencies that use a clinical ladder, serving as a preceptor may be a means of advancing professionally within the system or developing essential leadership and teaching skills. Additionally, working with students may be counted toward specialty recertification requirements. For example, the American Nurses Credentialing Center (2022) allows individuals renewing their certification to complete 120 hours as a preceptor providing direct clinical supervision/teaching to students related to the certification area as part of one of the renewal categories. For the clinical site, the preceptorship model also produces opportunities to recruit potential staff members for the clinical agency from among students who work with preceptors. The agency gets a "try before you buy" approach as they can assess the student, their performance, and fit with the staff and agency thus enabling informed hiring decisions.

Typically, one of the greatest drawbacks of preceptorships to agencies and preceptors is the expected time commitment. Some clinical agencies may not agree to provide preceptors because of increased patient acuity and staffing concerns. Additionally, potential preceptors may decline to participate because of the perception that guiding and evaluating a student would add to their workloads and be time intensive (Gaynor & Barnes, 2021; Henry-Okafor et al., 2023). Other factors such as compliance requirements; preceptor fatigue; institutional constraints and productivity demands; lack of incentives, recognition, and preceptor support; limited resources and time; and lack of experience or poor preparation for teaching are some of the reasons contributing to the difficulty in securing clinical sites and preceptors to work with students (Burt et al., 2022; Henry-Okafor et al., 2023; Videtech et al., 2022).

Students who participate in preceptorships enjoy several benefits. They have the advantage of working one-on-one with an expert who can coach them to increase clinical competence and performance. Preceptorships also provide opportunities for students to experience the realities of clinical practice, including scheduling learning activities on evening and night shifts and weekends to follow their preceptors' schedules. However, following their preceptors' schedules often creates conflicts with students' academic, work, and personal commitments. Additionally, a preceptor's clinical assignment may not always be appropriate or align with the student's clinical learning objectives.

Preceptorships offer many advantages for the educational program in which they are used. The use of preceptors provides rich educational experiences for students and more intensive, individualized guidance of students' learning activities. Working collaboratively with preceptors also helps teachers to stay informed about the current realities of practice; up-to-date clinical information benefits ongoing curriculum development.

Several disadvantages related to the use of preceptors may affect educational programs. Contrary to a common belief, teachers' responsibilities do not decrease when students work with preceptors. Initial identification of appropriate clinical sites, review and selection of preceptors, preparation of preceptors and students, and ongoing collaboration and communication with preceptors and students require as much or more time as the traditional clinical teaching model. The preceptorship model requires considerable indirect teaching time for the development of relationships with agencies and preceptors and the evaluation of preceptors and students. When preceptors are used as clinical teachers, faculty members may be responsible for more students in several clinical agencies and feel uncertain whether student learning aligns with course objectives. Additionally, with the growth of online graduate programs, clinical sites may not be easily accessible, yet site visits may be expected by staff and students. Conducting a traditional in-person site visit may require substantial time and financial expenditures, especially in remote or geographically distant areas. Lastly, educators report that it may be difficult to secure preceptors in specialty areas. Baccalaureate programs face challenges locating preceptors in pediatric, acute care, obstetric, and mental health sites. In graduate program, preceptors are difficult to secure in select advanced practice specialties such as pediatric primary care, women's health, and family practice/primary care and in rural and underserved areas (American Association of Colleges of Nursing [AACN] and the American Organization for Nursing Leadership [AONL], 2020; McInnis et al., 2021).

SELECTING PRECEPTORS

The success of preceptorships largely depends on the selection of appropriate preceptors; such selection is one of the teacher's most important responsibilities. Most faculty members consider the experience and educational preparation of the preceptor to be important. Most academic programs require the preceptor to have at least the degree for which the student is preparing, although insistence on this level of educational preparation does not guarantee that learners will be exposed only to appropriate professional role models. Nursing accreditors may also provide specific guidelines for preceptor selection. The Commission on Collegiate Nursing Education (CCNE, 2024) requires that preceptors be academically and experientially qualified for their role and have the expertise to support student achievement of expected outcomes. Similarly, the Accreditation Commission for Education in Nursing (ACEN, 2024) indicates that preceptors hold education qualifications required by regulatory agencies and that the nursing program preceptors be experientially qualified for their roles and responsibilities. They also add that preceptors should be oriented, mentored, and monitored and have clearly documented roles and responsibilities, which may include input into student evaluation. The accreditation standards for nursing programs provided by the National League for Nursing Commission for Nursing Education Accreditation (NLN CNEA, 2021) provides a quality indicator for preceptors suggesting that they are qualified and prepared for their role and responsibilities. They provide further interpretive guidelines and allow the nursing program to define the academic and experience qualifications ensuring that they align with regulatory agency rules and professional standards.

There is little standardization of regulations for nurse preceptors across the United States. The state board of nursing within each state may regulate qualifications, preparation, training, and role responsibilities for preceptors, yet there is little uniformity from state to state. According to a National Council of State Boards of Nursing (NCSBN) report providing member board profiles, 13 of the responding member boards do not regulate the use of preceptors for providing supervision and/or education to NP student; seven boards do not regulate preceptorships for RN students (NCSBN, 2024). States may specify requirements such as preceptors holding a state professional license, educational qualifications, years of experience, the amount of clinical time students can engage in the preceptorship experience, the number of students each preceptor can work with, and the faculty-to-student ratios. Nursing faculty should carefully review the state regulations that guide these experiences.

Regardless of the state mandated regulations, the desire to teach and willingness to serve as a preceptor are important qualities of potential preceptors. Nurses who feel obligated to enact this role may not make enthusiastic, effective preceptors. Additional attributes of effective preceptors, according to Ciocco (2021), include:

- *Clinical expertise or proficiency, depending on the level of the learner:* Preceptors should be able to demonstrate expert psychomotor, problem-solving, critical thinking, clinical reasoning, and decision-making skills in their clinical practice. Prelicensure nursing students need preceptors who are proficient clinicians; graduate students need preceptors who are expert clinicians.

- *Leadership abilities:* Good preceptors are change agents in the healthcare organizations in which they are employed. They demonstrate effective communication skills and are trusted and respected by their peers. Additionally, they are team players and work well with others.
- *Teaching interest and skill:* Preceptors must understand and use principles of adult learning. They should be able to communicate ideas effectively to learners and give descriptive positive and negative feedback.
- *Professional role behaviors and attitudes:* Preceptors must act as role models for learners, demonstrating accountability, maturity, and self-confidence. They approach learners nonthreateningly and nonjudgmentally, with effective communication and openness to questions. A positive attitude, flexibility, accessibility, and a sense of humor are also important traits. Preceptors who are enthusiastic, open-minded, and willing to work with diverse learners are particularly valuable (Chicca & Shellenbarger, 2020).

The selection of a preceptor and the clinical setting should also take into account the learner's interest in a specific clinical specialty, as well as the need for development of particular skills. The teacher may collaborate with nurse managers or other clinical staff to select appropriate preceptors. It may be unwise to choose preceptors from newly established practice areas or those areas with recent high staff turnover.

Potential preceptors for nursing students may be found in any clinical setting that meets the requirements of the nursing education program. There are variable approaches to the identification and selection of nurse preceptors. Doherty et al. (2020) report findings from a recent national survey of NP programs regarding the student clinical placement process. They identified the process for securing preceptors varied across programs. Thirty-one percent of survey respondents indicated that most preceptors are arranged by the school with some effort by the student. This was followed closely by the school securing all preceptors (29%). Another method used by 26% of nursing programs requires the student to locate the preceptor but having some assistance from the school. Lastly, only 14% of NP students needed to find their own preceptor. In Texas, a plurality of NPs who were surveyed indicated they needed to find their own clinical placements and were challenged in finding preceptors (Gigli & Gonzalez, 2022). Some states may have statutes preventing nursing students, particularly advanced practice nursing students, from finding their own preceptors. Therefore, prior to mandating students to self-identify preceptors independently and autonomously, it is important for the educational institution to check state regulations to ensure compliance with legal requirements. Regardless of the selection process, it appears that many schools and faculty are involved in the preceptor selection process.

Programs report a serious preceptor gap with as many as 60% of NP programs reporting an insufficient number of preceptors available to meet the demand (Henry-Okafor et al., 2023). Nursing programs may need to take proactive measures to identify and secure preceptors that will meet student and program needs. Established networks such as existing clinical partnerships and outreach to alumni groups may be a helpful approach to recruit potential preceptors. Other programs may wish to use marketing approaches using social media or program websites to recruit preceptors (Henry-Okafor et al., 2023).

Clinical teachers should carefully screen and select preceptors to ensure that the preceptor complies with program requirements and state board of nursing regulations. Graduate programs need to confirm that preceptors have the appropriate advanced nursing experience and qualifications. To facilitate preceptor identification and the matching process, some schools are using electronic modalities and algorithms for matching students with preceptors (Doherty et al., 2020). Independent companies have emerged to offer preceptor matching services and brokering of clinical placements. As the pay-to-precept model emerges, nursing programs will need to identify if they will use these services and if so, whether the student or the program pays for these services. Since these are relatively new services and many times have an associated cost, students, teachers, and nursing programs should carefully investigate the services offered, costs, quality, and the appropriateness of the match.

When trying to locate appropriate nurse preceptors within a healthcare agency, the staff development or education department is a good starting point. Some agencies designate a specific staff member as a gatekeeper for preceptor requests who can help identify appropriate matches. If applicable, students may also suggest potential preceptors based on their work experience or connections with nursing staff from previous clinical placements. Alumni of the nursing program are a rich source of potential preceptors. Many alumni are eager to give back to their alma mater and are honored to be asked to serve as preceptors. These potential preceptors can be recruited through alumni association events, phone or email outreach, professional social media groups, or alumni newsletters.

Another trend emerging, in part because of the difficulty in securing clinical preceptors, especially in hard-to-place advanced practice areas, involves paying preceptors. In the past, many nursing programs provided nonmonetary incentives for preceptors, but that may no longer be sufficient in acknowledging the work of the preceptor. The literature suggests that many preceptors believe that they should receive compensation for their precepting efforts due to lost productivity and as compensation for their time and increased workload associated with the precepting role. A large study of NP preceptors indicated compensation was important, but they were flexible in the format of compensation provided such as monetary disbursements or other types of honoraria or resources offered (Burt et al., 2022). Preceptor payment leads to questions pertaining to who pays this fee, displacement of students due to lack of fiscal resources, and inequities that may impact programs and students.

The preceptor payment trend is occurring in other health-related fields, with approximately 21% of physician assistant programs paying preceptors. The shift in compensation for preceptors in other related disciplines will generate increasing discussion in nursing education and should be carefully monitored to assess the impact upon students, preceptors, and nursing programs. At present, most schools report not paying for clinical preceptors; however, there are some program and regional differences (AACN & AONL, 2020). Graduate programs are more likely to pay for preceptors than baccalaureate programs. Additionally, baccalaureate programs in the North Atlantic region and graduate schools in the South and Midwest are more likely to pay clinical preceptors (AACN & AONL, 2020).

Funding to support preceptor payment is emerging in several ways. Some schools are charging students additional fees for clinical courses, while other schools allocate students a designated honorarium to distribute to preceptors. Preceptor compensation is also being tackled at the state level, with states such as Alabama, Colorado, Georgia, Hawaii, Louisiana, Maryland, South Carolina, and Washington offering income tax incentive credit programs or grants to nurse preceptors (Alabama Area Health Education Centers, 2024; George, 2023; National Advisory Council on Nurse Education and Practice, 2024; Stickel, 2023). Specific state guidelines and tax credit amounts vary by state. Regardless of the source of compensation or credit, this preceptor payment approach requires careful monitoring as it could significantly impact nursing programs, thereby creating financial pressure for the institution and competition among programs and possibly preceptors.

In addition to payment issues, nursing programs face additional challenges when offering nursing education through distance delivery modalities. Nursing programs are now reaching previously untapped student populations in remote settings through innovative delivery methods. However, these programs and students face added challenges when planning preceptor experiences. Online programs may need to work with boards of nursing and regulatory bodies to ensure compliance with appropriate approval processes. When students are working with preceptors at remote or distant sites, the board of nursing in those states will need to be aware of clinical experiences occurring in their jurisdiction and the program must comply with any approval regulations or state authorization requirements. Clinical teachers or clinical coordinators are advised to contact the appropriate state board of nursing as other requirements may vary from state to state. Additionally, to streamline distance education program delivery and ensure quality, nursing programs may also wish to explore the National Council for State Authorization Reciprocity Agreements (NC-SARA) at www.nc-sara.org. It is important to identify possible clinical sites and preceptors early in the planning process so that appropriate screening can occur, and programs can ensure compliance with all regulations is complete before the clinical experience begins.

Working with preceptors at clinical sites, particularly those at distant locations or involving advanced practice programs, can be challenging. Developing partnerships with preceptors and clinical agencies may be an effective approach to ensure that qualified and adequately prepared preceptors are available for students. Clinical teachers can work closely with the clinical site preceptors to understand the unique aspects of the clinical site, the populations served, the clinical role, and to ensure that clinical placements align with program and student needs.

PREPARING THE PARTICIPANTS

Thorough preparation, either formal or informal, of preceptors and students for their roles is key to the success of preceptorships. Teachers are responsible for initial orientation and continuing support of all participants.

Preceptor Preparation

Preparation of preceptors may begin with a general orientation, possibly for groups of potential preceptors at the selected clinical site or for all preceptors working with students from one nursing education program. Given the rapid rise in remote preceptorship experiences and restricted faculty and preceptor time, educators may also develop and implement an electronic orientation for preceptors. A preceptorship preparation program acknowledges the need for and commitment to collaboration in nursing education and helps to decrease feelings of isolation, anxiety, or uncertainty associated with the preceptor role. This preparation supports the learning needs of preceptors, enabling them to perform their role effectively and confidently, and may also help to prevent potential issues.

To ensure adequate preceptor training, a structured program offering resources and ongoing support can help to meet preceptor needs. Content of a general preceptorship preparation program may include the training topics and resources identified in **Exhibit 10.1**. Additionally, NP preceptors suggested topics such as differential diagnosis generation, note writing, physical assessment, handoffs, and history taking were necessary to guide their work with graduate students (Burt et al., 2022).

Additionally, nursing faculty will also need to ensure preceptors understand course and faculty expectations, the academic program structure, curriculum, program goals, and information about the student they will be working with such as prior experiences and level in the program. Consideration should be given to the format of the orientation information provided to the preceptor. Educators might consider a multimodal approach which may include written materials supplemented with face-to-face, telephone, videoconferencing, or electronic delivery. Preceptors appreciate having electronic access and the ability to add to the repository and share information (Videtech et al., 2022). NP preceptors indicated they would prefer technology-based resources such as those with smartphone access or website platforms to facilitate easy retrieval of information. Paper manuals and verbal information was reported as the least helpful orientation strategy (Burt et al., 2022). **Exhibit 10.2** offers an example of written guidelines for preceptors of graduate nursing students.

EXHIBIT 10.1 Sample Content for Preceptorship Training and Resources

- Understanding the preceptor role and preceptor core competencies
- Facilitating learning
- Principles of adult learning
- Strategies for creating a positive learning environment
- Establishing a professional identity
- Developing and using goals, objectives, and outcomes
- Effective communication approaches
- Coaching
- Use of instructional technology
- Understanding the needs of specific learner populations
- Assessing and addressing preceptee behaviors
- Pragmatics of precepting including management and leadership development
- Self-care for preceptors

Source: Ulrich, B. T. (2024). *Mastering precepting* (3rd ed.). Sigma Theta Tau.

EXHIBIT 10.2 Sample Guideline Material to Include for a Preceptor of a Graduate Nursing Student

The preceptor is expected to:

- Facilitate the student's entry into the healthcare organization
- Provide the student with an orientation to the organization
- After receiving the student's learning goals for the precepted experience, provide suggestions for how these goals can be accomplished
- Assist the student to identify activities that are consistent with organizational needs and the student's interests, abilities, and learning needs
- Meet with the student at regular intervals to discuss progress and achievement of individual and course objectives
- Provide the student with regular feedback regarding their performance
- Communicate regularly with the faculty member regarding the student's progress
- Serve as a role model and facilitate learning opportunities
- At the end of the preceptorship experience, the preceptor should provide a written evaluation of the student's performance related to goal achievement, clinical knowledge and skill, problem-solving and decision-making, communication, and interpersonal skills

Additionally, other materials used for orientation may include course and program-specific information such as:

- *The educational level and previous experience of the student*: Preceptors will find it helpful to understand what courses and content students previously completed so the preceptor can develop realistic performance expectations and select appropriate learning experiences. Beginning students may not have developed the knowledge and skill to participate in all of the preceptor's activities. Graduate students need learning activities that build on their previous learning and prior experiences to produce advanced practice outcomes.
- *Structure of the course:* Information about the course including the number of hours required for the experience.
- *How to choose specific learning activities based on learning objectives:* The teacher may share samples of learning contracts or lists of learning activities to guide the preceptor's selection of appropriate activities for the student.
- *Scheduling of clinical learning activities*: A common feature of preceptorships is the scheduling of the student's learning activities according to the preceptor's work schedule. Preceptors should be advised of dates that students and teachers may not be

available because of school holidays, examinations, and other course requirements.
- *Contacts:* How and under what circumstances to contact the course faculty member.

New preceptors have learning needs much like those of students and new staff nurses; supportive role models and coaching are essential to success.

Student Preparation

Learners also need to understand the purposes and processes of the preceptorship. They need an orientation to the process of planning individual learning activities, an explanation of teacher and preceptor roles, and a review of policies specific to student practice. Some faculty may require students to develop clinical learning objectives and may need guidance on the creation of these items. At the beginning of the preceptorship, teachers should clarify evaluation responsibilities and expectations such as dates for learning contract approval, frequency and format of site visits, and conferences with faculty members.

IMPLEMENTATION

Successful implementation of preceptorships depends on mutual understanding of the roles and responsibilities of the participants. The teacher, student, and preceptor collaborate to plan and implement learning activities that will facilitate the student's goal attainment. Key to these processes is frequent, clear, and effective communication among the participants.

Roles and Responsibilities of Participants

PRECEPTORS

Preceptors are responsible for patient care delivery in addition to clinical teaching of the student. The preceptor is expected to be a positive role model and a resource person for the student. The clinical teaching responsibilities of the preceptor include creating a positive learning climate, including the student in activities that relate to learning goals, and providing feedback to the student and teacher. The Preceptor Expectation Checklist, developed by the National Organization of Nurse Practitioner Faculties (NONPF) and the American Association of Nurse Practitioners (AANP), provides a guide that faculty can use to ensure clear preceptor expectations. A recent international literature review proposed seven essential preceptor competencies that can be used to define the role of preceptors. These preceptor competencies are found in **Figure 10.1**.

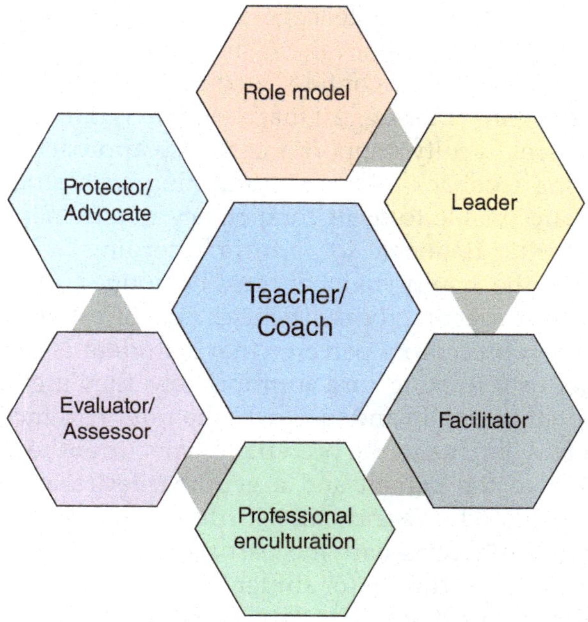

Figure 10.1. Seven RN preceptor competencies which together help facilitate clinical supervision of nursing students.

Source: Ryan, C. L. Cant, R., Hughes, L., Ahchay, D., & Strickland, K. (2024). Core competencies for registered nurse preceptors: A mapping review of quantitative studies. *Nursing Open, 11*(2), e2076. https://doi.org/10.1002/nop2.2076

Role model behaviors important for preceptors to demonstrate can be classified into four categories:

- *Technical and Technology Skills:* Demonstrates nursing care procedures; operation of equipment unique to that clinical setting; use of the electronic health record; and evidence-based, current nursing practices.
- *Interpersonal Skills:* Uses effective communication techniques with patients and family members; interacts with members of the interdisciplinary healthcare team in a collegial, confident manner; displays appropriate use of humor; demonstrates caring attitude toward patients; gives constructive feedback; uses questioning techniques.
- *Clinical Reasoning and Clinical Judgment:* Listens carefully during reporting and asks pertinent questions about patients' conditions; demonstrates proficient problem solving, critical thinking, and clinical reasoning; and incorporates skills of noticing, interpreting, responding, and reflecting as part of clinical decision making.
- *Professional Role Behaviors:* Keeps patient information confidential; encourages discussion of ethical issues; demonstrates enthusiasm about nursing; demonstrates accountability for own actions.

Sometimes preceptors experience conflict between the educator and evaluator roles. Preceptors play a key role as professional gatekeepers' ensuring the delivery of safe and competent care. Although preceptors may lack experience and confidence with the evaluator role and be hesitant to suggest that a student is failing, they must seek faculty support and devise approaches for offering feedback and communicating with students who are unable to meet competency requirements. If the learner is unable to perform according to expectations, the faculty member must be notified so that a plan for correcting the deficiencies may be established.

When preceptors perceive that a student is unable to perform nursing care appropriately, they are often tempted to step in and take over the care. This inclination may be due to the preceptor's concurrent responsibility to the patient and a genuine desire to share clinical knowledge and skill with the student. However, doing so interferes with the learning experience and is a missed opportunity for student development.

To support students as they learn their nursing role, preceptors should use a coaching process. In sports, coaches stand on the sidelines; they do not participate in or interfere with the game unless there is a risk of injury. For example, a soccer coach who notices lightning on the horizon may interrupt the game by alerting the referee to stop play and clear the field. A good preceptor, using coaching techniques, allows the learner to be in control of the patient situation and stands nearby, monitoring the unfolding situation, offering verbal cues when needed, asking questions to guide the student's problem solving and clinical reasoning, offering encouragement (e.g., "That's right," "Keep going"), and then giving immediate feedback for the student to reflect on. One effective feedback strategy that can be used by preceptors is the Ask, Respond, Tell method. The preceptor can ask the student how they felt during a clinical experience, respond with observations made during the experience, and then share or "tell" one teaching point (Johnson, et al., 2022). The coach's expression of belief in the student's capacity to succeed helps the student develop self-efficacy and self-confidence. Thus, effective coaching can help students feel more confident in their clinical abilities and see themselves as authentic care providers. However, if a student "freezes" because of overwhelming anxiety, an error, inadequate preparation, or an unexpected occurrence, the preceptor may need to intervene if this places the patient at risk. The preceptor may need to temporarily assume the nursing responsibilities the student was attempting to perform, beginning or taking the next step of the task, and then encouraging the student to continue while continuing to coach from the sidelines.

Another useful teaching tool that nurse preceptors have found effective is the use of the One-Minute Preceptor model. This microteaching strategy, taking 5 minutes or less, involves probing for supporting evidence, providing key teaching points, delivering positive feedback and reinforcing correct behaviors, and offering constructive approaches to correct mistakes (Liu et al., 2025). This strategy provides preceptors with a structured teaching approach that can enhance student learning

STUDENTS

The student is expected to actively participate in planning their own learning activities. Planning may take the form of a learning contract that specifies individualized objectives and clinical learning activities. Because the teacher is not always present during learning activities, the student must communicate frequently with the teacher. Communication may take many forms, such as a written assignment like a reflective journal or an electronic discussion. Graduate students will be expected to track their clinical hours and experiences. Some nursing programs use electronic data tracking systems to record clinical time logs, assignments, portfolio documents, and evaluations. Written assignments allow students to share experiences with the teacher on a regular basis throughout the semester. The pervasiveness and accessibility of mobile technology allow immediate access and regular communication with faculty during clinical time.

The student must notify the teacher immediately of any problems encountered during the preceptorship. Students may experience problems or conflict during their preceptor experiences but may hesitate to report them for various reasons. They might feel they are expected to fit into the practice setting with minimal disruption or may feel powerless, replying on the preceptor's evaluation to successfully complete the clinical practicum. The student's responsibilities also include self-evaluation and evaluation of the preceptor's teaching effectiveness, as will be discussed later in this chapter.

TEACHERS

As previously discussed, the teacher is responsible for making preceptor selections, pairing students with preceptors, and orienting preceptors and students. Gathering information about the site, either through a site visit or a conversation with the staff, prior to students beginning their experience, may be helpful for teachers to learn about the population served. These discussions can also help establish a relationship with the nursing staff. The teacher can use this time to provide an overview and/or orientation to the program and explain clinical expectations. The teacher is an important resource to preceptors and students and can assist in problem solving as issues arise. The teacher must be alert to any sign of conflict in the student–preceptor relationship and promptly take a proactive role in resolving it. If a conflict cannot be resolved to the satisfaction of student, preceptor, and faculty member, the student's well-being should take precedence, and, if necessary, the student should be reassigned.

Teacher availability is particularly important if a problem arises at the clinical site and the preceptor and student cannot resolve the issue independently. The teacher must plan for consultation via telephone, email, messaging, or electronic conferencing. The teacher also arranges individual and group conferences with students and preceptors and visits the clinical sites as needed or requested by any of the participants. During a clinical site visit, the teacher may observe student performance and ask questions of both the preceptor and the student. If problems are identified, the teacher may need to work collaboratively to strategize resolutions. However, teachers may need to initiate remediation plans if potentially unsafe practices are identified (Oermann et al., 2025). Close monitoring by the preceptor and/or faculty may be necessary to ensure both patient and student safety are maintained. Teachers are responsible for gathering input from the preceptor about the student's performance and incorporating this feedback into the overall evaluation of learner performance. Faculty should also seek input from the student about the effectiveness of the preceptor and the learning opportunities available at the clinical site.

EXHIBIT 10.3 Learning Contract Template

Student Information
Name and credentials:
Address:
Phone number:
Email address:

Teacher Information
Name and credentials:
Address:
Office phone number:
Mobile phone number:
Email address:

Preceptor Information
Name and credentials:
Address:
Phone number:
Email address:

Clinical Learning Objectives/Outcomes	Learning Activities and Resources	Evaluation Evidence, Responsibility, and Time Frame

Start date ______________ Completion date ________
Student Signature ______________ Date ________
Preceptor Signature ______________ Date ________
Teacher Signature ______________ Date ________

Planning and Implementing Learning Activities

A common strategy for planning and implementing students' learning activities in the preceptorship model of clinical teaching involves the use of an individualized learning contract. A learning contract is an explicit agreement between a teacher and student that clarifies expectations of each participant in the teaching–learning process. It specifies the learning goals that have been established, the learning activities selected to meet the objectives, and the expected outcomes and criteria by which they will be evaluated. In a preceptorship experience, the learning contract is negotiated among the teacher, student, and preceptor and guides the planning and implementation of the student's learning activities. Even though the learning contract is individualized to meet student and agency needs, it needs to be consistent with course learning outcomes. **Exhibit 10.3** is an example of a learning contract that could be adapted for any level of learner.

As discussed previously, effective communication among the preceptor, student, and teacher is critical to the success of the preceptorship. Communication between teacher and student may be facilitated by the student keeping a reflective journal and sharing it with the teacher on a regular basis. In the journal, the student describes and analyzes learning activities that relate to the objectives, reflecting on the meaning and value of the experiences. Journals provide an opportunity for students to review and record their thoughts, impressions, and reactions. They can also assist students to understand and clarify clinical situations, link clinical learning to theory, and examine their thinking and actions while helping to keep the teacher informed of the learning experiences. The journal entries may be recorded in a computer file, on paper, on audio recording, or posted to an online discussion board. Additionally, the student and teacher have telephone, email, or face-to-face contact as necessary for the teacher to give consultation and guidance. Similarly, the teacher and preceptor should have regular contact by telephone, email, messaging, or face-to-face meetings so that the teacher receives feedback about learner performance and offers guidance and consultation as needed.

One way to ensure regular contact with the student and preceptor is to conduct site visits or check-ins. Both students and preceptors report that site visits or virtual check-ins are valuable and worthwhile as they enhance connection with the faculty and program, provide real-time opportunities for feedback, and enhance student confidence (Burt et al., 2022; Chicca & Shellenbarger,

2021). It is recommended that faculty make site visit expectations clear and then spend adequate time with the student and preceptor during the visit to ensure mentoring and communication of progress and needs. It may be best to schedule site visits after the student has an opportunity to get comfortable in the setting. Several site visits throughout the semester will allow the faculty to assess progress and student development over time.

A growing trend, particularly with the growth of online program delivery, is the use of virtual site visits and teleprecepting. Given the cost and faculty time needed for conducting in-person site visits, virtual visits are becoming more popular. These remote visits can be conducted using interactive video technology that enables the teacher to observe student performance at the clinical site, provide real-time interaction, and enable the delivery of feedback to all parties. With the shortage of clinical sites and the shifts in access to care sites resulting from the COVID-19 pandemic, teleprecepting emerged as an alternative for NP preceptorships. **Exhibit 10.4** offers some suggestions for how preceptors, teachers, and students can work together to ensure that a virtual visit or teleprecepting is successful (Chicca & Shellenbarger, 2021; DeClerk et al., 2023; Diegel-Vacek et al., 2021; Harris et al., 2020; Johnson et al., 2022).

Experts suggest that precepted telehealth visits should augment learning experiences and not serve as the sole learning approach. Students are expected to demonstrate foundational knowledge and skills prior to participating in virtual activities. Faculty, students, and preceptors should also engage in ongoing monitoring to evaluate learning and satisfaction with this educational approach (DeClerk et al., 2023).

The realities of clinical and academic cultures present challenges to effective communication among teacher, preceptor, and student. Preceptors often work a variety of shifts; students often have complex academic, personal, and work demands; and teachers have multiple responsibilities in addition to clinical teaching. Flexibility and commitment to establishing and maintaining communication are essential to overcome these challenges.

EXHIBIT 10.4 Virtual Precepting

- Secure approval from the clinical site, preceptor, and client for a virtual visit
- Select a secure interactive video platform that ensures privacy, provides password protection, offers encryption, and complies with the Health Insurance Portability and Accountability Act (HIPAA)
- Orient faculty, preceptor, students, and client for device use
- Test the video platform prior to using to guarantee a quality transmission
- Seek permission from all parties including patients, family (if appropriate), and preceptors
- Ensure privacy during clinical experiences
- Position device, such as a laptop, tablet, or phone, so that the student and their actions can be observed
- Consider use of an adjustable technology stand, such as gooseneck holders, that allow for manipulation and movement of the recording device during an exam
- Provide adequate lighting and avoid positioning directly in front of windows that may create shadows or glare
- Look directly at the camera to ensure eye contact
- Remain alert to cues and use nonverbal behaviors to elicit responses
- Enable access to electronic health records
- Arrange for technology support to assist with problem troubleshooting and devise a backup plan for technology failure
- Test and practice with technology before clinical implementation
- Orient all parties and provide clear expectations for roles
- Plan for delivery of performance feedback

EVALUATING THE OUTCOMES

Students, teachers, and preceptors share responsibility for monitoring the progress of learning and for evaluating outcomes of the preceptorship. Student performance may be evaluated according to the terms specified in the learning contract or through the clinical evaluation methods used by the educational program. Throughout the clinical experiences, students should be encouraged to self-assess their performance to identify strengths and areas needing ongoing improvement (Oermann et al., 2025). If a learning contract is used, student self-evaluation is usually an important strategy for assessing outcomes. As discussed earlier, preceptors are expected to give feedback to the learner and to the teacher, but ultimately the teacher has the responsibility for the summative evaluation of learner performance.

An important aspect of evaluation concerns the teaching effectiveness of preceptors. Students are an important source of information about the quality of their preceptors' clinical teaching, but the teacher should also assess the degree to which preceptors were able to effectively guide the students' learning. A modified form of a teaching effectiveness tool used to evaluate clinical teachers may be used to collect data from students regarding their preceptors. **Exhibit 10.5** is an example of a form for student evaluation of preceptor teaching effectiveness. Because each preceptor may be assigned to only one student at a time, it is usually impossible to maintain anonymity of student evaluations. Therefore, teachers may wish to share a summary of the student's evaluation, instead of the raw data, with the preceptor.

EXHIBIT 10.5 Sample Tool for Student Evaluation of Preceptor Teaching Effectiveness

Directions: Rate the extent to which each statement describes your preceptor's teaching behaviors by circling a number following each item, using the following scale:

4 = to a large extent
3 = to a moderate extent
2 = to a small extent
1 = not at all

1. The preceptor was an excellent professional role model.	4	3	2	1
2. The preceptor guided my clinical problem solving.	4	3	2	1
3. The preceptor helped me to apply theory to clinical practice.	4	3	2	1
4. The preceptor was responsive to my individual learning needs.	4	3	2	1
5. The preceptor provided constructive feedback about my performance.	4	3	2	1
6. The preceptor communicated clearly and effectively.	4	3	2	1
7. The preceptor encouraged my independence.	4	3	2	1
8. The preceptor was flexible and open-minded.	4	3	2	1
9. Overall, the preceptor was an excellent clinical teacher.	4	3	2	1
10. I would recommend this preceptor for other students.	4	3	2	1

REWARDING PRECEPTORS

Preceptors make valuable contributions to nursing education programs, and they should receive appropriate rewards and incentives for their participation. At minimum, every preceptor should receive an individualized thank-you letter, specifying some of the benefits that the student received from the preceptorship. A copy of the letter may be sent to the preceptor's supervisor or manager to be used as evidence of clinical excellence. Some preceptors prefer nonmaterial rewards such as lighter workloads and support from managers and teachers; however, teachers may not be able to provide all these things as a reward and may use other methods of demonstrating appreciation.

Other formal and informal ways of acknowledging the contributions of preceptors for nursing students is provided in **Exhibit 10.6** (Doherty et al., 2020; Gaynor & Barnes, 2021; Videtech et al., 2022; Ulrich, 2024). Regardless of the recognition approach selected, preceptors also desire the development of a relationship and open communication with the faculty and program (Videtech et al., 2022).

EXHIBIT 10.6 Methods Used to Acknowledge Preceptors

- A name badge or pin that identifies the nurse as a preceptor
- A letter or certificate of appreciation, signed by the administrator of the nursing education program
- An annual preceptor recognition event, including refreshments and an inspirational speaker
- Free or reduced-price registration for continuing education programs offered by the nursing education program or clinical facility
- Documentation of hours for certification renewals
- Free or reduced-rate tuition for one or more academic courses or the opportunity to audit a nursing course
- A free meal
- Campus guest privileges such as library access
- Adjunct or affiliate faculty appointment
- Differential pay or adjustment of work schedule (e.g., exemption from weekend shifts)
- Nomination of preceptors for awards, providing letters of reference, and collaborating on research projects
- A small gift such as a fruit basket, plant, or gift certificate

SUMMARY

The use of preceptors is an alternative to the traditional clinical teaching model based on the assumption that a consistent relationship between an experienced nurse and a nursing student is an effective way to provide individualized guidance in clinical learning and professional socialization. Preceptorships have been used extensively with prelicensure as well as graduate nursing students preparing for advanced practice roles.

A preceptorship is a time-limited, one-to-one relationship between a learner and an experienced nurse. The teacher may not be physically present during the learning activities; the preceptor provides intensive, individualized learning opportunities that improve the learner's clinical competence and confidence. The teacher has overall responsibility for the quality of the clinical teaching and learning and provides the link between the educational program and the practice setting. The preceptor functions as a role model and provides individualized clinical instruction, coaching, support, and socialization for the learner.

The use of preceptors in clinical teaching has both advantages and disadvantages for the educational program, clinical agency, teachers, preceptors, and students. Benefits for preceptors and their employers include the stimulation of working with learners who raise questions about clinical practice, rewards through a clinical ladder system for participation as a preceptor, and opportunities to recruit potential staff members for the agency from among students who work with preceptors. The greatest drawback of preceptorships to agencies and preceptors is usually the expected time commitment.

Students experience the benefits of working one-on-one with clinical experts who can coach them to improved performance as well as opportunities to experience the realities of clinical practice. However, following their preceptors' schedules often creates conflicts with students' academic, work, and family commitments. Despite these challenges, preceptorships offer many advantages to teachers and educational programs. The use of preceptors provides more clinical teachers for students and thus more intensive guidance of students' learning activities. Working collaboratively with preceptors also helps teachers to stay informed about the current realities of practice. Disadvantages include the amount of indirect teaching time required to select, prepare, and communicate with preceptors and students.

Selection of appropriate preceptors is important to the success of preceptorships. Most academic programs require the preceptor to have at least the degree for which the student is preparing. Desire to teach and willingness to serve as a preceptor are very important qualities of potential preceptors. Additional attributes of effective preceptors include clinical expertise or proficiency, leadership abilities, teaching skills, and professional role behaviors and attitudes.

Teachers are responsible for the initial orientation and continuing support of all participants; preparation can be formal or informal. A general orientation for potential preceptors may include information about benefits and challenges of precepting, characteristics of a good preceptor, principles of adult learning, clinical teaching and coaching techniques, evaluation methods, and the structure and goals of the nursing education program. After preceptors have been selected, they need a specific orientation to their responsibilities, including information about the student's educational level and previous experience, choosing specific learning activities based on learning objectives, and scheduling of clinical learning activities. Learners also need an orientation that includes information about the purposes of the preceptorship, the process of planning individual learning activities, and an explanation of teacher and preceptor roles.

Successful implementation of preceptorships depends on mutual understanding of the roles and responsibilities of the participants. The preceptor is expected to be a positive role model and a resource person for the student. The responsibilities of the preceptor include creating a positive learning climate, including the student in activities that relate to learning goals, and providing feedback to the student and teacher. The student usually arranges the schedule of clinical learning activities to coincide with the preceptor's work schedule and is expected to participate actively in planning learning activities. Because the teacher is not always present during learning activities, the student must keep the teacher informed about progress through frequent communication. In addition to making preceptor selections and orienting preceptors and students, the teacher is an important resource to preceptors and students to assist in problem-solving. Teachers must make adequate arrangements for communication with participants.

A common strategy for planning and implementing students' learning activities is the use of an individualized learning contract—an explicit agreement among the teacher, student, and preceptor that specifies the learning goals, learning activities selected to meet the objectives, and the expected outcomes and criteria by which they will be evaluated. The learning contract guides the planning and implementation of the student's learning activities.

Students, teachers, and preceptors share responsibility for monitoring the progress of learning and for evaluating outcomes of the preceptorship. Student performance is assessed according to the terms specified in the learning contract or through the clinical evaluation methods used by the educational program, through self-evaluation, and through feedback from preceptors. The teacher is responsible for the summative evaluation of learner performance. Students are an important source of information about their preceptors' clinical teaching effectiveness, but the teacher should also assess the degree to which preceptors were able to effectively guide students' learning.

Preceptors should receive appropriate rewards and incentives for the contributions they make to the educational program. At minimum, every preceptor should receive an individualized thank-you letter, specifying some of the benefits that the student received from the preceptorship. Other formal and informal ways of acknowledging the contributions of preceptors were discussed.

CNE®cl EXAMINATION TEST BLUEPRINT CORE COMPETENCIES

1. **Function within the Education and Health Care Environments**
   A. **Function in the Clinical Nurse Educator Role**
      1. Integrate theory and practice in the clinical setting

2. Foster professional growth of learners (e.g., coaching, reflection, and debriefing)
3. Use technologies to support clinical teaching and learning

B. **Operationalize the Curriculum**

1. Assess congruence of the clinical environment with curriculum, course outcomes, and learner needs when evaluating clinical sites
2. Identify learner goals and outcomes
4. Prepare learners for clinical experiences (e.g., facility, clinical expectations, equipment, and technology-based resources)
5. Implement clinical activities to help learners develop interprofessional collaboration and teamwork skills
6. Provide opportunities for learners to develop clinical judgment related to course outcomes
7. Implement academic program's assigned models of clinical teaching consistent with course outcomes (e.g., traditional, preceptor, simulation, dedicated education units)
8. Engage in theory-based clinical instruction (e.g., constructivism, social cognitive theory, adult learning)

C. **Abide by Legal Requirements, Ethical Guidelines, Agency Policies, and Guiding Framework**

1. Apply ethical and legal principles to create a safe clinical learning environment (e.g., privacy laws, confidentiality, error/near-miss situation reporting, remediation, negligence, liability, scope/standards of practice)
2. Assess learner readiness prior to clinical learning experiences
3. Facilitate learning activities that support the mission, goals, and values of the academic institution and the clinical agency
4. Inform others of program and clinical agency policies, procedures, and practices
5. Adhere to program and clinical agency policies, procedures, and practices when implementing clinical experiences (e.g., due process, accommodations, academic integrity)

2. Facilitate Learning in the Healthcare Environment

D. Create opportunities for learners to develop critical thinking and clinical reasoning skills
E. Promote a culture of safety and quality in the delivery of health care
F. Create a positive and caring learning environment
G. Develop collegial working relationships with learners, faculty, and clinical environment personnel

3. Demonstrate Effective Interpersonal Communication and Collaborative Interprofessional Relationships

A. Foster the development of a collegial learning community
B. Facilitate opportunities to collaborate within the healthcare team
C. Support an environment of frequent, respectful, and civil communication within the healthcare team
D. Demonstrate respect for learners, healthcare team, colleagues, clients, families, and others
E. Use clear and effective communication in all interactions (e.g., written, electronic, verbal, non-verbal, virtual)
J. Function as an accessible resource to learners and the healthcare team in the clinical learning environment
L. Communicate performance expectations to learners and clinical staff

5. Facilitate Learner Development and Socialization

A. Mentor learners in professional nursing behaviors
B. Promote professional integrity and accountability
C. Assist learners to use self-assessment, self-reflection, and goal setting for ongoing professional development
D. Create learning environments that promote socialization to the role of the nurse
E. Empower learners to achieve professional and educational goals

6. Implement Effective Clinical and Assessment Evaluation Strategies

A. Employ a variety of strategies to determine achievement of learning outcomes
B. Conduct formative and summative evaluation specific to the learner and learning outcomes
D. Maintain integrity (e.g., ethical, non-biased) in the assessment and evaluation of learners
E. Provide timely, objective, and constructive feedback to learners
F. Document learner clinical performance, feedback, and progression
G. Evaluate the quality of the clinical learning experiences and environment

LEARNING ACTIVITIES

CourseConnect

To access self-assessment questions and interactive, competency-based learning activities for this chapter, visit www.springerpub.com/courseconnect. See inside front cover and tear-out card for CourseConnect details.

REFERENCES

Accreditation Commission for Education in Nursing. (2024). *ACEN standards and criteria*. https://resources.acenursing.org/space/SAC/1824227333/2023+Standards+and+Criteria

Alabama Area Health Education Centers. (2024). *Alabama preceptor tax incentive program (APTIP)* [Brochure]. https://www.alahec.org/aptip-brochure-2024/

American Association of Colleges of Nursing and the American Organization for Nursing Leadership. (2020). *AACN-AONL clinical preceptor survey summary report*. https://www.aacnnursing.org/Portals/42/Data/AACN-AONL-Clinical-Preceptor-Survey-May-2020.pdf

American Nurses Credentialing Center. (2022). *Certification renewal requirements*. https://www.nursingworld.org/globalassets/certification/renewals/ancc-certrenewal requirements.pdf

Burt, L., Sparbel, K., & Corbridge, S. (2022). Nurse practitioner preceptor resource needs and perceptions of institutional support. *Journal of the American Association of Nurse Practitioners, 34*(2022), 348–356. https://doi.org/10.1097.JXX.0000000000000629

Chicca, J., & Shellenbarger, T. (2020). Implementing successful clinical nursing preceptorships. *Nurse Educator, 45*(4), E41–E42. https://doi.org/10.1097/NNE.0000000000000750

Chicca, J., & Shellenbarger, T. (2021). Preparing, maintaining, and evaluating remote preceptorships: Considerations for nurse educators. *Teaching and Learning in Nursing, 16*(2021), 396–400. https://doi.org/10.1016/j.teln.2021.04.006

Ciocco, M. (2021). *Fast facts for the nurse preceptor* (2nd ed.). Springer Publishing Company.

Commission on Collegiate Nursing Education. (2024). *Standards for accreditation of baccalaureate and graduate nursing programs*. https://www.aacnnursing.org/Portals/0/PDFs/CCNE/CCNE-Education-Standards-2024.pdf

DeClerk, L., Wells, C., Chasteen, S., Baxter, J., Martinez, J., & Rojo, M. (2023). Preceptorship and telehealth: Nurse practitioner's perspectives. *The Journal for Nurse Practitioners, 19*(10), 104772. https://doi.org/10.1016/j.nurpra.2023.104772

Diegel-Vacek, L., Cotler, K., Reising, V., & Corbridge, S. J. (2021). Transition of nurse practitioner faculty practice and student clinical to telehealth: Response to the COVID-19 pandemic. *The Journal for Nurse Practitioners, 17*(3), 317–321. https://doi.org/10.1016/j.nurpra.2020.12.023

Doherty, C. L., Fogg, L., Bigley, M. B., Todd, B., & O'Sullivan, A. L. (2020). Nurse practitioner student clinical placement processes: A national survey of nurse practitioner programs. *Nursing Outlook, 68*(1), 55–61. https://doi.org/10.1016/j.outlook.2019.07.005

Gaynor, B., & Barnes, H. (2021). Nurse practitioner preceptor plan: A focus on preceptor rewards and preferences. *Nursing Education Perspectives, 43*(1), 35–37. https://doi.org/10.1097/01.NEP.0000000000000773

George, K., (2023). *States with preceptor tax credits*. National Council of State Legislatures. https://www.healthworkforceta.org/wp-content/uploads/2023/12/Preceptor-Tax-Credits.pdf

Gholizadeh, L., Shahbazi, S., Valizadeh, S., Mohammadzad, M., Ghahramanian, A., & Shohani, M. (2022). Nurse preceptors' perceptions of benefits, rewards, support, and commitment to the preceptor role in a new preceptorship program. *BMC Medical Education, 22*, 472. https://doi.org/10.1186/s12909-022-03534-0

Gigli, K. H., & Gonzalez, J. D. (2022). Meeting the need for nurse practitioner clinicals: A survey of practitioners. *Journal of the American Association of Nurse Practitioners, 34*(8), 991–1001. https://doi.org/10.1097/JXX.0000000000000749

Harris, M., Rhoads, S. J., Rooker, J. S., Kelly, M. A., Lefler, L., Lubin, S., Martel, I. L., & Beverly, C. J. (2020). Using virtual site visits in the clinical evaluation of nurse practitioner students: Student and faculty perspectives. *Nurse Educator, 45*(1), 17–20. https://doi.org/10.1097/NNE.0000000000000693

Henry-Okafor, Q., Chenault, R. D., & Smith, R. B. (2023). Addressing the preceptor gap in nurse practitioner education. *The Journal for Nurse Practitioners, 19*(10), 104818. https://doi.org/10.1016/j.nurpra.2023.104818

Johnson, D., Gatewood, E., Ling, A., & Kuo, A C. (2022). Teleprecepting: A timely approach to clinical education during COVID-19. *Journal of the American Association of Nurse Practitioners, 34*(1), 153–159. https://doi.org/10.1097/JXX.0000000000000567

Lerman, R., Jacoby, T. Nemil, D., & Colborn, J. (2024). *How community colleges can help scale US apprenticeships: Evidence from the field*. Apprenticeships for America.

Liu, L., Teunissen, P., Xie, H., Li, Z., Wang, J., & Tan, C. S. E. (2025). One-minute preceptor model: An ideal teaching tool for nurse preceptors? *Teaching and Learning in Nursing, 20*(2025), e205–e210. https://doi.org/10.1016.j.teln.2024.10.008

McInnis, A., Schlemmer, T., & Chapman, B. (2021). The significance of the NP preceptorship shortage. *OJIN: The Online Journal of Issues in Nursing 26*(1), Manuscript 5. https://doi.org/10.3912/OJIN.Vol26No01Man05

National Advisory Council on Nurse Education and Practice. (2024). *Mitigating nursing workforce challenges by optimizing learning environments* (19th Report). United States Department of Health and Human Services, Health Resources and Services Administration. https://www.hrsa.gov/sites/default/files/hrsa/advisory-committees/nursing/reports/nacnep-19th-report.pdf

National Center for the Apprenticeship Degree. (2024). *Apprenticeship degrees in nursing: State landscape analysis and implementation playbook*. Author.

National Council of State Boards of Nursing. (2024). *Member board profiles*. https://www.ncsbn.org/public-files/Education_Survey_2023.pdf

National League for Nursing Commission for Nursing Education Accreditation. (2021). *Accreditation standards for nursing programs*. https://cnea.nln.org/standards-of-accreditation

National Task Force on Quality Nurse Practitioner Education. (2022). *Standards for quality nurse practitioner education* (6th ed.). https://cdn.ymaws.com/www.nonpf.org/resource/resmgr/ntfstandards/ntfs_final.pdf

Oermann, M. H., Gaberson, K. B., & De Gagne, J. C. (2025). *Evaluation and testing in nursing education* (7th ed.). Springer Publishing Company.

Ryan, C. L. Cant, R., Hughes, L., Ahchay, D., & Strickland, K. (2024). Core competencies for Registered Nurse preceptors: A mapping review of quantitative studies. *Nursing Open, 11*(2), e2076. https://doi.org/10.1002/nop2.2076

Stickel, M. (2023). *Inside the beltway*. National Association of Pediatric Nurse Practitioners. https://www.napnap.org/inside-the-beltway-december-2023/

Ulrich, B. T. (2024). *Mastering precepting* (3rd ed.). Sigma Theta Tau.

Videtech, K., Moran, K., Zajac, L., & Myers, R. (2022). Changing the trajectory of clinical precepting for nurse practitioner students with the development of a preceptor resource network. *Journal of the American Association of Nurse Practitioners, 34*(2022), 909–917. https://doi.org/10.1097/jxx.0000000000000732

III

Evaluation Strategies in Clinical Teaching

Clinical Teaching at a Distance

11

OBJECTIVES:

1. Analyze effective strategies for clinical teaching in distance education, including structured mentorship, preceptor engagement, and competency-based assessment, to optimize student learning outcomes.
2. Discuss best practices for working with preceptors in distance education settings, with a focus on communication strategies, preceptor support, competency-based models such as apprenticeships, and evaluation of clinical performance.
3. Examine the role of innovative technologies in distance-based clinical education, including their application in student learning, preceptor training, faculty–preceptor–student communication, and methods for evaluating clinical teaching effectiveness.

Distance education has become an integral component of nursing education, offering students flexible, accessible, and innovative opportunities to engage in clinical learning. Although often contrasted with traditional on-campus instruction, distance education is not a one-size-fits-all approach; it encompasses synchronous, asynchronous, and hybrid models, each requiring intentional design and thoughtful implementation to maintain the rigor and effectiveness of experiential learning. Clinical teaching at a distance demands strategic approaches that foster active student engagement, structured mentorship, quality preceptor support, and robust assessment of clinical competencies.

The role of preceptors is a key consideration in distance-based clinical education, as preceptors provide essential mentorship and real-world guidance for students in remote clinical settings. Successful preceptorship in distance education depends on effective communication, structured support, and clearly defined roles and expectations. Apprenticeship-based models are emerging as promising alternatives to traditional preceptorships; these models offer students extended, competency-based learning experiences that facilitate a smoother transition from education to clinical practice. They also provide longitudinal mentorship to support progressive skill acquisition and continuity in student–preceptor relationships, even in distance-based settings.

Technology continues to reshape clinical education as telehealth, artificial intelligence (AI), and digital learning tools expand opportunities for remote patient encounters, competency-based simulations, and interactive learning experiences. These advancements not only support student competency development but also enhance preceptor training, faculty–preceptor communication, and clinical performance evaluation, thereby ensuring that clinical mentorship remains effective and sustainable in distance education.

Equally important to the success of distance-based clinical education is the evaluation of student learning, preceptor effectiveness, and clinical site quality. Assessment of student performance in remote clinical placements requires structured evaluation tools such as preceptor assessments, faculty site visits (both virtual and in-person), and technology-assisted competency evaluations. It is important to gather feedback on the quality of the mentorship and guidance provided by the preceptor and clinical site suitability to ensure that students receive consistent, high-quality learning experiences in distance settings.

This chapter examines strategies and best practices for optimizing clinical teaching at a distance, working with preceptors, integrating apprenticeship models, leveraging technology to enhance both student learning and preceptor support, and implementing structured evaluation processes. Educators can strategically implement these approaches to provide distance-based clinical experiences that remain engaging, rigorous, and aligned with the demands of modern nursing practice.

STUDENTS WHO SEEK DISTANCE LEARNING

The growing demand for distance learning raises an important question: *Why* do students choose this mode of education? The answer lies in accessibility, flexibility, and technological advancements (De Gagne & Oermann, 2025).

For some students, distance education is the only feasible option due to location constraints and life commitments. It is not practical for nursing students who are working professionals with families to relocate or commute long distances for their education.

Distance-based clinical education allows students to fulfill clinical requirements in their own communities through affiliated healthcare facilities, telehealth experiences, or virtual simulations, despite geographic separation from faculty. By eliminating the need for students to be physically present on campus, distance learning has overcome geographic barriers and expanded access to specialized clinical experiences that might otherwise be unattainable.

Flexibility is another key driver of distance learning. The accelerated adoption of online and remote clinical education, which began as an emergency response to the COVID-19 pandemic, reinforced the need for innovative, flexible training models and inspired a permanent transformation of how clinical education is delivered and experienced. As institutions rapidly transitioned to virtual and hybrid formats, both students and educators gained new insight into the effectiveness and sustainability of distance-based clinical training.

Although distance learning broadens access to clinical training, it also requires commitment, self-discipline, and strong time management skills. Balancing work, clinical experiences, and coursework can be overwhelming, particularly for those unfamiliar with the structure, expectations, and complexities of distance-based clinical training. Institutions must acknowledge these challenges and provide structured support, including virtual mentorship, academic advising, and resources for managing clinical learning at a distance. Similarly, by fostering a supportive and helpful environment, educators can ensure that distance learning, including clinical training, remains a powerful, effective, and sustainable option for preparing future nurses.

CLINICAL PRACTICE IN A DISTANCE LEARNING ENVIRONMENT

Faculty and students experience less stress and enhanced satisfaction when they understand the components (i.e., the roles of the institution, faculty, student, and preceptor) necessary for a successful clinical practicum offered at a distance from their nursing program. The educational institution's role comprises a commitment to deliver an effective and high-quality clinical practice experience by ensuring state authorization, establishing strong academic–clinical partnerships, and facilitating necessary contracts. Academic–clinical partnerships help bridge the gap between educational programs and clinical sites by fostering structured collaboration, resource sharing, and mentorship, all of which are essential for supporting distance-based clinical education (Toly et al., 2022).

State Authorization

State authorization is a critical requirement for institutions offering distance education, particularly when students engage in clinical practica across state lines. However, the process of obtaining authorization can be complex and requires thorough preparation to ensure compliance. The National Council for State Authorization Reciprocity Agreements (NC-SARA) facilitates this process through the State Authorization Reciprocity Agreement (SARA), a voluntary agreement among member states and territories that establishes comparable national standards for interstate postsecondary distance education (NC-SARA, 2025a, 2025b). SARA provides a streamlined approach to obtaining state authorization, allowing institutions to offer distance education programs across member states without seeking separate approvals (NC-SARA, 2025b). The NC-SARA website (nc-sara.org) provides resources, including the State Authorization Guide, which serves as a comprehensive tool for institutions navigating state authorization compliance (NC-SARA, 2025a). This guide compiles state laws, regulations, and requirements to assist institutions in understanding and adhering to the varying regulations across states (NC-SARA, 2025a).

In addition to state regulations, institutions must consider the varying requirements of state boards of nursing. Some states may mandate that all faculty hold a license within the state, require the identification of preceptors, necessitate an on-site presence, or demand detailed documentation such as educational expectations and syllabi. To maintain compliance, institutions often designate an individual to monitor and manage these requirements, as state regulations can change with minimal notice. Establishing a continuous review process ensures that institutions remain informed of any regulatory changes; faculty and students must be aware of these procedures to prevent inadvertent violations that could affect compliance. Failure to comply with state board of nursing regulations can result in severe consequences, including substantial fines, the prohibition of student placements in certain states, and denial of licensure for graduates of noncompliant programs. Therefore, conducting a thorough review of state board of nursing requirements before initiating a distance learning program is imperative (NC-SARA, 2025b).

Clinical Partnerships

Developing strong academic–clinical partnerships is essential for mitigating preceptor shortages and streamlining onboarding processes, both of which are frequently cited as barriers to clinical practica (Toly et al., 2022). Establishing effective partnerships requires intentional groundwork, including clearly defined expectations, mutual commitment, and ongoing evaluation to ensure sustainability. These partnerships should be initiated at the leadership level, such as by the dean or designee, and continuously nurtured by faculty members who work directly with students in clinical settings. Strong partnerships not only support student learning but also enhance collaboration between academia and clinical practice, ultimately strengthening the nursing workforce.

Clinical Contracts

Once academic–clinical partnerships are established, the next step is the development and management of clinical contracts. Most healthcare facilities require a formal contract between the educational institution and the clinical site that outlines key legal and operational responsibilities, such as liability coverage, student insurance, facility and institution obligations, and the role of the preceptor. Corporate lawyers often review these contracts for both parties. Some agreements are straightforward without extensive legal negotiations, but others may require multiple revisions to align with the interests of all stakeholders. In settings such as private clinical offices, a more streamlined contract is often sufficient; this may consist of a simple document signed by the office manager, ensuring that essential terms and conditions are met. Regardless of the setting, maintaining a structured contract-tracking system is critical for ensuring compliance and facilitating seamless clinical placements for students.

FACULTY ROLE

The faculty role in supporting students' clinical learning at a distance is multifaceted, encompassing both didactic coordination and the critical task of securing and vetting preceptors. Despite institutional support and structured preparation, preceptor shortages remain a significant challenge. Studies show that more than 40% to 50% of nurse preceptors report difficulty balancing their roles as educators, facilitators, and evaluators—especially in times of crisis, such as the COVID-19 pandemic (Rashwan et al., 2023). In distance education programs, students lack proximity to established preceptor networks, so the burden of securing clinical placements falls almost entirely on schools (McInnis et al., 2021).

To address these challenges, institutions have begun leveraging strategic partnerships with hospital systems, alumni networks, and professional organizations across state lines. Additionally, virtual preceptor recruitment and orientation strategies (e.g., informational webinars) have been implemented to expand access to qualified preceptors. These initiatives highlight the evolving nature of clinical education in a digital era and reinforce the importance of collaboration between academia and clinical practice.

Securing qualified preceptors has become a national challenge resulting in the emergence of for-profit third-party services that connect students with preceptors—for a fee (Gilmore & Nguyen, 2024). Some institutions have introduced preceptor stipends for which students absorb the additional cost. However, paying preceptors does not absolve institutions of their responsibility to vet them thoroughly. Faculty must ensure that preceptors meet educational, licensure, certification, and practice standards. In some cases, preceptors accept multiple students for financial compensation, creating suboptimal learning environments. Faculty must actively monitor these situations and intervene when necessary to protect the quality and integrity of clinical education.

Preceptors frequently cite lack of institutional support, unclear expectations, and minimal recognition as barriers to participation. These concerns are amplified in distance education settings, where faculty are not physically present to provide real-time guidance. Key strategies to enhance preceptor engagement and effectiveness include:

- preceptor orientation and training (e.g., providing concise, structured guidance on expectations, evaluation methods, and institutional resources);
- consistent faculty engagement (e.g., conducting regular check-ins to ensure support and accountability); and
- recognition and incentives (e.g., offering certificates, continuing education credits, adjunct faculty appointments, or awards for excellence in preceptorship) to acknowledge and enhance preceptor participation.

Once a preceptor is secured and vetted, faculty must proactively establish clear lines of communication among the student, preceptor, and faculty. This triadic model of communication is essential for student success in distance-based clinical experiences. Initial faculty contact with the preceptor should include:

- a warm welcome and expression of appreciation for their role;
- faculty contact information for accessibility;
- a course syllabus outlining learning objectives and clinical expectations;
- the clinical evaluation plan, including performance assessments and feedback mechanisms; and
- clear expectations for faculty, preceptors, and students.

Setting expectations early prevents miscommunication and ensures alignment throughout the clinical practicum. Faculty must emphasize active student engagement, as distance learners may be more prone to passivity. Encouraging students to ask questions, seek learning opportunities, and reflect on experiences fosters deeper clinical integration. Structured activities such as reflection assignments, discussion boards, and synchronous seminars facilitate peer engagement and knowledge sharing, even in a virtual setting. **Exhibit 11.1** outlines the core responsibilities of faculty, preceptors, and students in distance-based clinical education. These expectations can be tailored to align with institutional policies, program structures, and regulatory requirements to ensure quality clinical experiences across various synchronous, asynchronous, and hybrid models.

EXHIBIT 11.1 Responsibilities of Faculty Members, Preceptors, and Students in Distance-Based Clinical Learning

Faculty Responsibilities:

- Provide a course syllabus, introduction letter, and structured preceptor orientation outlining expectations.
- Conduct at least one structured virtual check-in or training session with preceptors to ensure alignment with course expectations and provide ongoing support.
- Establish and maintain clear and proactive communication with the preceptor and student.
- Approve students' clinical objectives within the first week.
- Conduct virtual or in-person site visits and confer with students and preceptors at least twice per term.
- Monitor student engagement through clinical logs, course assignments, and discussion forums to ensure active participation.
- Lead scheduled clinical seminars to discuss clinical role development, professional competencies, and student challenges.
- Provide timely feedback and intervention if issues arise pertaining to student performance or preceptor concerns.
- Complete a final evaluation of student performance incorporating feedback from the preceptor and student self-assessments.
- Send a thank-you letter to preceptors at the end of the practicum to acknowledge their contribution.

Preceptor Responsibilities:

- Orient students to clinical policies, procedures, and expectations to facilitate seamless integration into the clinical setting.
- Provide structured learning opportunities tailored to the student's level of competence and clinical objectives.
- Ensure that students engage in appropriate patient care experiences while adhering to ethical and professional standards.
- Offer ongoing feedback and model critical thinking, decision-making, and clinical reasoning skills.

(continued)

EXHIBIT 11.1 Responsibilities of Faculty Members, Preceptors, and Students in Distance-Based Clinical Learning (*cont.*)

- Validate and cosign student documentation per agency policies and regulations.
- Engage in regular communication with faculty, including at least two structured check-ins per term.
- Address student progress and areas for improvement in collaboration with faculty.
- Provide guidance in clinical decision-making, patient management, and interdisciplinary collaboration.
- Identify additional learning opportunities such as specialized cases, professional readings, or case discussions.
- Complete and submit midterm and final evaluations based on student performance.

Student Responsibilities:

- Develop personal learning objectives aligned with course outcomes and seek faculty and preceptor approval.
- Follow agency policies, dress code, and professional standards, and demonstrate punctuality, responsibility, and engagement.
- Maintain effective communication with preceptors and faculty, seeking feedback proactively.
- Prepare for clinical experiences by reviewing patient conditions, diagnoses, and evidence-based guidelines.
- Maintain confidentiality in all clinical documentation and ensure compliance with HIPAA regulations.
- Actively engage in patient care, assessments, and clinical decision-making, demonstrating initiative and critical thinking.
- Participate in clinical discussions, case reviews, and interdisciplinary collaborations as appropriate.
- Submit a clinical log and reflective journal to track learning progress and identify areas for growth.
- Complete self-assessment reflections at midterm and final evaluations to assess progress toward clinical competencies.
- Attend and participate in scheduled virtual seminars or discussion forums to enhance collaborative learning with peers.

HIPAA, Health Insurance Portability and Accountability Act

APPRENTICESHIP MODELS IN CLINICAL EDUCATION

Preceptors are essential to clinical education at both pre- and post-licensure levels. They serve as mentors who facilitate experiential learning and professional development, guide students through competency acquisition, and bridge the gap between theoretical knowledge and hands-on practice. In distance-based clinical education, where students and faculty are often geographically dispersed, preceptors carry an even greater responsibility for ensuring that students gain meaningful clinical experiences despite physical separation from academic institutions.

Given the challenges of preceptor shortages, inconsistent mentorship structures, and the need for continuous faculty support, apprenticeship models have emerged as competency-driven solutions that not only enhance student learning but also support preceptors in their mentorship role. Traditionally associated with skilled trades, these models are being applied to healthcare education as a means of addressing preceptor shortages and enhancing experiential learning (Gardiner, 2023). By emphasizing progressive skill acquisition, longitudinal mentorship, and competency-based assessment, apprenticeship models provide a structured alternative to traditional preceptorships. In distance-based clinical education, they offer a sustainable framework for student learning while ensuring that competency development remains the foundation of clinical practice (Cadmus et al., 2021).

Unlike traditional preceptorships, which often rely on short-term placements, apprenticeship models extend the learning experience over a longer duration, allowing students to develop clinical expertise incrementally. The emphasis on longitudinal mentorship strengthens professional relationships, deepens engagement with clinical learning, and promotes competency-based progression (Hosseinpour et al., 2024). Rather than relying on fixed-hour requirements, students advance based on demonstrated proficiency, ensuring that learning is tailored to individual progress rather than the number of training hours completed (Gardiner, 2023). Research suggests that structured feedback mechanisms, such as planned meetings where faculty and preceptors provide constructive feedback to students, significantly enhance student performance and confidence in clinical settings (Hosseinpour et al., 2024). These models provide consistent, structured feedback that reinforces clinical reasoning and professional growth throughout the training process.

For successful implementation in nursing education, apprenticeship models must follow one of three primary structures: time-based, competency-based, or hybrid (Gardiner, 2023). The time-based model, the most traditional, requires students to complete a set number of clinical hours before advancing. Although this approach ensures broad clinical exposure, it does not accommodate individual learning differences. In contrast, competency-based apprenticeships focus on skill mastery and allow students to progress based on demonstrated proficiency in key competencies. This learner-centered approach aligns with evidence-based assessment strategies and is increasingly favored in nursing education (Gardiner, 2023). A hybrid model incorporates elements of both approaches, ensuring competency-based progression while maintaining a minimum hour requirement to balance flexibility and clinical exposure.

Institutions can integrate apprenticeship models into distance-based clinical education to create sustainable preceptorship structures, reduce faculty burden, and maintain high-quality clinical training. The intentional incorporation of technology, competency-driven assessments, and faculty oversight ensures that students receive structured, high-quality experiential learning, even in remote clinical placements.

INTEGRATING TECHNOLOGY IN PRECEPTOR TRAINING AND SUPPORT

As clinical education evolves, the integration of technology-enhanced mentorship has become increasingly important for supporting preceptors, particularly in distance-based learning environments. Technology and telehealth modalities are discussed in Chapter 9, but their specific application in preceptor training and support deserves further exploration. These tools not only bridge geographic gaps but also enhance faculty–preceptor–student communication to ensure consistency in clinical oversight. Virtual learning platforms, AI, and telehealth-based assessment tools enable structured preceptor training and a high standard of mentorship and clinical supervision.

One of the primary challenges of distance-based clinical education is providing adequate preceptor orientation and training, particularly when their work is independent of faculty oversight. A practical solution to this challenge is the use of virtual learning management systems (LMS) offering asynchronous training modules that preceptors can access at their convenience (De Gagne & Oermann, 2025). These platforms provide self-paced educational content on topics such as competency assessment, evaluation strategies, and effective remote mentorship techniques. Additionally, interactive webinars and discussion forums allow preceptors to engage with faculty and peers, thus fostering collaborative learning and problem-solving.

Beyond initial training, maintaining consistent communication between faculty and preceptors is critical for monitoring student progress and addressing challenges. Advances in teleconferencing and virtual site visits allow faculty to conduct scheduled remote check-ins to confirm that students are receiving appropriate clinical guidance and preceptors feel supported. Through secure telehealth platforms, faculty can observe student–patient interactions in real time and provide immediate feedback on clinical decision-making, patient communication, and procedural skills (Kleib et al., 2024). Moreover, interdisciplinary virtual learning experiences allow preceptors, students, and other healthcare professionals to collaborate in team-based discussions and case reviews, thereby enriching the clinical training process (Al Nufaiei et al., 2024).

The integration of AI and data-driven learning analytics has transformed preceptor support and student assessment in distance-based programs. AI-driven tools can analyze clinical logs, case documentation, and student performance metrics to provide real-time insights into competency development (Cary et al.,

2024). Preceptors can generate individualized student performance reports so as to tailor feedback to specific learning needs and provide students with targeted interventions to strengthen their clinical proficiency (Wittler et al., 2025). AI-powered simulations allow preceptors to assess students' communication and reasoning skills in virtual patient encounters, offering an innovative approach to evaluating telehealth competencies and clinical decision-making (Yalcinkaya et al., 2024).

Simulated case-based learning, an essential aspect of preceptor development in distance-based clinical education, has been widely recognized for its role in enhancing clinical reasoning, feedback delivery, and decision-making skills (Forneris, 2023). Although traditionally used for student learning, simulation-based approaches can benefit preceptor training by providing structured opportunities for mentoring students effectively in remote settings. Institutions can adapt these evidence-based simulation strategies to better equip preceptors with the skills and confidence necessary to mentor students in distance-based clinical learning environments.

Given that preceptors in distance-based education models often work in isolation, institutions should establish online peer networks to create a sense of community and shared learning. Virtual platforms enable preceptors to connect with colleagues, share mentorship strategies, and engage in discussions on best practices. A digital repository of resources, including recorded webinars, evidence-based mentorship guidelines, and competency assessment tools, can serve as an accessible reference for preceptor development and support. By leveraging these technological innovations, institutions can create a structured, responsive, and engaging preceptor training experience and ensure that distance-based clinical education remains rigorous and student centered.

EVALUATION

Evaluation is a critical component of clinical learning at a distance as it provides an objective measure of student progress, preceptor effectiveness, and clinical site suitability. A comprehensive evaluation process should assess multiple dimensions of the learning experience, including student performance, preceptor contributions, and the quality of the clinical site.

Student Evaluation

The evaluation of student performance in distance-based clinical education must be structured, competency-driven, and aligned with learning outcomes. Faculty should design evaluation tools that reflect expected competencies and behaviors so that both students and preceptors understand the criteria for assessment (Oermann et al., 2024). Preceptors play a key role in evaluating student performance, and their feedback should be formally documented using structured evaluation tools deployed at midterm and final assessments. These tools should include both quantitative rating scales and free-text comment sections to capture subtle aspects of student progress.

Evaluation tools are often administered electronically through LMS or third-party software, although some programs may still use evaluations that preceptors submit via email or upload to a digital platform. Regardless of format, preceptors should be encouraged to review evaluations with students to ensure that feedback is clear, constructive, and actionable. A transparent evaluation process prevents unexpected performance concerns and allows students to address areas for improvement in a timely manner.

When student performance concerns arise, a well-structured communication plan is essential for timely intervention. Preceptors should be encouraged to report concerns to faculty as they emerge, rather than waiting until the end of the term. For example, if a student consistently arrives late to a clinical site, faculty should be notified early so that corrective measures can be implemented. Proactive communication ensures that students have an opportunity to remediate issues, and it prevents minor concerns from escalating into significant academic challenges. Faculty must also determine how preceptor evaluations contribute to student grading within the clinical practicum. In some programs, preceptor evaluations account for a percentage of the student's overall grade, while in others, they serve as a pass/fail requirement. Transparency in grading policies both ensures that preceptors understand the weight of their evaluations and reinforces the importance of their feedback in student assessment.

A critical component of student evaluation is the assessment of clinical competencies, which may include performing a physical assessment, patient education, procedural skills, or interdisciplinary communication. These competencies may be assessed through clinical intensives during which students demonstrate skills either in-person or virtually in a structured, supervised environment (Oermann et al., 2024). Although on-campus assessments offer valuable hands-on experience, virtual evaluations provide greater accessibility for students in fully online programs. Faculty should ensure that logistical challenges, such as scheduling and resource availability, are considered when integrating intensive skill-based assessments.

Faculty site visits serve as an additional strategy for evaluating student performance and clinical learning environments. Site visits allow faculty to observe the physical environment, interact with students and preceptors, and assess clinical site operations. Although in-person visits are ideal, virtual site visits using platforms such as Zoom®, Webex®, or Microsoft® Teams provide a viable alternative for geographically dispersed students. During these visits, faculty can observe student–preceptor interactions, discuss student progress, and address concerns in real time. Virtual site visits should be structured yet non intrusive and respect preceptor time while maintaining faculty oversight and engagement in clinical education.

Preceptor and Site Evaluation

The evaluation process must assess preceptor effectiveness and the quality of the clinical site. Student feedback on their preceptors and clinical experiences provides valuable insight into the learning environment. Preceptors must meet technical qualifications but also possess the critical ability to foster a positive and supportive clinical learning experience. Students should have the opportunity to evaluate preceptors and clinical sites and provide feedback on mentorship quality, communication, and overall supportiveness of the learning environment. Although students are encouraged to report issues throughout the term, some may hesitate due to fear of retaliation or concerns about losing a clinical placement. Faculty should create a safe, confidential mechanism that allows students to share honest feedback about their clinical experiences.

In some cases, faculty may need to remove students from a clinical site due to safety concerns, inadequate learning opportunities, or conflicts between the student and preceptor. These situations are not ideal, but faculty must prioritize the student's education and well-being. Maintaining open communication within the faculty–preceptor–student triad is critical to resolving issues early and ensuring that students have a successful clinical practicum experience. Establishing an ongoing evaluation system will help to ensure that the institution maintains high standards for clinical education in distance-based settings. **Exhibit 11.2** provides an example of a structured student evaluation form for preceptors and clinical sites, which can be adapted to institutional needs and accreditation requirements.

SUMMARY

Clinical teaching at a distance requires intentional design, structured mentorship, technology integration, and comprehensive evaluation to ensure that students receive high-quality experiential learning in remote clinical settings. Institutions play a critical role in state authorization, clinical partnerships, contract management, and preceptor support. Faculty serve as both educators and facilitators, assisting students in securing preceptors, establishing clear communication pathways, and implementing competency-based assessments to evaluate student progress.

EXHIBIT 11.2 Student Evaluation of Preceptor and Clinical Setting

Preceptor/Setting ___________
Semester: Fall Spring Summer Year______
Practicum Course No.___________ Title________________
____

Directions: This evaluation form is designed to provide you with the opportunity to evaluate the preceptor and clinical site. Please indicate your response in the appropriate column on the scoring sheet. Please provide any additional written comments at the bottom or back of the page.

Items	Consistently				Never
Overall this preceptor stimulated my learning.	5	4	3	2	1
Clinical activity was presented at an appropriate pace.	5	4	3	2	1
The preceptor was well prepared for my visits and organized in guiding my experiences.	5	4	3	2	1
The preceptor used a variety of teaching methods to ensure that I learned the rationale for the management of patients.	5	4	3	2	1
I felt challenged to master the clinical practice.	5	4	3	2	1
The client population was appropriate to my learning goals.	5	4	3	2	1
The preceptor handled questions appropriately.	5	4	3	2	1
I felt respected as a student practitioner.	5	4	3	2	1
I had the opportunity to actively participate during clinical.	5	4	3	2	1

(continued)

EXHIBIT 11.2 Student Evaluation of Preceptor and Clinical Setting (*cont.*)

Items	Consistently				Never
The preceptor offered feedback to guide my progress throughout the experience.	5	4	3	2	1
The preceptor specified the criteria for managing patients in that setting.	5	4	3	2	1
The preceptor related current research and professional issues to the practice experience.	5	4	3	2	1
The clinical setting offered rich experiences for the student.	5	4	3	2	1
The preceptor promoted an atmosphere that fostered critical thinking.	5	4	3	2	1
The preceptor provided opportunities to develop effective written and/or oral communication needed for practice.	5	4	3	2	1
Comments:					

The preceptor–student–faculty relationship is central to distance-based clinical education, which requires structured mentorship, ongoing engagement, and clearly defined expectations. Apprenticeship models offer a competency-driven alternative to traditional preceptorships, providing students with longitudinal mentorship, progressive skill development, and competency-based progression. These models promote sustainable student-preceptor relationships while alleviating some of the burden placed on preceptors by integrating structured learning frameworks into clinical education.

Technology continues to reshape distance-based clinical learning to enhance student learning, preceptor training, and faculty oversight. Telehealth, AI, virtual simulations, and data-driven learning analytics expand opportunities for competency-based assessment, remote mentorship, and interactive learning experiences. Faculty can observe clinical interactions through virtual site visits, track competency development with AI-assisted assessments, and support preceptors via digital training modules. These advancements allow continuous communication, effective feedback mechanisms, and real-time oversight of student learning outcomes.

Evaluation is a critical component of distance-based clinical education encompassing student performance, preceptor effectiveness, and clinical site quality. Preceptor evaluations should be structured, competency-driven, and aligned with institutional learning outcomes to ensure consistency and accuracy in student assessment. Faculty oversight—through virtual or in-person site visits, teleconferencing, and structured communication—allows for early intervention and remediation, if needed. Additionally, student feedback on preceptors and clinical site suitability supports high-quality mentorship and learning environments for future students.

This chapter explored effective strategies for clinical teaching at a distance, including structured mentorship, apprenticeship models, and technology-enhanced learning. It has provided practical guidance for educators on supporting preceptors, implementing competency-based assessments, and utilizing digital tools to enhance remote clinical education. Additionally, the chapter has emphasized the importance of systematic evaluation of students, preceptors, and clinical sites to ensure high-quality learning experiences. As distance-based clinical education continues to evolve, these strategies will help maintain rigor, engagement, and effectiveness in an increasingly digital healthcare landscape.

CNE®cl EXAMINATION TEST BLUEPRINT CORE COMPETENCIES

1. Function within the Education and Health Care Environments

A. Function in the Clinical Nurse Educator Role

1. Integrate theory and practice in the clinical setting
3. Use technologies to support clinical teaching and learning
4. Act as a role model of professional nursing within the clinical learning environment
5. Create a diverse, equitable, and inclusive learning environment

B. Operationalize the Curriculum

1. Assess congruence of the clinical environment with curriculum, course outcomes, and learner needs when evaluating clinical sites

2. Identify learner goals and outcomes
3. Facilitate meaningful and relevant clinical learning activities to promote optimal learning
7. Implement academic program's assigned models of clinical teaching consistent with course outcomes (e.g., traditional, preceptor, simulation, dedicated education units)

C. Abide by Legal Requirements, Ethical Guidelines, Agency Policies, and Guiding Framework
3. Facilitate learning activities that support the mission, goals, and values of the academic institution and the clinical agency
4. Inform others of program and clinical agency policies, procedures, and practices
5. Adhere to program and clinical agency policies, procedures and practices when implementing clinical experiences (e.g., due process, accommodations, academic integrity)
6. Comply with current program and clinical agency policies, procedures, and practices related to personal protective equipment and other infection control measures for self and learners
7. Demonstrate ethical and legal behaviors in the clinical nurse educator role

2. Facilitate Learning in the Healthcare Environment

A. Implement a variety of clinical teaching strategies congruent with learner needs, desired learner outcomes, course outcomes, setting, and context (e.g., virtual, telehealth, in-person, simulation)

C. Use academic and client-care technology to support the teaching-learning process

D. Create opportunities for learners to develop clinical judgment

G. Develop collegial working relationships with learners, faculty, and clinical environment personnel

3. Demonstrate Effective Interpersonal Communication and Collaborative Interprofessional Relationships

F. Use clear and effective communication in all interactions (e.g., written, electronic, verbal, non verbal, virtual)

J. Function as an accessible resource to learners and the healthcare team in the clinical learning environment

N. Communicate performance expectations to learners and clinical staff

6. Implement Effective Clinical and Assessment Evaluation Strategies

B. Conduct formative and summative evaluation specific to the learner and learning outcomes

C. Communicate learner clinical performance to course faculty in a timely manner

E. Provide timely, specific, objective, and constructive feedback to learners

F. Use situational assessment data to facilitate learning in the clinical environment

G. Document learner clinical performance, feedback, and progression

H. Evaluate the quality of the clinical learning experiences and environment

This chapter was prepared based on work by Christine Lind Colella in the sixth edition of the book.

LEARNING ACTIVITIES

CourseConnect

To access self-assessment questions and interactive, competency-based learning activities for this chapter, visit www.springerpub.com/courseconnect. See inside front cover and tear-out card for CourseConnect details.

REFERENCES

Al Nufaiei, Z. F., Bukhari, A. A., Abalkhail, N. A., Melebari, R. M., Alluhibi, R., Al Zhranei, R. M., Allhadian, F., Turkestani, F. A., Alsulami, M., Alshamrani, K. M., Abdelrahman, E. I., & Zipp, G. P. (2024). Health care clinical preceptors' attitudes towards interprofessional education in Saudi Arabia: A cross-sectional study. *Advances in Medical Education and Practice*, *15*, 343–355. https://doi.org/10.2147/AMEP.S451938

Cadmus, E., Roberts, M. L., & Olson, E. (2021). Creating a statewide nurse residency: Using an apprenticeship model. *Journal of Nursing Administration*, *51*(11), 568–572. https://doi.org/10.1097/NNA.0000000000001065

Cary, M. P., Jr., De Gagne, J. C., Kauschinger, E. D., & Carter, B. M. (2024). Advancing health equity through artificial intelligence: An educational framework for preparing nurses in clinical practice and research. *Creative Nursing*, *30*(2), 154–164. https://doi.org/10.1177/10784535241249193

De Gagne, J. C., & Oermann, M. H. (2025). *Teaching in nursing and role of the educator: The complete guide to best practice in teaching, evaluation, and curriculum development* (4th ed.). Springer Publishing Company.

Forneris, S. (2023). Teaching and learning using simulation. In D. M. Billings & J. A. Halstead (Eds.), *Teaching in nursing: A guide for faculty* (7th ed., pp. 422–448). Elsevier.

Gardiner, K. (2023). *Time-based, competency-based, or hybrid programs? Considerations for selecting an approach to registered apprenticeship*. Urban Institute. https://www.urban.org/research/publication/time-based-competency-based-or-hybrid-programs

Gilmore, D. M., & Nguyen, C. (2024). *Partnering with online program managers for distance education: Approaches to policy, quality, and leadership* (1st ed.). Routledge. https://doi.org/10.4324/9781003387138

Hosseinpour, A., Nasiri, M., Keshmiri, F., Arabzadeh, T., & Sharafi, H. (2024). Comparison of the effects of apprenticeship training by sandwich feedback and traditional methods on final-semester operating room technology students' perioperative competence and performance: a randomized, controlled trial. *BMC Medical Education*, *24*(1), 578. https://doi.org/10.1186/s12909-024-05598-6

Kleib, M., Arnaert, A., Nagle, L. M., Ali, S., Idrees, S., Costa, D. D., Kennedy, M., & Darko, E. M. (2024). Digital health education and training for undergraduate and graduate nursing students: Scoping review. *JMIR Nursing*, *7*, e58170. https://doi.org/10.2196/58170

McInnis, A., Schlemmer, T., & Chapman, B. (2021). The significance of the NP preceptorship shortage. *OJIN: The Online Journal of Issues in Nursing*, *26*(1). https://ojin.nursingworld.org/table-of-contents/volume-26-2021/number-1-january-2021/the-significance-of-the-np-preceptorship-shortage-/

National Council for State Authorization Reciprocity Agreements. (2025a). *The state authorization guide.* https://nc-sara.org/guide/state-authorization-guide

National Council for State Authorization Reciprocity Agreements. (2025b). *What is SARA?* https://nc-sara.org

Oermann, M. H., Gaberson, K. B., & De Gagne, J. C. (2024). *Evaluation and testing in nursing education* (7th ed.). Springer Publishing Company.

Rashwan, Z. I., Busebaia, T. J., Khonji, L. M., Eweida, R. S., Matooq, A. A., & Bayoumi, M. M. (2023). Between challenges and support: Preceptors run clinical nursing training amidst unprecedented crisis. *International Journal of Educational Research Open*, *4*, 100260. https://doi.org/10.1016/j.ijedro.2023.100260

Toly, V. B., Eliades, A., Miller, A., Sidora, S., Kracker, J., Fiala, M., & AlShammari, T. (2022). Collaborative development of an innovative virtual research recruitment strategy through an academic/clinical partnership. *Applied Nursing Research*, *68*, 151626. https://doi.org/10.1016/j.apnr.2022.151626

Wittler, A., Perez, A., & Griffin, V. (2025). Telehealth virtual simulation across the family nurse practitioner curriculum. *Nursing Education Perspectives*, *46*(1), 52–54. https://doi.org/10.1097/01.NEP.0000000000001262

Yalcinkaya, T., Ergin, E., & Yucel, S. C. (2024). Exploring nursing students' attitudes and readiness for artificial intelligence: A cross-sectional study. *Teaching and Learning in Nursing*, *19*(4), e722-e728. https://doi.org/10.1016/j.teln.2024.07.008

Clinical Evaluation and Grading 12

OBJECTIVES:

1. Analyze the role of clinical evaluation in fostering students' competencies, including clinical judgment, technical skills, and professional attitudes, within diverse healthcare settings.
2. Compare and contrast various methods of clinical evaluation, highlighting their suitability for assessing knowledge, cognitive skills, and performance in practice.
3. Describe strategies for grading and providing feedback in clinical practice, including approaches for addressing student challenges or potential failures.

Nursing practice requires the development of clinical judgment and higher-level thinking skills, psychomotor and technological skills, attitudes and values, and other competencies for care of patients across settings. Through clinical evaluation, the teacher arrives at judgments about students' competencies—their performance in practice. After establishing a framework for evaluating students in clinical practice and exploring one's own values, attitudes, and biases that may influence evaluation, the teacher identifies a variety of methods for collecting data on student performance. Clinical evaluation methods are strategies for assessing competencies in clinical practice. Some evaluation methods are most appropriate for use by faculty members or preceptors who are on-site with students and can observe their performance; other evaluation methods assess students' knowledge, cognitive skills, and other competencies but do not involve direct observation of their performance.

This chapter describes the process of clinical evaluation in nursing, use of competencies and entrustable professional activities (EPAs) for assessment of performance, and giving feedback to students. Multiple methods for evaluating clinical performance are described with some examples: observation, checklists, varied rating scales, simulations, standardized patients (SPs), objective structured clinical examinations (OSCE), writing assignments, cases, e-portfolios, conferences, group projects, and self-assessment. How to grade students in clinical courses, examples of grading systems, and principles to follow in evaluating and grading clinical practice, including guidelines to follow if a student is failing a clinical practicum or has the potential for failing it, also are discussed in the chapter.

CONCEPT OF CLINICAL EVALUATION

Clinical evaluation is a process by which judgments are made about learners' competencies in practice. This practice may involve care of patients, families, and communities; other types of learning activities in the clinical setting; simulation activities; performance of varied skills in learning laboratories; or activities using technologies. Most frequently, clinical evaluation involves observing performance and arriving at judgments about the student's competence. Judgments influence the data collected—that is, the specific types of observations made to evaluate the student's performance—and the inferences and conclusions drawn from the data about the quality of that performance. Teachers may collect different data to evaluate the same competencies, and when presented with a series of observations about a student's performance, there may be minimal consistency in their judgments about how well that student performed.

Clinical evaluation is not an objective process; it involves subjective judgments by the clinical educator, preceptor, and others involved in the process. This is most apparent in judging clinical performance, where the educator's values may influence the observations made of students and the judgments about the quality of performance. Thus, it is important for educators and nurses in other roles to be aware of their own values that might bias their judgments of students. For example, if the teacher prefers students who initiate discussions and participate actively in conferences, this value should not influence the assessment of students' competencies in other areas.

Clinical Evaluation Versus Grading

Clinical evaluation is not the same as grading. In evaluation, the teacher makes observations of performance and collects other types of data, then compares this information to a set of standards to arrive at a judgment. From this assessment, a quantitative symbol or grade may be applied to reflect the evaluation data and judgments made about performance. The clinical grade, such as pass–fail or A through F, is the symbol to represent the evaluation. Clinical performance may be evaluated and not graded, such as with formative evaluation or feedback to the learner, or it may be graded. Grades, however, should not be assigned without sufficient data about clinical performance. Grades are important to students at all educational levels in nursing (Poorman & Mastorovich, 2019).

Formative and Summative Clinical Evaluation

Clinical evaluation may be formative or summative. Formative evaluation in clinical practice provides feedback to learners about their progress in developing the clinical competencies. The purposes of formative evaluation are to enable students to develop further their clinical knowledge, skills, and values; indicate areas in which learning and practice are needed; and provide a basis for suggesting additional instruction to improve performance. Feedback is critical to learning in the clinical setting: The teacher provides specific information that fills gaps in learning and helps students improve their performance. Formative evaluation is assessment *for* learning: It is diagnostic and should not be graded (Oermann, 2022).

Summative clinical evaluation, however, is designed for determining clinical grades because it determines the competencies that students have developed in clinical practice. It is done at the end of a period of time—for example, at midterm or at the end of the clinical practicum—to assess the extent to which learners have achieved the clinical competencies. Summative evaluation is assessment *of* learning. Summative evaluation is not diagnostic; it summarizes the performance of students at a particular point in time. For much of clinical practice in a nursing program, summative evaluation comes too late for students to have an opportunity to improve performance.

Any protocol for clinical evaluation should include extensive formative evaluation and periodic summative evaluation. Formative evaluation is essential to provide feedback to improve performance while practice experiences are still available.

FEEDBACK IN CLINICAL EVALUATION

For clinical evaluation to be effective, the teacher should provide continuous feedback to students about their performance and how they can improve it. Giving constructive feedback helps learners to bridge the gap between their current performance and the competencies to be achieved (Orsini et al., 2022). Feedback may be verbal, by describing observations of performance and explaining what to do differently, or visual, by demonstrating correct performance. Feedback should be accompanied by further instruction from the teacher or by working with students to identify appropriate learning activities.

The ultimate goal is for students to progress to a point at which they can judge their own performance, identify resources for their learning, and use those resources to further develop competencies. Students must have an underlying knowledge base and beginning skills to judge their own performance. Sometimes students are not able to perform at the expected level because they lack the prerequisite knowledge and skills for developing the new competencies. As such, it is important to begin the clinical instruction by assessing whether students have learned the necessary concepts and skills and, if not, to start there.

Principles of Providing Feedback

There are four principles for providing feedback to students as part of the clinical evaluation process. First, the feedback should be precise and specific. General information about performance, such as, "You need to work on your assessment" or "You need more practice in the simulation laboratory," does not indicate what behaviors need improvement or how to develop them. Instead of using general statements, the teacher should indicate what specific areas of knowledge are lacking, where there are problems in clinical judgments, and what particular competencies need more development. Rather than saying to a student, "You need to work on your assessment," the student would be better served if the teacher identified the specific areas of data collection omitted and the physical examination techniques that need improvement. Specific feedback is more valuable to learners than a general description of their behavior.

Second, for procedures and any psychomotor skills, the teacher should provide both verbal and visual feedback to students. This means that the teacher should explain first, either orally or in writing, where the errors were made in performance and then demonstrate the correct procedure or skill. This should be followed by deliberate practice; that is, repetitive practice of a skill with assessment of performance and instruction to guide performance (Ericsson, 2008; Johnson et al., 2020). This practice is essential to retain skills and develop proficiency in them.

Third, feedback about performance should be given to students at the time of learning or immediately following it. Providing prompt and rich feedback is equally important when teaching nurses and other learners. The longer the period of time between performance and feedback from the teacher, the less effective the feedback becomes. As time passes, neither student nor teacher may remember specific areas of clinical practice to be improved. This principle holds true whether the performance relates to cognitive learning, a procedure or clinical skill, or an attitude or value expressed by the student, among other areas.

Whether working with a group of students in a clinical setting, communicating with preceptors about students, or teaching an online course, the teacher needs to develop a strategy for giving focused and immediate feedback to students and following up with further discussion as needed. Recording short notes about observations of students' performance for later discussion with individual students helps remember important points about performance.

Fourth, students need different amounts of feedback and positive reinforcement. In beginning practice and with clinical situations that are new to learners, most students will need frequent and extensive feedback. As students progress through the program and become more competent, they should be able to assess their own performance and identify personal learning needs.

Ossenberg et al. (2023) developed an educational intervention designed to provide feedback to students in the clinical setting that incorporated best practices of feedback. Clinical performance data were collected at three time points, demonstrating that the feedback improved students' performance during the practicum. The authors recommended that students have an active role in feedback conversations related to their learning goals.

RELATIONSHIP OF EVALUATION TO CLINICAL COMPETENCIES

The competencies provide the basis for clinical evaluation. Competencies are the observable abilities of the student; that is, what the student can do (Oermann, 2022). The American Association of Colleges of Nursing (AACN) defines competency as the ability of a healthcare professional that integrates multiple components, including knowledge, skills, values, and attitudes (AACN, 2021). The AACN *The Essentials: Core Competencies for Professional Nursing Education* identify 10 domains or areas of nursing competence that include broad competencies and multiple subcompetencies. Because competencies are observable, they can be assessed to ensure that students have developed these abilities at the end of their program. Competency-based education focuses on the end point and allows variable times for achievement (Jones-Schenk, 2025).

Table 12.1 provides a list of competencies that students should achieve by the end of their program. These competencies are stated broadly and can be used to identify subcompetencies for clinical assessment for prelicensure and nurse practitioner (NP) and other advanced practice nursing (APRN) students. Integrated in this list are core competencies for interprofessional collaborative practice that are needed by all healthcare professionals. **Exhibit 12.1** identifies the four areas of core competencies. **Table 12.1** also includes the domains or areas of competency from the AACN *Essentials*.

These competencies provide a framework for faculty to use in planning their clinical courses and in deciding how to assess student performance. Not all competencies are developed in every nursing course; for example, some courses may not call for the acquisition of technological or delegation skills. However, overall most courses will move students toward achievement of these competencies as they progress through the nursing program.

For nurses in practice, competencies reflect the expected level of performance to care for patients in the healthcare setting. Competencies for nurses are assessed as part of the initial employment and orientation to the healthcare setting and on an ongoing basis.

In some nursing programs, outcomes or objectives to be met in clinical practice are indicated for clinical learning and evaluation instead of competencies. For example, each course in the curriculum might have an outcome on communication. In a beginning clinical course, the outcome might be, "Identifies verbal and nonverbal techniques for communicating with patients." In a later course, the communication outcome might be, "Collaborates with other healthcare providers in care of patients."

Regardless of the format used, caution should be exercised in developing clinical competencies to avoid having too many for evaluation when considering the number of learners for whom the teacher is responsible, types of clinical learning opportunities available, and time allotted for clinical learning. Nurse educators should keep in mind that they need to collect sufficient data about students' performance of each competency specified for that course. The clinical competencies should reflect safe and effective practice, be realistic, and be useful for guiding the assessment.

Entrustable Professional Activities

NPs need to achieve competencies identified in the AACN *Essentials* and those established by the National Organization of Nurse Practitioner Faculties (NONPF). NONPF has identified competencies and subcompetencies that NPs must achieve for entry into practice regardless of their population focus (NONPF, 2024). NONPF also provides a guide with behaviors that indicate achievement of each subcompetency and examples of strategies for assessment that can be used. Key to this assessment is the ability of the NP student to perform activities that demonstrate these subcompetencies (Moore et al., 2024). EPAs are discrete workplace tasks that NPs and other learners are entrusted to perform unsupervised once they demonstrate their competence (Ten Cate et al., 2015; Wagner et al., 2018). EPAs are observable and measurable so they can be used for evaluating the competencies of

TABLE 12.1 COMPETENCIES TO BE DEVELOPED IN CLINICAL PRACTICE

Competencies	Related Domain in AACN *Essentials* With Sample Competency[a]
Apply concepts, theories, and other knowledge to clinical practice	Domain 1: Knowledge for Nursing Practice (1.2 Apply theory and research-based knowledge from nursing, the arts, humanities, and other sciences)
Use higher level thinking and clinical judgment in patient care	Domain 1: Knowledge for Nursing Practice (1.3 Demonstrate clinical judgment founded on a broad knowledge base)
Provide comprehensive and evidence-based care for patients with varied health problems and needs	Domain 2: Person-Centered Care (2.3 Integrate assessment skills in practice, 2.4 Diagnose actual or potential health problems and needs, 2.5 Develop a plan of care, 2.7 Evaluate outcomes of care)
Care for patients, families, and populations across the health continuum	Domain 3: Population Health (3.1 Manage population health)
Use research and other evidence in clinical practice	Domain 4: Scholarship for the Nursing Discipline (4.2 Integrate best evidence into nursing practice)
Apply knowledge, skills, and values continuously improving the quality and safety of healthcare	Domain 5: Quality and Safety (5.1 Apply quality improvement principles in care delivery)
Communicate effectively with patients, families, communities, and interprofessional teams	Domain 2: Person-Centered Care (2.2 Communicate effectively with individuals) Domain 6: Interprofessional Partnerships (6.1 Communicate in a manner that facilitates a partnership approach to quality care delivery)
Demonstrate leadership skills within complex healthcare systems	Domain 7: Systems-Based Practice (7.1 Apply knowledge of systems to work effectively across the continuum of care)
Demonstrate competencies in psychomotor skills, information and communication technology, informatics, and other technologies	Domain 8: Informatics and Healthcare Technologies (8.2 Use information and communication technology to gather data, create information, and generate knowledge)
Demonstrate knowledge and values essential for providing care to a culturally and ethnically diverse patient population	Domain 9: Professionalism (9.6 Integrate diversity, equity, and inclusion as core to one's professional identity)
Accept responsibility for actions and decisions	Domain 9: Professionalism (9.3 Demonstrate accountability to the individual, society, and the profession)
Demonstrate continued learning and self-development	Domain 10: Personal, Professional, and Leadership Development (10.2 Demonstrate a spirit of inquiry that fosters flexibility and professional maturity)

[a]Some of these competencies are also integrated in other domains.

Source: American Association of Colleges of Nursing. (2021). *The essentials: Core competencies for professional nursing education.* American Association of Colleges of Nursing. Oermann, M. H., Gaberson, K. B., & De Gagne, J. C. (2025). *Evaluation and testing in nursing education* (7th ed., p. 244). Springer Publishing Company.

NP students in clinical practice. By using EPAs, the evaluation of students' performance can be explicit, competency-based, and standardized (Corrigan et al., 2022).

Moore developed a list of eight EPAs that describe the core professional activities that all NPs should be able to perform and validated these EPAs in a Delphi study. These EPAs, in **Table 12.2**, provide a framework for the evaluation of the competencies of NP students. Anthamatten and Pitts (2024) integrated EPAs into their clinical evaluation tool and found that it collected critical information about student performance in their clinical practicum.

CLINICAL EVALUATION METHODS

There are many evaluation methods for use in nursing education. Some methods, such as journals, are most appropriate for formative evaluation, while others are useful for either formative or summative evaluation.

Selecting Clinical Evaluation Methods

There are several factors to consider when selecting clinical evaluation methods to use in a course. First, the evaluation methods should provide information on student performance of the clinical competencies

EXHIBIT 12.1 Interprofessional Education Collaborative (IPEC) Core Competencies for Interprofessional Collaborative Practice

1. Values and Ethics: Ability to work with members of the healthcare team
2. Roles and Responsibilities: Ability to use knowledge of one's own role and the expertise of team members to meet patient and population health outcomes
3. Communication: Ability to communicate responsibly, respectfully, and compassionately with team members
4. Teams and Teamwork: Ability to apply values and principles of teamwork in a variety of settings.

Source: Adapted from Interprofessional Education Collaborative. (2023). *IPEC core competencies revision: Version 3 (2021–2023).* https://www.ipecollaborative.org/2021-2023-core-competencies-revision

associated with the course. With the evaluation methods, the teacher collects data on performance to judge whether students are developing the clinical competencies or have achieved them by the end of the course.

Second, for many competencies, different strategies can be used, thereby providing flexibility in choosing methods for evaluation. Varying the methods maintains student interest and takes into account learners' individual needs, abilities, and characteristics. Some students may be more proficient in methods that depend on writing, while others prefer strategies such as conferences and other discussions. Using multiple evaluation methods in clinical practice takes into consideration these differences among students. It also avoids relying on one method, such as a rating scale, for determining the entire clinical grade.

Third, the teacher should select evaluation methods that are realistic considering the number of students to be evaluated, available practice or simulation activities, and constraints such as the teacher's or preceptor's time. Planning for an evaluation method that depends on patients with specific health problems or particular clinical situations is not realistic considering the types of experiences with actual or simulated patients available to students. Some methods are not appropriate because of the number of students who would need to use them within the time frame of the course. Others may be too time consuming for educators to provide feedback to students. Discussions with students one-to-one or in small groups, cases analyzed by students in postclinical conferences, group writing activities, and similar methods might replace strategies that require more teacher time for assessment and accomplish the same purposes.

Fourth, evaluation methods can be used for formative or summative evaluation. In the process of deciding how to evaluate students' clinical performance, the teacher should identify whether the methods will be used to provide feedback to learners (formative) or for grading (summative). In clinical practice, students should know ahead of time whether the assessment by the teacher is for formative or summative purposes. Some of the methods designed for clinical evaluation provide feedback to students on areas for improvement and should not be graded. Other methods, such as rating scales and written assignments, can be used for summative purposes and can be included as part of the clinical grade.

Fifth, before finalizing the plan for how students will be evaluated in a course, the teacher should review the purpose and number required of each assignment completed by students. What are the purposes of these assignments, and how many are needed to demonstrate competency? In some clinical courses, students

TABLE 12.2 NURSE PRACTITIONER CORE ENTRUSTABLE PROFESSIONAL ACTIVITIES

Number	Title	Description
1	Gather a History	Gathers a patient-centered history tailored to the healthcare concern, setting, and type of visit.
2	Perform a Physical Exam	Performs a patient-centered physical exam tailored to the patient's history, setting, and type of visit.
3	Perform a Clinical Procedure	Performs clinical procedures following standards of care.
4	Document a Clinical Encounter	Documents a clinical encounter following professional standards.
5	Formulate a Diagnosis	Integrates clinical data to formulate a prioritized differential diagnosis list and identify the most likely/working diagnosis.
6	Order and Interpret Diagnostic and Screening Tests	Order and interpret results of diagnostic and screening tests.
7	Present Orally a Clinical Encounter	Deliver a clear, accurate, and well-organized oral summary of a clinical encounter to a healthcare professional.
8	Develop and Manage a Plan of Care	Develop and manage an evidence-based plan of care for diagnosis(es) identified during a wellness, episodic, and/or chronic visit.

Source: Moore, J., Chan, T., Doucette, J., Lipps, T., & Slager, D. (2024). Defining nurse practitioner core entrustable professional activities: Essential step toward competency-based education. *Nurse Educator, 49*(5), 237. Reprinted by permission Wolters Kluwer Health Inc, January 6, 2025.

complete an excessive number of written assignments. Students benefit from continuous feedback from the teacher, not from repetitive assignments that contribute little to their development of clinical knowledge and skills.

Observation

The main strategy for evaluating clinical performance is observing students in clinical practice, simulation and learning laboratories, and other settings. Although observation is widely used, there are threats to its validity and reliability. First, observations of students may be influenced by the teacher's values and biases, as discussed earlier. There may also be overreliance on first impressions, which might change as the teacher or preceptor observes the student over a period of time and in different situations. In any performance evaluation, there needs to be a series of observations made before drawing conclusions about performance. Every observation in the clinical setting reflects only a sampling of the learner's performance. An observation of the same student at another time may reveal a different level of performance.

Second, in clinical practice, there are many aspects of performance on which the educator may focus attention. For example, while observing a student change a surgical wound dressing, the teacher may focus mainly on the technique and not how the student interacts with the patient, while another educator observing this same student may zero in on the interaction. The competencies should guide the teacher on what to observe, but all observations about performance should be shared with the students.

Third, the teacher may arrive at incorrect judgments about the observation, such as inferring that a student is inattentive during conference when, in fact, the student is thinking about the comments made by others in the group. It is important to discuss observations with students, obtain their perceptions of their performance, and be willing to modify one's own judgments when new data are presented.

Fourth, it is difficult, if not impossible, to remember the observations made of each student for each clinical activity. For this reason, clinical educators need some type of notes that describe the observations made of students. Notes about the student's performance should be recorded as close to the time of the observation as possible and should be shared frequently with students.

Checklists

Multiple types of tools are available to guide and structure observations and assessments of clinical performance such as checklists and rating scales (Ekman et al., 2020). A checklist contains specific behaviors or activities to be observed with a place for marking whether they were present during the performance (Brookhart & Nitko, 2019). A checklist often lists the steps to be followed in performing a procedure or demonstrating a skill. Checklists guide the teacher's observation of procedures performed by learners and provide a way for them to assess their own performance.

For common procedures, teachers can often find checklists already prepared that can be used for evaluation. When these resources are not available, teachers can develop their own checklists but should avoid including every possible step, which makes the checklist too cumbersome and prescriptive. Instead, the focus should be on critical behaviors for safe performance of the procedure or skill.

Rating Scales

Rating scales, also referred to as clinical evaluation tools, forms, or instruments, provide a means of recording judgments about the observed performance of students in clinical practice. A rating scale has two parts: (a) a list of competencies (or outcomes and behaviors) the student is to demonstrate in clinical practice and (b) a scale for rating their performance of them. Rating scales are most useful for summative evaluation of performance. After observing students over a period of time, the teacher determines if the competencies were achieved and, for tools with multiple levels, rates the quality of the performance.

The same rating scale can be used for multiple purposes. **Exhibit 12.2** shows sample competencies from a rating scale that is used midway through a course and at the end for the final summative rating.

TYPES OF RATING SCALES

Many types of rating scales are used for evaluating clinical performance. The scales may have multiple levels for rating performance, such as 1 to 5 or exceptional to below average, or have two levels, such as pass–fail. Types of scales with multiple levels for rating performance include:

- Letters: A, B, C, D, E or A, B, C, D, F
- Numbers: 1, 2, 3, 4, 5
- Qualitative labels: Excellent, very good, good, fair, poor; or exceptional, above average, average, below average
- Frequency labels: Always, usually, frequently, sometimes, never
- Combinations of these scales

A short description included with the letters, numbers, and labels for each of the competencies rated improves objectivity and consistency (Brookhart &

EXHIBIT 12.2 Sample Competencies from Rating Scale

Student Name ____________ Faculty Name ____________
Date ________

	Midterm			Final	
Competencies	**S**	**NI**	**U**	**S**	**U**
1. Provides patient-centered care for patients with chronic health problems across the lifespan					
A. Completes a comprehensive assessment using multiple sources of data					
B. Develops an individualized plan of care reflecting patient values, preferences, and needs					
C. Implements nursing interventions based on evidence					
D. Evaluates the outcomes of care					
E. Demonstrates caring behaviors					
2. Collaborates with nurses, the interprofessional team, and others in the healthcare system and community					
A. Demonstrates effective communication skills (with patients, families/caregivers, nurses, and other healthcare providers)					
B. Communicates relevant information about the patient and clinical situation using SBAR					
C. Collaborates with members of intra- and interprofessional teams					
D. Identifies resources for patients and caregivers for discharge and transitions of care					
3.					

NI, needs improvement; S, satisfactory; SBAR, situation–background–assessment–recommendation; U, unsatisfactory.

Source: Oermann, M. H., Gaberson, K. B., & De Gagne, J. C. (2025). *Evaluation and testing in nursing education* (7th ed., p. 259). Springer Publishing Company.

Nitko, 2019). For example, with a scale based on numbers, short descriptions of each level in the scale could be written to clarify the expected performance. For the competency "Collects relevant data from patients," the descriptors might be:

1. Differentiates relevant from irrelevant data, analyzes multiple sources of data, collects comprehensive data, identifies data needed for evaluating possible patient problems.
2. Collects significant data from patients, uses multiple sources of data as part of assessment, identifies possible patient problems based on the data.
3. Collects significant data from patients, uses data to develop main patient problems.
4. Does not collect significant data and misses important cues in data; unable to explain relevance of data for patient problems.

However, even with descriptors the level of performance is often not clear cut, and there may be inconsistency in clinical nurse educator and preceptor interpretations of the quality of performance. What is the difference between a 2, 3, or 4 level of performance? Do all clinical educators in the course agree? Scales based on frequency labels are often difficult to implement because of limited experiences for students to practice and demonstrate a level of skill rated as "always, usually, frequently, sometimes, and never." How should teachers rate students' performance in situations in which they practiced the skill perhaps only once or twice? With rating scales that have two levels (e.g., pass–fail, satisfactory–unsatisfactory, and met–did not meet the competency), there is less variability in the judgments to be made by educators, but even two-dimensional scales present room for variability. It is critical that everyone involved in the evaluation has an opportunity to discuss each of the competencies on a rating tool, what each means, the expected performance, and the rating for that performance level, and come to an agreement.

RATING ERRORS

Brookhart and Nitko (2019) identified common errors that can occur with rating scales applicable to rating clinical performance. The first three errors can occur with tools that have multiple points on the scale for rating performance, such as 1 to 5 or below average to exceptional. The other errors can occur with any type of clinical performance rating scale.

1. Leniency error results when the teacher tends to rate all students toward the high end of the scale.
2. Severity error is the opposite of leniency, tending to rate all students toward the low end of the scale.
3. Central tendency error is hesitancy to mark either end of the rating scale and instead use only the midpoint of the scale.
4. Halo effect is a judgment based on a general impression of the student. With this error, the teacher lets an overall impression of the student influence the ratings of specific aspects of the student's performance. The halo may be positive, giving the student a higher rating than is deserved, or negative, letting a general negative impression of the student result in lower ratings of performance.
5. Personal bias occurs when the teacher's biases influence ratings.
6. Logical error results when similar ratings are given for items on the scale that are logically related to one another. This is a problem with rating scales that are too long and too detailed. For example, there may be multiple competencies on communication to be rated. The teacher observes some of these but not all of them. In completing the clinical evaluation form, the teacher gives the same rating to all competencies related to communication on the tool. When this occurs, some of the items on the rating scale can often be combined.
7. Rater drift occurs when the clinical nurse educators and others involved in the evaluation redefine the competencies to be observed and assessed. Initially, in developing a clinical evaluation form, all agree on the competencies to be rated and the scale to be used. However, over time, the competencies may be interpreted differently, drifting away from the original intent. For this reason, discussion of the tool is critical at the beginning and midpoint of a course.
8. Reliability decay is a similar issue. Brookhart and Nitko (2019) indicated that immediately following training on using a rating tool, educators tend to use the tool consistently across students and with each other. As the course continues, though, educators may become less consistent in their ratings. Discussion of the tool among evaluators, as indicated earlier, may improve consistency in its use.

Although there are issues with rating scales, they allow clinical educators, preceptors, and others to rate performance over time and to assess patterns of performance. **Exhibit 12.3** provides guidelines for using rating scales for clinical evaluation in nursing.

EXHIBIT 12.3 Guidelines for Using Rating Scales for Clinical Evaluation

1. Be alert to the possible influence of your own values, attitudes, and biases in observing performance and drawing conclusions about it.
2. Use the clinical competencies to focus your observations. Give students feedback on your observations.
3. Collect sufficient data on students' performance before rating it summatively. Students should be observed more than one time. Rating scales, when used for clinical evaluation, are intended for assessing performance over a period of time.
4. Do not rely on first impressions; they may not be accurate.
5. Always discuss observations with students, obtain their perceptions of performance, and be willing to modify judgments and ratings when new data are presented.
6. Avoid using rating scales as the only source of data about a student's performance—use multiple evaluation methods for clinical practice.
7. Rate each competency individually based on the observations made of performance. If you have insufficient information about achievement of a particular competency, do not rate it—leave it blank.
8. If the rating form is not useful for judging student performance, then revise and reevaluate it. Consider these questions: Does the form yield data that can be used to make valid decisions about students' competence? Does the form yield reliable, stable data? Is it easy to use? Is it appropriate considering the types of learning activities that students have in their clinical settings or can obtain in simulation or skills laboratory?
9. Discuss as a group (with other educators, preceptors, and others involved in the evaluation) each competency on the rating scale. Come to agreement about the meaning of the competencies and what a student's performance would look like at each rating level in the tool. Share examples of performance, how you would rate them, and your rationale. As a group exercise, observe a video clip or other simulation of a student's performance, rate it with the tool, and come to agreement about the rating. Such exercises and discussions should be held before the course begins and periodically during it to ensure reliability across teachers and settings.

Simulations for Clinical Evaluation

Simulations are not only effective for instruction in nursing, but they are also useful for clinical evaluation. Students can demonstrate skills, conduct assessments, analyze scenarios and make decisions about actions to take, carry out interventions, and evaluate the effects of their decisions. Simulation can be used to guide students' development of clinical judgment skills and can be used for assessment of clinical judgment (Bussard & Jacobs, 2024; Bussard et al., 2025). Bussard et al. (2025) evaluated the development of students' clinical judgment from the beginning to the end of a BSN program using the Lasater Clinical

Judgment Rubric (LCJR). Eighteen simulations were analyzed; LCJR scores increased progressively from the first to the last semester.

Most nursing programs have simulation laboratories with human patient simulators, manikins and models for skill practice and assessment, areas for SPs, clinically equipped examination rooms, and a wide range of multimedia that can be used to facilitate performance evaluations. Virtual simulations are becoming widely used in nursing programs and can be used for assessment. Video conferencing and other technology can be used to conduct clinical evaluations of students in settings at a distance from the nursing education program, effectively replacing on-site performance evaluations by faculty members.

The same principles for evaluating student performance in the clinical setting apply to using simulations. The first task is to identify which clinical competencies will be assessed with simulation. Is the aim simply to provide feedback to students, or is the assessment for making high-stakes decisions where students need to pass the assessment to progress in the course? For high stakes, more than one evaluator should observe and rate performance. Evaluators should be trained and use a valid and reliable tool and should not know the students being evaluated (Alsulimani, 2021; Dupre & Naik, 2021; Holland et al., 2020; Oermann et al., 2025). Simulation-based assessments, however, are resource-intensive and may be best suited for individualized feedback (Sinz et al., 2021).

Standardized Patients

One type of simulation for clinical evaluation uses SPs—individuals who have been trained to accurately portray the role of a patient with a specific diagnosis or condition. With simulations using SPs, students can be evaluated on a history and physical examination, related skills and procedures, and communication techniques, among other competencies. SPs are effective for evaluation because the actors are trained to re-create the same patient condition and clinical situation each time they are with a student, providing for consistency in the performance evaluation.

When SPs are used for formative evaluation, they provide feedback to the students on their performance, an important aid to their learning. Because SPs are trained for their role, however, they are well suited for summative evaluation of students' clinical and communication skills, verifying performance competency. Chua et al. (2023) conducted a mixed-studies systematic review of 20 studies to examine the use of SPs in APRN programs. Students benefited from SPs in terms of refining their knowledge, clinical skills, and communication skills, and felt more confident in their competencies.

Objective Structured Clinical Examination

An OSCE provides a means of evaluating performance in a simulation laboratory rather than in the clinical setting. In an OSCE, students rotate through a series of stations; at each station, they complete an activity or perform a task, which is then evaluated. Some stations assess the student's ability to take a patient's history, perform a physical examination, and implement other interventions while being observed by the teacher or an examiner. The student's performance can then be rated using a rating scale or checklist. At other stations, students might be tested on their knowledge and clinical judgment—they might be asked to analyze data, identify patient problems, select interventions and treatments, and manage the patient's condition. There may also be postencounter stations to facilitate the evaluation of cognitive skills such as interpreting lab results and other data, developing management plans, and making other types of judgments and decisions about patient care. In a scoping review of 204 studies, Goh et al. (2019) found that OSCEs were valid, reliable, and an acceptable method for evaluating performance in nursing. OSCEs were used across various nursing specialties in 33 countries. OSCEs are typically used for summative clinical evaluation but can also be used formatively to assess performance and provide feedback to students.

Written Assignments

Written assignments accompanying the clinical practicum are effective methods for assessing students' higher-level learning, understanding of concepts and content relevant to the assignment, use of resources to support ideas in papers, and ability to express ideas in writing. Written assignments may be evaluated formatively or summatively. Periodic assessment of drafts of papers and work in progress is formative in nature and is not intended for arriving at a grade. For written assignments that are not graded, the teacher's role is to give prompt and sufficient feedback for students to learn from the assignment. If the assignment will be graded (summative evaluation), then criteria for grading and the rubric to be used should be shared with students. Some writing assignments, such as concept maps and reflective journals, do not lend themselves to grading and instead are best used for formative evaluation only. Other assignments such as short written assignments, nursing care plans, and analyses of patient data and clinical scenarios can be evaluated to provide feedback to learners or can be graded. Types of written assignments were described in Chapter 7.

Feedback on assignments should be specific and guide revisions, not general statements such as "unclear introduction." Instead, tell students exactly what was unclear and needs to be revised. This is especially important if drafts of papers are submitted first for feedback. For example, "The introduction is about noise reduction strategies rather than the problem on the unit with noise. Revise the introduction to explain the problem with noise on the unit, supporting data on noise levels, and why we need strategies to reduce noise for both patients and staff."

CRITERIA FOR EVALUATION

The criteria for evaluation of a paper should relate to the learning outcomes or competencies to be met. For example, if students write a short paper to meet the outcome, "Compare interventions for nausea associated with chemotherapy," criteria should relate to the appropriateness and evidence for the interventions selected for critique, how effectively the student compared them, the rationale developed for the analysis, and the like. General criteria for evaluating written assignments in clinical courses are presented in **Exhibit 12.4**. For assignments that are graded, students should have the criteria for evaluation and rubric (scoring guide) before they begin writing so they know what will be assessed.

EXHIBIT 12.4 General Criteria for Evaluating Papers in Clinical Courses

Content

Content is relevant to patient or clinical situation.
Content is accurate.
Significant information is presented.
Concepts and theories are used appropriately for analysis.
Content is comprehensive.
Content reflects current research and evidence.
Hypotheses, conclusions, and decisions are supported.

Organization

Content is organized logically.
Ideas are presented in logical sequence.
Paragraph structure is appropriate.
Headings are used appropriately to indicate new content areas.

Process

Process used to arrive at approaches, decisions, judgments, and so forth is adequate.
Consequences of decisions are considered.
Sound rationale is provided.
For papers analyzing issues, the rationale supports position taken.
Multiple perspectives and new approaches are considered.

Writing Style

Ideas are described clearly.
Sentence structure is clear.
There are no grammatical errors.
There are no spelling errors.
Appropriate punctuation is used.
Writing does not reveal bias.
Length of paper is consistent with requirements.
Literature used in paper is up to date (within the past 5 years).
References are cited appropriately throughout paper.
References are accurate and prepared according to required format.

GRADING ASSIGNMENTS

In grading written assignments, a rubric, which is a scoring guide, should be developed based on the criteria established for evaluation. The rubric includes the areas to be evaluated and points allotted for each one, and keeps the evaluation focused on the criteria, not some other standard. Some teachers tend to be more lenient and others tend to be more critical in their review of papers. Use of a rubric to guide the assessment of a paper can lead to more reliable scoring. DeCoux Hampton and Chafetz (2021) developed a rubric to measure general and scientific writing skill proficiency in nursing. They found that the rubric was effective for distinguishing the specific skills needed for health science writing, and it also led to higher rater consistency.

There are different types of rubrics. With a holistic rubric, the teacher scores the paper as a whole without assessing individual parts. An analytic rubric guides the assessment of separate parts of the paper and then sums them for a total score. **Exhibit 12.5** is an example of an analytic rubric that was developed using the general criteria in **Exhibit 12.4**.

PRINCIPLES FOR ASSESSING WRITTEN ASSIGNMENTS

Written assignments that are graded should be read anonymously if possible although this is often difficult to do with small groups of students. There is a tendency in evaluating written assignments, similar to essay items, for the teacher to be influenced by a general impression of the student. This is called the halo effect. The teacher may have positive or negative feelings about the student or other biases that may influence evaluating and grading the assignment.

Another reason to read papers anonymously is to avoid a carryover effect, in which the teacher carries an impression of the quality of one written assignment to the next one that the student completes. If the student develops an outstanding paper, the teacher may be influenced to score subsequent written assignments at a similarly high level; the same situation may occur with a poor paper. The impression of the student is carried from one written assignment to the next (Oermann et al., 2025). Papers should be read in random order to avoid scoring papers read early higher than those read near the end. Many of the assignments in a clinical course, however, are not graded, and the educator instead provides feedback for further learning.

EXHIBIT 12.5 Sample Scoring Rubric for Papers in Clinical Courses

Content		
Content relevant to patient or clinical situation, comprehensive, and in-depth 5	Content relevant to patient or clinical situation with critical information included 4–3	Some content not relevant to patient or clinical situation, critical information missing, lacks depth 2–1
Content accurate 5	Most of content accurate 4–3	Major errors in content 2–1
Sound background developed from peer-reviewed articles and wide range of information sources 5	Textbook and websites predominant sources of information for developing background 4–3	Background not developed, limited support for ideas 2–1
Current research and evidence synthesized and integrated effectively 10–7	Current research and evidence summarized 6–4	Limited research and evidence in paper, not used to support ideas 3–1
Organization		
Purpose of paper well developed and clearly stated 3	Purpose apparent but not developed sufficiently 2	Purpose poorly developed, not clear 1
Content well organized and logically presented, organization supports arguments and development of ideas 10–7	Clear organization of main points and ideas 6–4	Poorly organized, content not developed adequately 3–1
Effective conclusions based on analysis 3	Conclusions based on summary of content, limited analysis 2	Poor conclusions, not based on content in paper 1
Writing Style and Format		
Sentence structure clear, smooth transitions, correct grammar and punctuation, no spelling errors 10–7	Adequate sentence structure and transitions; few grammar, punctuation, and spelling errors 6–4	Poor sentence structure and transitions; errors in grammar, punctuation, and spelling 3–1
Writing Style and Format		
Professional appearance of paper, all parts included, length consistent with requirements 3	Paper legible, some parts missing or too short or too long considering requirements 2	Unprofessional appearance, missing sections, paper too short or too long considering requirements 1
References used appropriately; references current, no errors in references, correct use of APA style 6–5	References used appropriately but limited, most references current, some citations or references with errors or some errors in APA style 4–3	Few references and limited breadth, old references (not classic), errors in references, errors in APA style 2–1
Total score ______ (sum points for total score; maximum score 60)		

APA, American Psychological Association.

Cases

Cases for clinical learning were described in Chapter 7. Cases can be completed by students individually or as a group activity. They are effective methods for group discussion and analysis in postclinical conferences and for online discussions. In an online course, the case scenario can be presented with open-ended questions, and, based on student responses, other questions can be introduced for discussion. Using this approach, cases are effective for encouraging higher-level thinking. By discussing cases as a clinical group, students are exposed to other possible approaches and perspectives they may not have identified themselves. With this method, the teacher can provide feedback on the content and thought process used by students to arrive at their answers. One advantage of cases is they can be done for instructional purposes and not graded, or they can be graded.

Electronic Portfolio

An electronic portfolio (e-portfolio) is a collection of projects and materials (also referred to as artifacts) developed by the student that documents achievement of the competencies or outcomes of the clinical course. E-portfolios are valuable for clinical evaluation because students provide evidence in their e-portfolios on their competencies and new learning and skills acquired in a course.

E-portfolios can be used in prelicensure, RN-BSN, APRN, and doctor of nursing practice (DNP) programs to document the student's achievement of competencies and program outcomes practice (Chang et al., 2019; Melander et al., 2018; Sidebotham et al., 2018; Waldrop et al., 2023). They can be evaluated and graded by faculty members or clinical educators, or used for students' self-assessment of their progress in meeting personal and professional goals and not be evaluated by the teacher.

Brookhart and Nitko (2019) identified two types of portfolios: best work and growth. Best-work portfolios contain the students' best final products. These provide evidence that the students have demonstrated certain competencies and met the outcomes of the course, and thus are appropriate for summative evaluation. Growth portfolios are designed for monitoring students' progress and providing feedback, and for self-reflection on learning (Brookhart & Nitko, 2019). Steps for planning an e-portfolio for clinical evaluation are in **Exhibit 12.6**.

EXHIBIT 12.6 Steps for Planning an Electronic Portfolio for a Clinical Practicum

1. Identify the purpose of the e-portfolio. (Provide evidence of students' best work in clinical practice, their learning over a period of time, or both? Used for formative or summative evaluation, or both? Provide assessment data for a clinical course or for program evaluation and accreditation?)
2. Identify the type of documents and content to be included in the e-portfolio. (Required types of documents? Minimum number required? How to organize?)
3. Decide on the evaluation of the e-portfolio including criteria for evaluation. (How will the e-portfolio be integrated within the grade, if at all? Develop rubric for scoring the e-portfolio and/or individual documents.)

Source: Brookhart, S. M., & Nitko, A. J. (2019). *Educational assessment of students* (6th ed.). Pearson.

Conferences

The ability to present ideas orally is an important outcome of clinical practice. Sharing information about a patient, leading others in discussions about clinical practice, presenting ideas in a group format, and giving presentations are skills that students need to develop in a nursing program. Working with nursing staff members and the interprofessional team requires the ability to communicate effectively. Conferences provide a method for developing oral communication skills and for evaluating competency in this area. Discussions also can lead to higher-level thinking if questions are open ended and used as prompts for clinical judgment.

Criteria for assessing conferences include the ability of students to:

- present ideas clearly and in a logical sequence to the group;
- participate actively in the group discussion;
- offer ideas relevant to the topic;
- demonstrate knowledge of the content discussed in the conference;
- offer different perspectives on the topic, engaging the group in critical thinking; and
- assume a leadership role, if relevant, in promoting group discussion and arriving at group decisions.

Most conferences are evaluated for formative purposes, with the teacher giving feedback to students as a group or to the individual who led the group discussion. **Exhibit 12.7** provides a sample form that can be used to evaluate how well a student leads a clinical conference.

Group Projects

Most of the clinical evaluation methods presented in this chapter focus on individual student performance, but group projects also can be assessed as part of the clinical evaluation in a course. Some group work is short term—only for the time it takes to develop a product, such as a teaching plan or group presentation. Other groups may be formed for the purpose of cooperative learning, with students working in small groups or teams in clinical practice over a longer period of time. With any of these group formats, both the products developed by the group and the ability of the students to work cooperatively can be assessed.

EXHIBIT 12.7 Evaluation of a Clinical Conference

Student's name ____________________
Conference topic ____________________
Date ________

Rate the behaviors by circling the appropriate number. Some behaviors will not be applicable depending on the student's role in the conference; mark those as not applicable (na).

Behaviors	Rating					
	Poor				Excellent	
States goals of conference	1	2	3	4	5	na
Leads group in discussion	1	2	3	4	5	na
Asks thought-provoking questions	1	2	3	4	5	na
Uses strategies that encourage all students to participate	1	2	3	4	5	na
Participates actively in discussion	1	2	3	4	5	na
Includes important content	1	2	3	4	5	na
Includes evidence for practice	1	2	3	4	5	na
Offers new perspectives to group	1	2	3	4	5	na
Considers different points of view	1	2	3	4	5	na
Assists group members in recognizing biases and values	1	2	3	4	5	na
Is enthusiastic about topic	1	2	3	4	5	na
Is well prepared for discussion	1	2	3	4	5	na
Monitors time	1	2	3	4	5	na
Develops quality materials to support discussion	1	2	3	4	5	na
Summarizes major points at end of conference	1	2	3	4	5	na

There are different approaches for grading group projects. The same grade can be given to every student in the group (i.e., a group grade), although this does not take into consideration individual student effort and contribution to the group product. Another approach is for the students to indicate in the finished product the parts to which they contributed, providing a way of assigning individual student grades, with or without a group grade. Students can also provide a self-assessment of how much they contributed to the group project, which can then be integrated into their grade. Alternatively, students can prepare both a group and an individual product.

Rubrics should be used for assessing group projects and should be geared specifically to the project. To assess students' participation and collaboration in the group, the rubric also needs to reflect the goals of group work. With small groups, the teacher can observe and rate individual student cooperation and contributions to the group. However, this is often difficult because the teacher is not a member of the group, and the group dynamics change when the teacher is present. As another approach, students can assess the participation and cooperation of their peers. These peer evaluations can be used for the students' own development and shared among peers but not with the teacher, or they can be incorporated by the teacher in the grade for the group project. Students can also be asked to assess their own participation in the group.

Self-Assessment

Self-assessment is the ability of students to assess their own competencies and identify where further learning is needed. Self-evaluation begins with the first clinical course and develops throughout the nursing program, continuing into professional practice. Using students' own assessments, teachers can develop plans to assist students in gaining the knowledge and skills they need to meet the outcomes of the course. Self-evaluation is appropriate only for formative evaluation and should never be graded.

CLINICAL EVALUATION IN DISTANCE EDUCATION

Nursing programs use different strategies for offering the clinical component of distance education courses. One of the predominant strategies, widely used in APRN programs, is for schools in collaboration with students to identify clinical sites and preceptors in the settings to work one-to-one with students to guide their learning and evaluate performance. The course syllabus, competencies to be developed, rating forms, guidelines for clinical practice, and other materials associated with the course and clinical practicum need to be available to preceptors. Preceptors are carefully selected and should be prepared by the school to guide students' learning in the clinical setting and to assess their competencies. Faculty might also conduct virtual site visits using telehealth and other technologies (Harris et al., 2020).

GRADING CLINICAL PRACTICE

Grading systems for clinical practice are often two-dimensional, such as pass–fail, satisfactory–unsatisfactory, and met–did not meet the clinical competencies. Some nursing programs add a third category, honors, to acknowledge performance that exceeds the level required. Other grading systems are multidimensional; for example, using letter grades A through F; integers 1 through 5; and percentages. With any of these grading systems, it is not always easy to summarize the multiple types of evaluation data collected about the student's performance into a symbol representing a grade. This is true even in a pass–fail system; it may be difficult to arrive at a judgment to pass or fail based on the evaluation data and the circumstances associated with the student's clinical and simulated practice.

Categories for grading clinical practice such as pass–fail have advantages over a system with multiple levels, although there are some disadvantages as well. Pass–fail places greater emphasis on giving feedback to the learner because only two categories of performance need to be determined. With a pass–fail grading system, clinical educators may be more inclined to provide continual feedback to learners because they do not have to ultimately differentiate performance according to four or five levels of proficiency such as with a multidimensional system.

A pass–fail system requires only two types of judgment about clinical performance. Do the evaluation data indicate that the student has demonstrated satisfactory performance of the competencies to indicate a pass? Or do the data suggest that the performance of those competencies is not at a satisfactory level? Deciding whether the learner has passed or failed is often easier for the teacher than using the same evaluation information for deciding on multiple levels of performance. A letter system for grading clinical practice, however, acknowledges the different levels of clinical proficiency students may have demonstrated in their clinical practicum.

A disadvantage of pass–fail for grading clinical practice is the inability to include a clinical grade into the course grade. One strategy is to separate nursing courses into two components for grading: one for theory and the second for clinical practice (designated as pass–fail). Typically, guidelines for the course indicate that the students must pass the clinical component to pass the course. A second mechanism is to offer two separate courses with the clinical course graded on a pass–fail basis.

Methods for Assigning the Clinical Grade

Once the grading system is determined, there are varied ways of using it to arrive at the clinical grade. The grade can be assigned based on the competencies achieved by the student. To use this method, faculty can designate some of the competencies as critical for achievement in the course. For example, an A might be assigned if all of the clinical competencies were met; a B might be assigned if all of the competencies designated by the faculty as critical behaviors and at least half of the others were met. For pass–fail grading, the faculty might indicate that all of the competencies must be met to pass the course or can designate critical ones required for passing the course. For both of these grading systems, the clinical evaluation methods provide the data for determining whether the student's performance reflects achievement of the competencies. These evaluation methods may or may not be graded separately as part of the course grade.

Another way of arriving at the clinical grade is to base it on the clinical evaluation methods. In this system, the clinical grade is computed based on the evaluation methods. The rating on the clinical evaluation tool is only a portion of the clinical grade as shown in **Table 12.3**. An advantage of this approach is that it incorporates into the grade the summative evaluation methods completed by students. If pass–fail is used for grading clinical practice, the grade might be computed as shown in **Table 12.4**.

FAILING CLINICAL PRACTICE

Clinical teachers, preceptors, and educators in other roles may be faced with students not demonstrating sufficient competence to pass the clinical course. There are principles that should be followed in evaluating and grading clinical practice, which are critical if a student fails a clinical practicum or course or has the potential for failing it.

Communicate Evaluation and Grading Methods in Writing

The evaluation methods used in a course, how each will be graded if at all, and how the clinical grade will be assigned should be in writing and communicated to the students. The teacher's practices in evaluating and grading clinical performance must reflect this written

TABLE 12.3 EXAMPLE OF CLINICAL GRADE BASED ON EVALUATION METHODS WITH PERFORMANCE GRADED

Assignment	Percent of Grade
Paper on analysis of clinical practice issue	10
Analysis of clinical case	5
Online conference presentation	15
Community resource paper	5
Electronic portfolio	25
Rating scale (of performance)	40
Total	100

TABLE 12.4 EXAMPLE OF CLINICAL GRADE BASED ON EVALUATION METHODS WITH PASS–FAIL GRADING

Assignment	Percent of Grade
Paper on analysis of clinical practice issue	10
Analysis of clinical case	5
Online conference presentation	15
Community resource paper	5
Electronic portfolio	25
OSCE	40
Rating scale (of performance)	Pass required
Total	100

OSCE, objective structured clinical examination.

information. It is critical for adjunct faculty, part-time clinical educators, preceptors, and clinicians who are supervising students in practice to understand the competencies to be achieved and outcomes of the course, the evaluation methods, how to observe and rate performance, and responsibilities when students are not performing adequately.

Develop a Learning Plan

Students need continuous feedback on their clinical performance. Observations made by the clinical nurse educator or preceptor should be shared with the student for discussion. Students may have different perceptions of their performance and, in some cases, may provide new information that influences the teacher's judgment about clinical competencies.

In courses where the clinical instruction is provided by preceptors, adjunct and part-time faculty, or clinicians who are supervising students, and not by the faculty member, the performance problems of students should be shared immediately with the academic faculty member who is responsible for the course. Typically, a conference will be held with the student to discuss areas of concern and the faculty member, clinical educator or preceptor, and student will collaboratively develop a plan for remediation. It is critical that these conferences focus on problems in performance combined with specific learning activities for addressing them. The conferences should not be the teacher telling the student everything that is wrong with clinical performance: The student needs an opportunity to respond to these concerns and identify how to address them.

One of the goals of the conference is to develop a plan with learning activities for the student to correct deficiencies and develop competencies further. The plan should indicate that (a) completing the remedial learning activities does not guarantee that the student will pass the course, (b) one satisfactory performance of the competencies will not constitute a passing clinical grade (the improvement must be sustained), and (c) the student must demonstrate satisfactory performance of the competencies by the end of the course. A template is provided in **Exhibit 12.8** that can be used to develop a learning plan for students. It is important to remember that students have until the end of the clinical practicum (the course) to improve their performance unless they are unsafe in the clinical setting. In that case, the student may be removed from the clinical course depending on the policies of the nursing program, which every clinical educator, preceptor, and student should understand.

Any discussions with students at risk of failing clinical practice should focus on the student's inability to meet the outcomes of the course and perform the specified competencies, not on the teacher's perceptions of the student's intelligence and overall ability. In addition, opinions about the student's ability in general should not be discussed with others.

Conferences should be held in private, and a summary of the discussion should be prepared. The summary should include the date and time of the conference, who participated, areas of concern about clinical performance, and the learning plan with a time

EXHIBIT 12.8 Template of a Learning Plan

1. List of clinical competencies and areas of performance to be improved.
2. For each of the competencies/areas, identify specific learning activities to be completed by the student with due dates.
3. List the process to be used for evaluating the student's progress and performance. Include dates for achieving competencies and specific meeting times for feedback on progress.

frame for completion. The summary should be signed by all participants including the student. Related policies of the nursing education program might specify other requirements.

Students who are at risk of failing clinical practice may have other problems affecting their performance. Teachers should refer students to counseling and other support services and not attempt to provide these resources themselves. Attempting to counsel the student and help the student cope with other problems may bias the clinical educator and influence judgment of the student's clinical performance.

Identify Effect of Failing Clinical Practicum on Course Grade

If failing clinical practice, whether in a pass–fail or a letter system, means failing the nursing course, this should be stated clearly in the course syllabus and policies. By stating it in the syllabus, which all students receive, they have it in writing before clinical learning activities begin. A sample policy statement for pass–fail clinical grading is:

> The clinical component of NUR XXX is evaluated with a pass or fail. A failing grade in the clinical component results in failure of the course, even if the theory grade is 75% or higher.

In a letter grade system, the policy should include the letter grade representing a failure in clinical practice—for example, below a C grade. A sample policy statement is:

> Students must pass the clinical component of NUR XXX with the grade of C or higher. A grade lower than a C in the clinical component of the course results in failure of the course, even if the theory grade is 75% or higher.

Ask Students to Sign Rating Forms and Evaluation Summaries

Students should sign any written clinical evaluation documents—rating forms (of clinical practicum, clinical examinations, and performance in simulations), notes, and any other narrative comments about the student's performance, and summaries of conferences—in which performance was discussed. Their signatures do not mean they agree with the ratings or comments, only that they have read them. Students should have an opportunity to write in their own comments. These materials are important because they document the student's performance and indicate that the educator provided feedback and shared concerns about that performance.

Follow Policy on Unsafe Clinical Performance

There should be a policy in the nursing program about actions to be taken if a student is unsafe in clinical practice. Students who have problems performing some of the competencies can continue in the clinical practicum as long as they demonstrate safe care. This is because the clinical competencies and outcomes of a course are identified for achievement at the end of the course, not during it. If the student demonstrates performance that is potentially unsafe, however, the teacher can remove the student from the clinical site, following the policy of the nursing program. Specific learning activities outside of the clinical setting need to be offered for students to develop the knowledge and skills they lack; practice in the skills laboratory and in simulation may be valuable in these situations. A learning plan should be prepared and implemented as described earlier.

In all cases, the teacher must follow the policies of the nursing program. If the student fails the clinical course, the student must be notified of the failure and its consequences as indicated in these policies. In some nursing programs, students are allowed to repeat only one clinical course, and there may be other requirements to be met. If a student is to be dismissed from the program due to failure, they must be informed in writing. Generally, there is a specific time frame for each step in the process, which must be adhered to by the faculty, administrators, and students.

SUMMARY

Through clinical evaluation, a teacher arrives at judgments about students' performance in clinical practice. The competencies to be demonstrated or outcomes to be met in the clinical practicum provide the framework for learning and the basis for evaluating performance. Competencies are the observable abilities of the student: what the student can do. The AACN defines competency as the ability of a healthcare professional that integrates knowledge, skills, values, and attitudes. The AACN *Essentials* identify 10 domains or areas of nursing competence that include broad competencies and multiple subcompetencies. Because competencies are observable, they can be assessed to ensure that students have developed these abilities at the end of their program. NPs need to achieve competencies identified in the AACN *Essentials* and competencies established by NONPF. EPAs are discrete workplace tasks that NPs and other learners are entrusted to perform unsupervised once they demonstrate their competence. EPAs are observable and measurable so they can be used for evaluating the competencies of NP students in clinical practice. Clinical nurse educators, preceptors, and other clinicians involved in teaching students need to understand these competencies and methods for evaluating their achievement.

Many clinical evaluation methods are available for assessing student competencies. The predominant method for clinical evaluation is observing the performance of students in clinical practice. Although observation is widely used, there are threats to its validity and reliability. In observing clinical performance, there are many aspects of that performance on which the teacher may focus attention. Every observation reflects only a sampling of the student's performance during a clinical learning activity. Such issues point to the need for a series of observations before drawing conclusions about performance. There are several ways of recording observations of students (e.g., checklists and rating scales). Other methods for clinical evaluation are simulations, SPs, OSCEs, written assignments, cases, e-portfolios, conferences, group projects, and self-evaluation. Some methods are appropriate only for formative evaluation and providing feedback to students. Other methods can be used for both formative and summative evaluation.

Important guidelines for grading clinical practice and working with students who are at risk of failing a clinical course were discussed in the chapter. These guidelines give direction to teachers in establishing sound grading practices and following them when working with students in clinical practice.

CNE®cl EXAMINATION TEST BLUEPRINT CORE COMPETENCIES

6. Implement Effective Clinical Assessment and Evaluation Strategies

A. Employ a variety of strategies to determine achievement of learning outcomes
B. Conduct formative and summative evaluation specific to the learner and learning outcomes
C. Communicate learner clinical performance to course faculty in a timely manner
D. Maintain integrity (e.g., ethical, non-biased) in the assessment and evaluation of learners
E. Provide timely, specific, objective, and constructive feedback to learners
F. Use situational assessment data to facilitate learning in the clinical environment
G. Document learner clinical performance, feedback, and progression
H. Evaluate the quality of the clinical learning experiences and environment

LEARNING ACTIVITIES

CourseConnect

To access self-assessment questions and interactive, competency-based learning activities for this chapter, visit www.springerpub.com/courseconnect. See inside front cover and tear-out card for CourseConnect details.

REFERENCES

Alsulimani, L. K. (2021). The feasibility of simulation-based high-stakes assessment in emergency medicine settings: A scoping review. *Journal of Education and Health Promototion, 10*, 441. https://doi.org/10.4103/jehp.jehp_1127_20

American Association of Colleges of Nursing. (2021). *The essentials: Core competencies for professional nursing education*. American Association of Colleges of Nursing.

Anthamatten, A., & Pitts, C. (2024). Integration of entrustable professional activities in a competency-based clinical assessment tool in a nurse practitioner program. *Nurse Educator, 49*(5), 241–245. https://doi.org/10.1097/nne.0000000000001697

Brookhart, S. M., & Nitko, A. J. (2019). *Educational assessment of students* (6th ed.). Pearson.

Bussard, M. E., & Jacobs, L. (2024). Assessing clinical judgment and AACN domains in self-reflection of video recorded high-fidelity simulation scenarios. *Nurse Educator, 49*(6), 327–332. https://doi.org/10.1097/nne.0000000000001704

Bussard, M. E., Jacobs, L. A., Mahoney, S. A., Davis, L. L., Oberhaus, A. M., & Lavoie, P. (2025). Development of clinical judgment in prelicensure nursing students through simulation: A longitudinal study. *Nurse Educator, 50*(3), 117–122. https://doi.org/10.1097/nne.0000000000001790

Chang, C. P., Lee, T. T., Mills, M. E., & Hsieh, Y. P. (2019). E-portfolio functional requirements for the final semester baccalaureate practicum course: A qualitative research study. *Journal of Professional Nursing, 35*(5), 405–411. https://doi.org/10.1016/j.profnurs.2019.04.004

Chua, C. M. S., Nantsupawat, A., Wichaikhum, O. A., & Shorey, S. (2023). Content and characteristics of evidence in the use of standardized patients for advanced practice nurses: A mixed-studies systematic review. *Nurse Education Today, 120*, 105621. https://doi.org/10.1016/j.nedt.2022.105621

Corrigan, C., Moran, K., Kesten, K., Conrad, D., Manderscheid, A., Beebe, S. L., & Pohl, E. (2022). Entrustable professional activities in clinical education: A practical approach for advanced nursing education. *Nurse Educator, 47*(5), 261–266. https://doi.org/10.1097/nne.0000000000001184

DeCoux Hampton, M., & Chafetz, L. (2021). Evaluating scientific writing skill in DNP program students. *Nurse Educator, 46*(3), 164–169. https://doi.org/10.1097/nne.0000000000000883

Dupre, J., & Naik, V. N. (2021). The role of simulation in high-stakes assessment. *BJA Education, 21*(4), 148–153. https://doi.org/10.1016/j.bjae.2020.12.002

Ekman, N., Taft, C., Moons, P., Mäkitalo, Å., Boström, E., & Fors, A. (2020). A state-of-the-art review of direct observation tools for assessing competency in person-centred care. *International Journal of Nursing Studies, 109*, 103634. https://doi.org/https://doi.org/10.1016/j.ijnurstu.2020.103634

Ericsson, K. A. (2008). Deliberate practice and acquisition of expert performance: A general overview. *Academic Emergency Medicine, 15*(11), 988–994. https://doi.org/10.1111/j.1553-2712.2008.00227.x

Goh, H. S., Zhang, H., Lee, C. N., Wu, X. V., & Wang, W. (2019). Value of nursing objective structured clinical examinations: A scoping review. *Nurse Educator, 44*(5), E1–E6. https://doi.org/10.1097/nne.0000000000000620

Harris, M., Rhoads, S. J., Rooker, J. S., Kelly, M. A., Lefler, L., Lubin, S., Martel, I. L., & Beverly, C. J. (2020). Using virtual site visits in the clinical evaluation of nurse practitioner students: Student and faculty perspectives. *Nurse Educator, 45*(1), 17–20. https://doi.org/10.1097/nne.0000000000000693

Holland, A. E., Tiffany, J., Blazovich, L., Bambini, D., & Schug, V. (2020). The effect of evaluator training on inter- and intrarater reliability in high-stakes assessment in simulation. *Nursing Education Perspectives, 41*(4), 222–228. https://doi.org/10.1097/01.Nep.0000000000000619

Interprofessional Education Collaborative. (2023). *IPEC core competencies revision: Version 3 (2021–2023)*. https://www.ipecollaborative.org/2021-2023-core-competencies-revision

Johnson, C. E., Kimble, L. P., Gunby, S. S., & Davis, A. H. (2020). Using deliberate practice and simulation for psychomotor skill competency acquisition and retention: A mixed-methods study. *Nurse Educator, 45*(3), 150–154. https://doi.org/10.1097/nne.0000000000000713

Jones-Schenk, J. (2025). Competency-based education coming to a nursing program near you. *The Journal of Continuing Education in Nursing, 56*(1), 8–9. https://doi.org/doi:10.3928/00220124-20241213-03

Melander, S., Hampton, D., Hardin-Pierce, M., & Ossege, J. (2018). Development of a rubric for evaluation of the DNP portfolio. *Nursing Education Perspectives, 39*(5), 312–314. https://doi.org/10.1097/01.Nep.0000000000000381

Moore, J., Chan, T., Doucette, J., Lipps, T., & Slager, D. (2024). Defining nurse practitioner core entrustable professional activities: Essential step toward competency-based education. *Nurse Educator, 49*(5), 235–240. https://doi.org/10.1097/nne.0000000000001673

National Organization of Nurse Practitioner Faculties. (2024). *NONPF's role core competencies*. https://cdn.ymaws.com/www.nonpf.org/resource/resmgr/competencies/nonpf_np_role_core_competenc.pdf

Oermann, M. H. (2022). Some principles to guide assessment of competencies. *Nurse Educator, 47*(1), 1. https://doi.org/10.1097/NNE.0000000000001143

Oermann, M. H., Gaberson, K. B., & De Gagne, J. C. (2025). *Evaluation and testing in nursing education* (7th ed.). Springer Publishing.

Orsini, C., Rodrigues, V., Tricio, J., & Rosel, M. (2022). Common models and approaches for the clinical educator to plan effective feedback encounters. *Journal of Educational Evaluation for Health Professions, 19*, 35. https://doi.org/10.3352/jeehp.2022.19.35

Ossenberg, C., Mitchell, M., Burmeister, E., & Henderson, A. (2023). Measuring changes in nursing students' workplace performance following feedback encounters: A quasi-experimental study. *Nurse Education Today, 121*, 105683. https://doi.org/10.1016/j.nedt.2022.105683

Poorman, S. G., & Mastorovich, M. L. (2019). The meaning of grades: Stories of undergraduate, master's, and doctoral nursing students. *Nurse Educator, 44*(6), 321–325. https://doi.org/10.1097/nne.0000000000000627

Sidebotham, M., Baird, K., Walters, C., & Gamble, J. (2018). Preparing student midwives for professional practice: Evaluation of a student e-portfolio assessment item. *Nurse Education in Practice, 32*, 84–89. https://doi.org/10.1016/j.nepr.2018.07.008

Sinz, E., Banerjee, A., Steadman, R., Shotwell, M. S., Slagle, J., McIvor, W. R., Torsher, L., Burden, A., Cooper, J. B., DeMaria, S., Jr., Levine, A. I., Park, C., Gaba, D. M., Weinger, M. B., & Boulet, J. R. (2021). Reliability of simulation-based assessment for practicing physicians: performance is context-specific. *BMC Medical Education, 21*(1), 207. https://doi.org/10.1186/s12909-021-02617-8

Ten Cate, O., Chen, H. C., Hoff, R. G., Peters, H., Bok, H., & van der Schaaf, M. (2015). Curriculum development for the workplace using entrustable professional activities (EPAs): AMEE guide No. 99. *Medical Teacher, 37*(11), 983–1002. https://doi.org/10.3109/0142159x.2015.1060308

Wagner, L. M., Dolansky, M. A., & Englander, R. (2018). Entrustable professional activities for quality and patient safety. *Nursing Outlook, 66*(3), 237–243. https://doi.org/10.1016/j.outlook.2017.11.001

Waldrop, J., Reynolds, S. S., McMillian-Bohler, J. M., Graton, M., & Ledbetter, L. (2023). Evaluation of DNP program essentials of doctoral nursing education: A scoping review. *Journal of Professional Nursing, 46*, 7–12. https://doi.org/10.1016/j.profnurs.2022.11.009

Appendices:
Resources for Nurse Educators

A. Selected Nursing And Higher Education Organization Resources

Organization	Mission	Website
American Academy of Nursing	Serves the public and nursing profession by advancing health policy and practice. Academy members, known as Fellows, are nursing's most accomplished leaders in education, practice, administration, and research.	www.aannet.org/page/about
American Association of Colleges of Nursing	Represents baccalaureate and higher-degree nursing programs. Promotes quality nursing education. Offers faculty development programs and webinars. Collects data about nursing education programs, faculty, and students, and analyzes trends in nursing education. Publishes position papers.	https://www.aacnnursing.org
American Association of Community Colleges	Provides advocacy for community colleges at the national level. Works closely with states on policy.	https://www.aacc.nche.edu
American Association of University Professors	Focuses on advancing academic freedom and shared governance. Defines fundamental professional values and standards for higher education and faculty.	https://www.aaup.org/
American Association of University Women	Promotes equity and education for women and girls. Advocates for fundamental educational, social, economic, and political issues.	https://www.aauw.org/
American Council on Education	Represents presidents of accredited, degree-granting institutions (2- and 4-year colleges, private and public universities, and nonprofit schools) in the United States. Focuses on higher education challenges, with the goal to improve access and better prepare students.	https://www.acenet.edu
American Nurses Credentialing Center	Provides a variety of services for practitioners, including certification in Nursing Professional Development. Addresses APRN regulatory requirements resulting in the Consensus Model for APRN Regulation: Licensure, Accreditation, Certification, and Education (LACE).	https://www.nursingworld.org /certification/aprn-consensus-model/
Association for Nurses in Professional Development	Advances quality healthcare by promoting nursing professional development practice. Is the leading resource for nursing professional development and offers a variety of resources and education for nurses in this specialty.	https://www.anpd.org/About/About-Us
Association of Standardized Patient Educators	A global network for human simulation education that provides resources, conferences, and professional development information for standardized patient educators	https://www.aspeducators.org/
Association of American Colleges and Universities	Focuses on promoting high-quality undergraduate liberal education. Website contains links to resources on liberal education, general education, curriculum, faculty work, assessment, diversity, and more.	https://www.aacu.org/about

(*Continued*)

A. SELECTED NURSING AND HIGHER EDUCATION ORGANIZATION RESOURCES (*continued*)

Organization	Mission	Website
Association of Black Nursing Faculty, Inc.	A group for Black professional nurses with similar interests and concerns to promote health-related issues and nursing education. Assists members in professional development and provides continuing education.	https://abnf.net
Association of Community Health Nursing Educators	Focuses on promoting excellence in community and public health nursing education, research, and practice.	https://www.achne.org/aws/ACHNE/pt/sp/home-page
EDUCAUSE	Advances higher education through the use of information technology. Focuses on issues and emerging trends and technologies affecting higher education.	https://www.educause.edu/
International Nursing Association for Clinical Simulation and Learning	A worldwide association dedicated to the science of healthcare simulation. Provides special interest groups, education opportunities, and resources such as the Healthcare simulation standards.	https://www.inacsl.org
Interprofessional Education Collaborative	Collaborative of schools of health professions that advance interprofessional learning experiences to prepare future health professionals for team-based care and improved population health outcomes. These organizations represent higher education in medicine, dentistry, nursing, pharmacy, and public health and created core competencies for interprofessional collaborative practice to guide curricula development across health professions schools.	https://www.ipecollaborative.org/
Multimedia Educational Resource for Learning and Online Teaching	Includes repository of resources and information for faculty development and to download for use in teaching. Publishes *Journal of Online Learning and Teaching.*	https://www.merlot.org/merlot/
National League for Nursing	Promotes excellence in nursing education at all levels. Offers faculty development programs, webinars, and annual educational conferences. Sponsors certifications for academic nurse educators and academic clinical nurse educators. Publishes vision series statements on nursing education. The Commission for Nursing Education Accreditation (CNEA) accredits nursing programs.	https://www.nln.org
National League for Nursing vSim for Nursing	Provides online virtual simulation materials.	https://solution.lww.com/vsim
National Organization of Nurse Practitioner Faculties	Focuses on promoting quality nurse practitioner (NP) education at national and international levels. Leading organization for NP faculty in the United States and globally.	https://www.nonpf.org
National Student Nurses Association	Serves as an organization for nursing students with the goal of enhancing their professional development and promoting transition into the profession.	https://www.nsna.org
Organization for Associate Degree Nursing	Is dedicated to enhancing the quality of associate degree (AD) nursing. Advocates for AD nursing and promotes academic progression of AD nursing graduates in furthering their education.	https://oadn.org

(*Continued*)

A. SELECTED NURSING AND HIGHER EDUCATION ORGANIZATION RESOURCES (*continued*)

Organization	Mission	Website
Quality and Safety Education for Nurses	Collaborative of nurses and other healthcare professionals focused on education, practice, and scholarship to improve quality and safety of healthcare. Identified knowledge, skills, and attitudes (KSAs) necessary to continuously improve quality and safety of healthcare. Website is a central repository of information on core Quality and Safety Education for Nurses (QSEN) competencies, KSAs, teaching strategies, and faculty development resources. The QSEN Institute was in place from 2012-2022.	https://www.qsen.org/about-qsen/
Sigma	Supports learning and professional development of nurses worldwide. Membership is by invitation to baccalaureate and graduate nursing students with excellence in scholarship and to nurse leaders with exceptional achievements in nursing. Offers conferences for sharing research and publishes *Journal of Nursing Scholarship*, among other resources.	https://www.sigmanursing.org/
Society for Simulation in Healthcare	An international society serving a global community interested in enhancing healthcare and advanced medical simulation in healthcare. The organization offers accreditation, certification, education, training, and other resources related to healthcare simulation.	https://www.ssih.org/
U.S. Department of Education	Official agency of the federal government that establishes policies and coordinates federal assistance to education. Website includes links to legislation, regulations, guidance, and other policy documents related to education.	https://www.ed.gov/about
U.S. Department of Justice, Civil Rights Division	Americans with Disabilities Act (ADA) website provides access to information about the ADA, regulations, and other resources.	https://www.ada.gov

B. Academic Clinical Nurse Educator (CNE®cl) Examination Test Blueprint

The National League for Nursing recognizes the knowledge and expertise of clinical educators through certification as a Certified Academic Clinical Nurse Educator (CNE®cl). Additional information can be found at https://www.nln.org/certification/Certification-for-Nurse-Educators/cne-cl

Category	Major Content Areas
1	Function within the Education and Health Care Environments
2	Facilitate Learning in the Health Care Environment
3	Demonstrate Effective Interpersonal Communication and Collaborative Interprofessional Relationships
4	Apply Clinical Expertise in the Health Care Environment
5	Facilitate Learner Development and Socialization
6	Implement Effective Clinical Assessment and Evaluation Strategies

Accessed April 6, 2025

The test blueprint is subject to revision and the most current version can be obtained in the CNE®cl Candidate Handbook, which can be obtained on the NLN website.

Index